Gastrointestinal Cancer

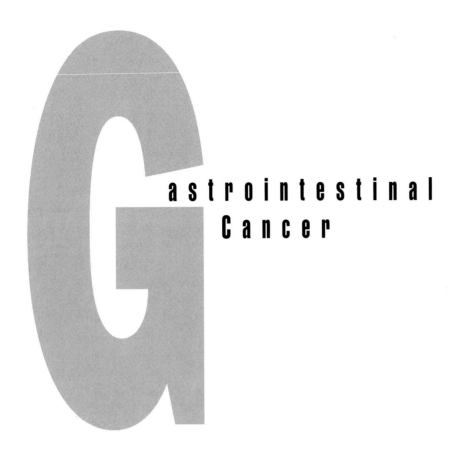

Gastrointestinal Cancer

Edited by

Sidney J. Winawer, MD
Chief, Gastroenterology and Nutrition Service
Attending Physician and Member
Memorial Sloan–Kettering Cancer Center
Professor of Medicine
Cornell University Medical College
New York, New York

Robert C. Kurtz, MD
Associate Attending Physician
Director, Gastrointestinal Endoscopy Unit
Memorial Sloan–Kettering Cancer Center
New York, New York

Gower Medical Publishing ▸ **New York** ▸ **London**

Distributed in the USA and Canada by:
Raven Press
1185 Avenue of the Americas
New York, NY 10036
USA

Distributed in Japan by:
Nankodo Company Ltd.
42-6, Hongo 3-Chome
Bunkyo-Ku
Tokyo 113
Japan

Distributed in the rest of the world by:
Gower Medical Publishing
Middlesex House
34-42 Cleveland Street
London W1P 5FB
UK

ISBN 1-56375-020-1

Library of Congress Cataloging-in-Publication Data
Gastrointestinal cancer / edited by Sidney J.
Winawer, Robert C. Kurtz.
    p. cm.
    Includes bibliographical references and index.
    ISBN 1-56375-020-1 :
    1. Gastrointestinal system—Cancer. I.
    Winawer, Sidney J.
II. Kurtz, Robert C.
    [DLNM: 1. Gastrointestinal Neoplasms—
diagnosis.
2. Gastrointestinal Neoplasms—therapy. WI 149
G2566]
RC280.D5G36 1992
616.99'433—dc20
DNLM/DLC
for Library of Congress   92-1527
                      CIP

British Library Cataloging-in-Publication Data
A catalogue record for this book is available from
the British Library.

Editors: Leah Kennedy, William Millard
Assistant Editor: David Yoon
Illustration Director: Laura Pardi Duprey
Illustration Supervisor: Sue Ann Fung Ho
Illustrators: Sue Ann Fung Ho, Gary Welch,
Hilda R. Muinos, Vantage Art, Inc. (charts)
Art Director: Jill Feltham
Cover Design: Enrique Sevilla
Interior Design & Layout: Tom Tedesco,
Lori Thorn, Jeff Brown, Enrique Sevilla,
Kathryn Greenslade
Typesetting Supervisor: Erick H. Rizzotto

Printed in Singapore by Imago Productions (FE)
Pte Ltd.

10 9 8 7 6 5 4 3 2 1

Dedication

To our wives, Andrea and Linda, and our children—
Daniel, Jonathan, Joanna, Scott, and Caren—with
love, for making everything possible.

Preface

This unique text was designed with the goal of providing those interested in the management of patients with gastrointestinal cancer with an educational instrument that is focused on the physician–patient encounter. Each chapter is devoted to management in a very practical, specific, and concise way. To supplement this practical management approach, a clear and comprehensive insight into diagnostic options is presented, as well as a clear understanding of all aspects of the disease, including its epidemiology and pathophysiology.

There exists a huge amount of new information about pathophysiology, diagnosis, and treatment of gastrointestinal cancer that can easily overwhelm readers. We decided, therefore, to cut through this enormous body of information and to concentrate on the major problem areas confronted on a daily basis. This text makes no attempt to cover rare gastrointestinal cancers in detail, nor is there an attempt to make the references encyclopedic. Rather, the focus of this text is always kept on the physician–patient encounter. The subject covered is luminal GI cancer, with liver cancer being left to the domain of hepatology.

This book utilizes a graphic presentation to guide readers through the large amount of available information. It is in full color and averages more than one illustration per page of text. Illustrations are not supplementary but rather are integrated for a full understanding of the material presented. The schematic artwork includes algorithms, renderings of surgical procedures, and various types of graphs. The extensive photographic artwork includes radiographs, gross and microscopic specimens, and endoscopic photos. Many of these images are accompanied by line drawings which are used to articulate and label areas of interest in the photographs.

The editors and authors hope that physicians and students involved in the day-to-day management of patients with gastrointestinal cancer will find this textbook a valuable, dynamic resource, one that they will use often when they need clear, concise information. We also hope that the graphic presentation of material will serve as a basis for many educational endeavors.

Acknowledgments

First and foremost, the editors would like to thank all of the contributors for working with enthusiasm toward the goals set forth for this textbook. Requirements for writing a chapter were special and quite demanding. Each chapter included not only a comprehensive narrative but also an extensive and detailed illustrative series. We feel that the authors responded so well because they wanted to participate in this creative work.

We are also grateful to Gower and its staff: to Abe Krieger who generated the initial enthusiasm for the book; to Leah Kennedy and Bill Millard who successfully guided it to completion; and to the design and illustration staff for their creativity and commitment to high-quality presentations.

Encouragement and many suggestions were made by our own Gastroenterology and Nutrition Service. In addition, we would like to thank Nancy Daley for help with manuscripts, logistics, and communications. We are also indebted to many individuals who generously made available to us prior materials published by Gower including Drs. Misiewicz (and co-authors Bartram, Cotton, Mee, Price, and Thompson), Mitros, Silverstein, Tytgat, Kassner, McNeil, Waye, Geenan, Venu, Fleisher, Lambert, and Farrar.

Finally, we would like to acknowledge the role of Paul Sherlock not only in our personal lives and careers but in the ever more important and growing field of gastrointestinal cancer. Paul would have been delighted to see the worldwide emphasis now being placed on GI cancer, the increasing number of participating clinicians and scientists, and this textbook, which we hope helps illuminate his life's work and love.

Contributors

Nasser K. Altorki, MD
Assistant Professor of Surgery
New York Hospital–Cornell Medical Center
New York, New York

Murray F. Brennan, MD
Chair, Department of Surgery
Memorial Sloan–Kettering Cancer Center
New York, New York

Eugene P. DiMagno, MD
Consultant in Gastroenterology
   and Internal Medicine
Mayo Clinic
Professor of Medicine
Mayo Medical School
Rochester, Minnesota

Warren E. Enker, MD
Attending Surgeon, Colorectal Service
Memorial Sloan–Kettering Cancer Center
Associate Member
Sloan–Kettering Institute
New York, New York

Robert C. Kurtz, MD
Associate Attending Physician
Director, Gastrointestinal Endoscopy Unit
Memorial Sloan–Kettering Cancer Center
New York, New York

Bernard Levin, MD
Professor of Medicine
Chief, Section of Digestive Diseases and
   Gastrointestinal Oncology
M.D. Anderson Hospital and Tumor Institute
Houston, Texas

Charles J. Lightdale, MD
Attending Physician
Memorial Sloan–Kettering Cancer Center
New York, New York

Michael O'Brien, MD
Associate Director
Mallory Institute of Pathology
Professor of Pathology
Boston University
Boston, Massachusetts

Man-Hei Shiu, MB, BS, FRCS, FACS
Consultant, Department of Surgery
Memorial Sloan–Kettering Cancer Center
New York, New York
Visiting Surgeon
Hong Kong Adventist Hospital
Hong Kong Sanatorium and Hospital
Hong Kong

David B. Skinner, MD
President and Chief Executive Officer
New York Hospital
Professor of Surgery
Cornell University Medical College
New York, New York

Jerome D. Waye, MD
Chief, Endoscopy Unit
Clinical Professor of Medicine
Mount Sinai Hospital
New York, New York

Sidney J. Winawer, MD
Chief, Gastroenterology and Nutrition Service
Attending Physician and Member
Memorial Sloan–Kettering Cancer Center
Professor of Medicine
Cornell University Medical College
New York, New York

Table of Contents

Tumors of the Esophagus

Nasser K. Altorki, Charles J. Lightdale, and David B. Skinner

Esophageal neoplasms are rare. The incidence of malignant tumors of the esophagus far exceeds that of benign tumors. Among malignant tumors, epithelial malignancies are the most common. Mesenchymal tumors, both benign and malignant, account for fewer than 1 percent of cases.

MALIGNANT TUMORS
Epidemiology and Etiology

SQUAMOUS CELL CARCINOMA
Squamous cell carcinoma of the esophagus demonstrates remarkable variability in incidence worldwide. While the disease is uncommon in most of western Europe and the U.S., clusters of high incidence occur in northern China, Iran, and South Africa. A high-incidence belt extends from the Caspian littoral region of Iran across the southern republics of the Soviet Union and into mainland China (Fig. 1.1). Variability occurs even within each country within these high-incidence areas. Esophageal squamous cell carcinoma is most common in northern China, where the incidence is over 300 per 100,000 population, almost 30 times the Chinese national average (1). Clusters of high-incidence areas are also seen in the Transkei region of South Africa, the Indian subcontinent, Sri Lanka, and among subjects of Chinese descent in Singapore. The U.S. has a low incidence, averaging five per 100,000 per year (2). In the

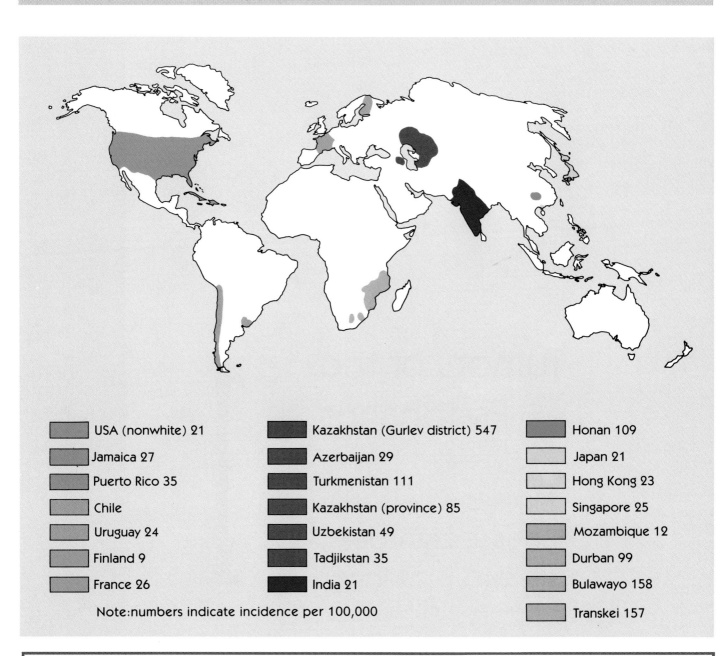

	USA (nonwhite) 21		Kazakhstan (Gurlev district) 547		Honan 109
	Jamaica 27		Azerbaijan 29		Japan 21
	Puerto Rico 35		Turkmenistan 111		Hong Kong 23
	Chile		Kazakhstan (province) 85		Singapore 25
	Uruguay 24		Uzbekistan 49		Mozambique 12
	Finland 9		Tadjikstan 35		Durban 99
	France 26		India 21		Bulawayo 158

Note:numbers indicate incidence per 100,000

Transkei 157

FIGURE 1.1 An esophageal cancer belt extends across mid-Asia with scattered high incidence foci worldwide. (Adapted from DeMeesler TR, Beulow AP. Surgery and current management for cancer of the esophagus and cardia: part I. *Curr Probl Surg* 25(7):477–531, 1988.)

continental U.S., the incidence is highest in Washington, D.C., and in the low country of the Carolinas, where the incidence is 28 per 100,000 (3).

Esophageal cancer is generally a disease of mid- to late adulthood, with a peak incidence between 50 and 70 years. The disease predominates in males, in whom the mortality rate is four to six times higher than females. The incidence of esophageal cancer among whites in the U.S. has remained relatively stable over the last 30 years. The age-adjusted mortality rate in blacks, however, has increased threefold over the same period of time. Esophageal cancer is now the leading cause of cancer death among black males less than 55 years of age (4).

Several epidemiologic studies implicate smoking and alcohol consumption as predisposing factors for esophageal cancer. Tobacco is one of the main sources of nitrosamines affecting humans (5). Many nitrosamine products contain potent carcinogens. Several cohort and case-control studies performed in the U.S. and England leave little doubt that smokers have a significantly elevated risk for cancer of the esophagus (6–8). The findings from these studies were not restricted to cigarettes; cigar and pipe smokers incurred a fourfold increase in esophageal cancer risk. The effect is especially prominent among heavy smokers. In a recent case-controlled study comparing 275 incident cases of carcinoma of the esophagus with 275 neighborhood controls, tobacco use (mainly cigarette smoking) was a significant risk factor for carcinoma of the esophagus (9). Ex-smokers had a reduced risk relative to those who continued to smoke, and current smokers of two or more packs per day had a higher risk than those who smoked less. Smoking, on the other hand, is not a major risk factor for esophageal cancer in the high-risk areas of the world. Smoking local tobacco in northern China has not been identified as a major risk factor for esophageal cancer. Chewing opium residues, known to contain potent mutagens, has been suggested as a risk factor in northern Iran (10). Morphine metabolites were detected by urinalysis in a significant number of the households of cancer patients.

The association of alcohol with esophageal carcinoma is based on compelling epidemiologic evidence. Both prospective and retrospective analyses revealed a high mortality from esophageal cancer among drinkers. Studies in Washington, D.C., and the New York area attributed a high incidence of esophageal cancer in blacks to drinking habits (11,12). Case-control studies in Brittany and Calvados in northwestern France showed a dose-response relation between alcohol intake and the risk of esophageal carcinoma (13,14). The same studies demonstrated the synergy between alcohol intake and tobacco smoking in the etiology of esophageal cancer. Within each category of smokers, the risk of esophageal cancer increased with the amount of alcohol consumed. The risk seems highest with spirits and lowest with beer, with sweet wines occupying an intermediate position. The multiplicative effect of smoking and drinking has also been recently redemonstrated. Among 275 patients with incident cases of esophageal cancer in the Los Angeles area, 93 percent were both drinkers and smokers (9). This synergy between alcohol and tobacco may be due in part to the facilitated diffusion of carcinogens present in tobacco to the basal cell layers in the esophagus, or to the poor nutritional status occasionally associated with heavy drinking.

Tobacco and alcohol consumption are unlikely causal agents in the high-incidence areas of Iran and northern China. In the Linxian province of China, smoking of locally grown tobacco is common, but no correlation has been found with the incidence of esophageal cancer. Drinking does not appear to be a problem in that part of the world. The dietary habits, however, are notable for the consumption of large amounts of pickled vegetables known to be contaminated by fungi. The mutagenicity of pickled vegetables has been tested at the National Cancer Institute in Tokyo, and extracts fed to rats could induce cancer (15). Furthermore, food samples from high-incidence areas demonstrated a higher level of secondary amines than those from low-incidence areas (16). Although dietary habits are different in various areas of the "esophageal cancer belt," the population in the high-risk areas generally manifests a poor nutritional status. Wheat and corn are the staple foods in these areas, and there is a low intake of fresh fruit and vegetables. Similar findings have been shown among the black population in the U.S. and are thought to account, together with smoking and drinking habits, for the threefold higher incidence of cancer in that group (9). Frank nutritional deficiencies are rare, but marginally low levels of vitamins A, B, and C and several trace elements are noted on biochemical analysis. Environmental factors such as asbestos, radiation, and ingested silica fragments have been implicated, but the evidence so far remains sparse (17–20).

The role of a viral agent in the causation of esophageal cancer is unknown. A few cases have been reported in which papillomavirus has been identified within tumor cells (21). Papillomavirus has been known to be associated with carcinoma of the uterine cervix (22). The clustering of high-incidence areas around the world and the steep fall in mortality rates as one moves away from these areas suggest a certain genetic predisposition. A familial predisposition is noted mostly in patients with tylosis, a rare autosomal-dominant disorder in which almost a third of the family members develop esophageal cancer by age 45 (23).

ADENOCARCINOMA

Adenocarcinoma of the esophagus has previously been reported to account for 5 percent of all esophageal tumors. More recent reports, however, estimate that adenocarcinoma accounts for 40 percent to 50 percent of all esophageal malignancies (24,25). The tumor occasionally originates from mucous glands in the esophageal wall or from heterotropic gastric epithelium. More commonly, however, tumors originate from abnormal columnar epithelium lining the esophagus in association with severe gastroesophageal reflux. This latter condition, which was described by Barrett in the early fifties, is now a well-recognized premalignant condition. Adenocarcinomas of the lower esophagus in the absence of Barrett's epithelium have generally been grouped with carcinomas of the stomach. This view disregards the histologic fact that the distal 2 to 3 cm of the normal esophagus is lined by glandular epithelium that could undergo malignant degeneration. Some contend that adenocarcinomas of the cardia are in fact Barrett's cancers in which all remnants of the abnormal epithelium have been replaced by tumor (26). This view is based on epidemiologic similarities between patients with carcinoma of the cardia and those with Barrett's adenocarcinoma (27). Morphologic comparisons of the tumor have shown close similarity in their pathologic features as well. The true incidence of esophageal adenocarcinoma may thus be largely underestimated. Several retrospective and prospective studies placed the incidence of Barrett's adenocarcinoma between one in 72 to one in 400 patient-years (28–31). These estimates represent a 30- to 40-fold increase in the incidence of esophageal carcinoma, compared with that noted among white males in North America.

We diagnose adenocarcinoma of the esophagus in our clinic either when remnants of metaplastic columnar epithelium are present within the esophagus or when more than 50 percent of the tumor is located within the tubular peristaltic esophagus. Using these criteria, adenocarcinomas of confirmed esophageal origin account for about 50 percent of cases seen at our institution. Perhaps some of the variability in the incidence figures between adenocarcinoma and squamous cell carcinoma could be explained by the different patient populations seen at different institutions or by some pathologists' arbitrary inclusion of all adenocarcinomas of the lower esophagus with gastric primaries.

In our series, adenocarcinomas are seen almost exclusively in Caucasians, with a male-to-female ratio exceeding 9:1 (32). Patients are generally in

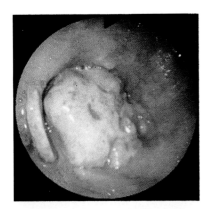

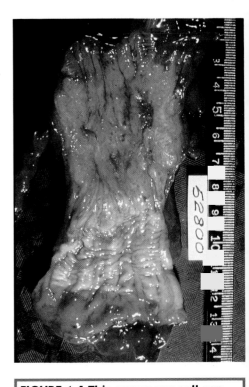

FIGURE 1.2 Endoscopic view of a fungating squamous cell carcinoma. (From Silverstein FE, Tytgat GNJ. *Atlas of gastrointestinal endoscopy.* New York: Gower Medical Publishing, 1987.)

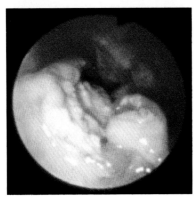

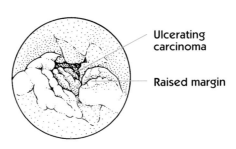

Ulcerating carcinoma

Raised margin

FIGURE 1.3 Squamous cell carcinoma of the esophagus presenting as a typical malignant ulcer. (From Silverstein and Tytgat, 1987.)

FIGURE 1.4 This squamous cell cancer infiltrated the esophageal wall with minimal mucosal irregularity. (From Mitros FA. *Atlas of gastrointestinal pathology.* New York: Gower Medical Publishing, 1988.)

the fifth decade of life—in contrast to those with squamous cell cancer—and most have a long-standing history of severe gastroesophageal reflux. The exact role of gastroesophageal reflux in the initiation or promotion of malignancy remains unknown. Several investigators reported on carcinoma arising in Barrett's esophagus even after antireflux surgery (33,34). These reports, however, suffer from a lack of data demonstrating objective control of reflux. The role of smoking and alcohol ingestion as potential promoters of carcinogenesis is supported by the fact that 30 percent to 50 percent of patients are both drinkers and smokers.

Pathogenesis

Studies in high-incidence areas in Iran and China suggested that atrophic esophagitis, a condition common to both areas, is a precancerous lesion (35). Mass screening projects in different geographic areas in China demonstrated a close correlation between the incidence of dysplasia and that of esophageal squamous cell cancer (36). Among 125,000 subjects surveyed, the ratio of dysplasia to carcinoma was 2:1. Furthermore, the average age of patients with severe dysplasia was about seven to eight years younger than that of the cancer patients. These data suggest a dysplasia/carcinoma in situ/invasive cancer sequence. Follow-up studies of 327 Chinese patients with severe dysplasia showed a progression to cancer at the rate of about 4 percent per year (37). Although such progression from dysplasia to squamous cell carcinoma is not observed in Western countries, careful pathologic examination of resected specimens revealed the presence of dysplasia or carcinoma in situ in more than 90 percent of cases (38).

More information is available in the West on the genesis of adenocarcinoma. Dysplasia and carcinoma in situ, often multifocal, are observed in over 85 percent of esophagi resected for adenocarcinoma

(39). Several reports described the progression from high-grade dysplasia to invasive carcinoma discovered on careful follow-up (40). Reports from various institutions on patients undergoing esophagectomy solely on the basis of high-grade dysplasia, without any preoperative evidence of invasive carcinoma, show that in almost 50 percent of cases, invasive cancer was found in the resected specimen (41,42). The dysplasia/carcinoma sequence in adenocarcinoma of the esophagus seems sufficiently well documented that esophagectomy is now indicated for high-grade dysplasia in suitable surgical candidates.

Pathology

SQUAMOUS CELL CARCINOMA

This histologic type accounts for 50 percent to 60 percent of esophageal tumors. The tumor is located in the middle third of the thoracic esophagus in almost 50 percent of patients, in the distal third in 30 percent, and in the proximal third in 10 percent. Carcinoma arising in the cervical esophagus is seen in 10 percent of patients. Sixty percent of squamous cell cancers are of the fungating type with an extrophytic ulcerating mass (Fig. 1.2). A malignant ulcer with a necrotic, hemorrhagic base and rolled, indurated edges is seen in 25 percent of patients (Fig. 1.3). An infiltrative variety, where the tumor grows extensively intramurally without breaking through the overlying mucosa, is noted in 15 percent of patients (Fig. 1.4). Microscopically, the tumor is composed of sheets of polygonal or polyhedral cells with varying degrees of differentiation. Well-differentiated tumors display keratin pearls (Fig. 1.5), while poorly differentiated tumors are occasionally recognized by individual cell keratinization and intercellular bridges. The majority of tumors, however, are moderately differentiated. A considerable number of tumors show either a substantial degree of extension along the submucosal lymphatics or synchronous noncontiguous foci of carcinoma in situ within 2 to 10 cm of the

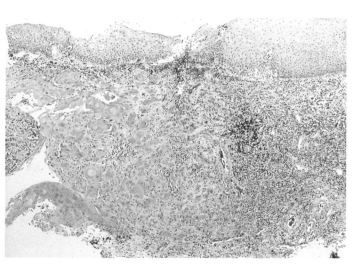

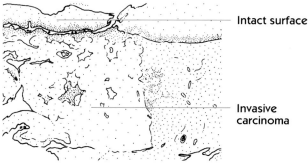

FIGURE 1.5 **Invasive well-differentiated squamous cell carcinoma** displaying keratin pearls.
(From Mitros, 1988.)

Intact surface

Invasive carcinoma

primary lesion (Fig. 1.6) (38). These findings suggest the need for subtotal esophagectomy in most cases, as well as frozen-section examination of the proximal resection margin at operation.

SQUAMOUS CELL VARIANTS

Two unusual variants of squamous cell carcinoma are occasionally seen. Verrucous carcinoma presents as a papillary intraluminal exophytic growth with low metastatic potential. The surface of the tumor is composed of well-differentiated squamous epithelium, and thus only deep biopsies demonstrating submucosal invasion prove its malignant nature. Another variant is carcinosarcoma of the esophagus, where in addition to the epithelial component there is a prominent spindle-cell component with interlacing spindle-shaped cells demonstrating pleomorphism, hyperchromatism, and frequent mitosis (Fig. 1.7). Misconceptions regarding the metastatic potential of the sarcomatous element resulted in the misnomer *pseudosarcoma*. Grossly, the tumor presents a predominantly intraluminal growth with a

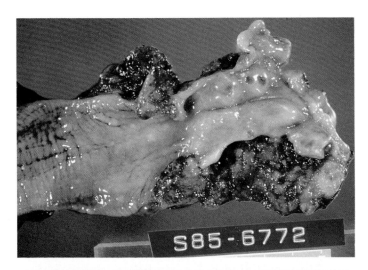

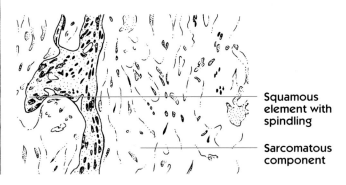

FIGURE 1.6 Underlying an intact mucosa, this tumor shows extensive spread along submucosal lymphatics. (From Mitros, 1988.)

Mucosal-covered carcinoma

Extension in submucosa beyond main tumor mass

FIGURE 1.7 A carcinosarcoma of the esophagus, showing both squamous and spindle cell components. (From Mitros, 1988.)

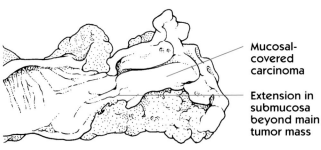

Squamous element with spindling

Sarcomatous component

FIGURE 1.8 Carcinosarcomas generally have little propensity for full wall penetration. (From Mitros, 1988.)

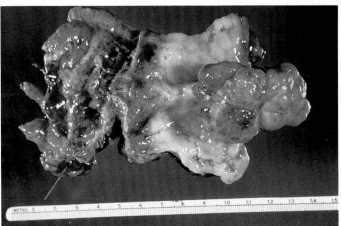

wide or narrow pedicle and little propensity toward full wall penetration of the esophagus (Fig. 1.8).

ADENOCARCINOMA

Esophageal adenocarcinoma may originate from the columnar mucosal lining of the distal 2 cm of the esophagus, from the esophageal mucous glands, or from abnormal glandular epithelium lining the esophagus (either associated with gastroesophageal reflux or representing remnants of embryonic columnar epithelium, particularly in the proximal esophagus). In 42 cases with confirmed Barrett's adenocarcinoma, the tumor was located in the distal esophagus in 25 patients and in the proximal or middle esophagus in 15 patients (32). Two patients developed carcinoma in heterotopic columnar mucosa in the cervical esophagus. Grossly, the tumors are commonly fungating or polypoid in appearance (Fig. 1.9), but flat, ulcerating lesions or annular stenosing types (Fig. 1.10) are occasionally encoun-

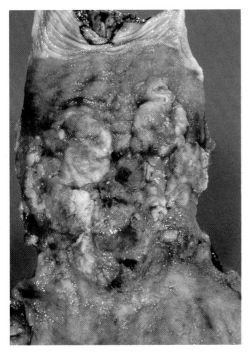
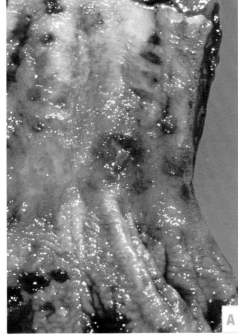

FIGURE 1.10 A small ulcer in this columnar-lined esophagus **(A)** harbored an invasive adenocarcinoma, as revealed in histologic examination of the epithelium **(B)**. Extensive biopsies of any abnormality are mandatory. (From Mitros, 1988.)

FIGURE 1.9 A large, fungating adenocarcinoma arising in a columnar-lined distal esophagus. Note the squamocolumnar junction. (From Mitros, 1988.)

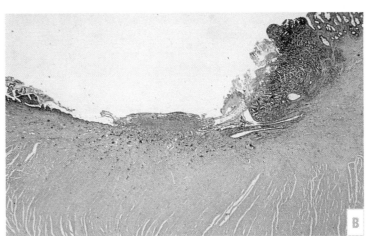

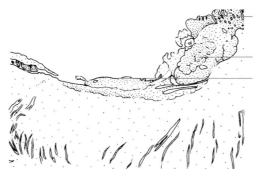

Specialized form of Barrett's with dysplasia

Focus of carcinoma

Surface of ulcer

tered. Histologically, various degrees of glandular differentiation are noted, but well-differentiated tumors predominate (Fig. 1.11). The surrounding mucosa shows evidence of intraepithelial neoplasia in 80 percent to 100 percent of cases. A variety of other tumors are occasionally included in some reports on adenocarcinoma of the esophagus and include adenocystic carcinoma and mucoepidermoid carcinoma. These are exceedingly rare tumors, with less than 50 cases collectively reported in the English literature. The tumors histologically resemble their salivary counterparts, and both are indistinguishable clinically and prognostically from the more common types of cancer of the esophagus.

SMALL CELL CARCINOMA

Originally described in 1952, this tumor accounts for fewer than 2 percent of esophageal tumors (43). Only 64 cases are reported in the literature, and the survival after diagnosis is generally less than six months. The tumor, like its pulmonary counterpart, originates from the APUD cell system present in the basal part of the esophageal squamous lining (43). The origin of these cells is controversial, although current opinion suggests that they arise from a totipotential stem cell (44). The tumor is formed of sheets of small, round, fusiform cells with a high nuclear-cytoplasmic ratio and with hyperchromatic nuclei (Fig. 1.12). Neurosecretory granules are demonstrated in a significant number of cases.

MALIGNANT MELANOMA

Primary malignant melanoma of the esophagus is exceedingly rare. The tumor is more common in males and is clinically indistinguishable from other esophageal neoplasms. Grossly, the tumor appears as a polypoid, bulky mass with some mucosal ulceration (Fig. 1.13). The melanin content determines its color on cut section; it may be black or totally amelanotic. Microscopically, the tumor is composed of sheets of polygonal or spindle-shaped cells with abundant eosinophilic cytoplasm that stains positively for melanin granules. The presence of atypical melanocytic proliferation in its radial component is essential for a definite diagnosis of primary esophageal melanoma (45). The prognosis is dismal even after complete surgical resection, with the five-year survival being less than 5 percent.

ESOPHAGEAL SARCOMA

Among malignant esophageal tumors of mesenchymal origin, leiomyosarcoma is the most common. Nonetheless, leiomyosarcoma accounts for fewer than 1 percent of all esophageal tumors. The disease occurs more frequently in males than females and has its peak incidence in the sixth to eighth decade of life. The gross pathologic appearance is usually that of a bulky, polypoid intraluminal mass, greyish-white on cut section, with occasional areas of hemorrhage and necrosis. Microscopically, there are interlacing spindle-shaped pleomorphic cells ar-

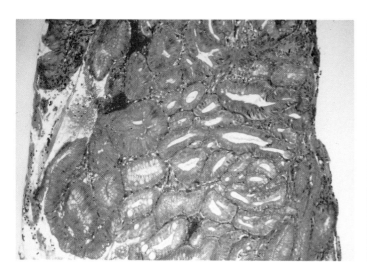

FIGURE 1.11 Well-differentiated adenocarcinoma.

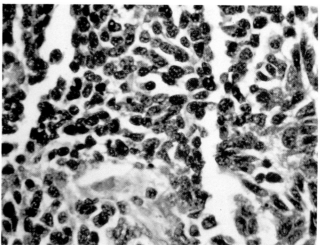

FIGURE 1.12 A classic oat cell tumor with small, spindly cell showing increased N/C ratio. (From Mitros, 1988.)

ranged in a prominent fascicular pattern with numerous mitotic figures. The reliance on frequent mitosis as an indication of malignancy has been challenged, and the emphasis is now on the paucity or absence, on electron microscopy, of cellular organelles present in normal smooth muscles (46). At times the operative findings and eventual biologic behavior are the sole determinants of the malignant character of the tumor. Leiomyosarcomas are generally large tumors that either ulcerate through the mucosa or are firmly attached to it, precluding any enucleation of the tumor from within the muscle layer.

Clinical Presentation

Most patients with carcinoma of the esophagus present with advanced disease and are beyond the realm of curative therapy. Delay in both presentation and diagnosis is responsible for the poor survival rates reported in Europe and North America.

The survival rate of patients with early cancer of the esophagus has been reported from China to be 90 percent at five years and 60 percent at ten years (47). Detection of these early lesions, which include carcinoma in situ and carcinoma invading the submucosa, was made possible through mass screening projects in the high-incidence counties of northern China. A clinical study of patients with early cancer of the esophagus showed that 90 percent had mild but definite symptoms related to swallowing, such as burning, discomfort, or slow passage of food (48). These symptoms were transient in nature and caused no immediate concern to the patient; they were distinctly different from those caused by esophagitis in being related only to food intake. Patients over 40 years of age with minimal symptoms should be fully evaluated for evidence of early esophageal cancer. The diagnosis of early lesions in entirely asymptomatic patients, however, is more problematic. Mass screening is unlikely to be cost-effective in low-incidence areas such as the U.S. and western Europe. Screening in such areas should more reasonably be directed toward groups of patients at high risk for cancer of the esophagus. Such patients include those with achalasia, Barrett's esophagus, or lye stricture, as well as those with a history of oral or airway cancer. Hereditary disorders such as tylosis, celiac disease, and the Plummer–Vinson syndrome should also be included in the high-risk category. The expertise required for radiographic or endoscopic screening dramatically decreases the cost-effectiveness of these modalities. There is a consensus, however, that cytologic screen-

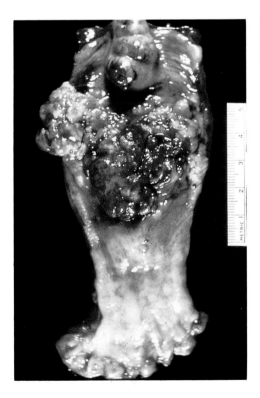

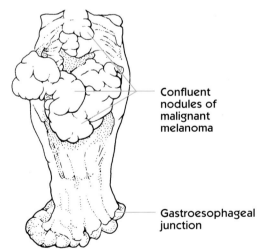

FIGURE 1.13 Polypoid melanoma of the esophagus. (From Mitros, 1988.)

Confluent nodules of malignant melanoma

Gastroesophageal junction

ing is both reliable and cost-effective. Various methods are available for the retrieval of esophageal cells for cytology. Abrasive balloon cytology has been widely used in China, while the sponge-and-capsule method has been reported by Nabeya from Japan, with equally good results (49). Our own preference is a modification of a system previously employed in northern Iran and later evaluated by our group (Fig. 1.14) (50).

Follow-up studies in 23 Chinese patients with early cancer of the esophagus who refused thera-py for a variety of reasons showed that the disease remained stable in half of the patients at five years and progressed in the remainder within 33 to 48 months (51). These data suggest that esophageal cancer has a prolonged preclinical latency period, permitting surveillance of high-risk groups as infrequently as once a year.

As previously stated, most Western patients present with far advanced disease. Dysphagia is a universal presenting symptom, occurring in over 95 percent of patients. Unfortunately, it is a late symp-

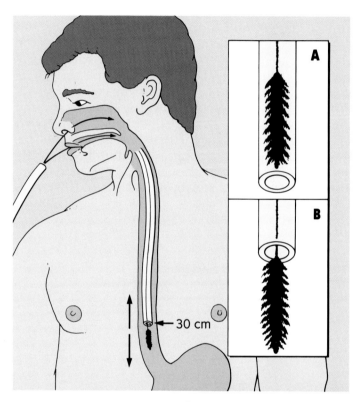

FIGURE 1.14 Abrasive brush cytology. The tip of a nasogastric tube is slit, and a cytology brush is inserted through it. The assembly is advanced to the desired location in the esophagus and the brush advanced to abrade the mucosa. The brush is pulled back into the tube and the process is repeated at 5-cm intervals.

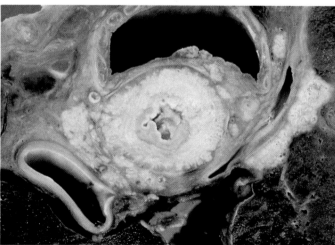

FIGURE 1.15 The esophagus abuts the membranous trachea and bronchi, and tumors of the cervical and proximal esophagus are likely to invade into these structures. (From Mitros, 1988.)

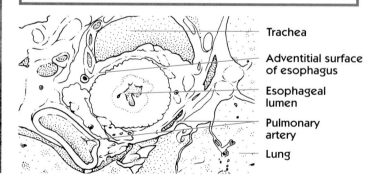

Trachea

Adventitial surface of esophagus

Esophageal lumen

Pulmonary artery

Lung

tom in the natural history of the disease. Lack of a serosal covering permits the esophagus to distend, accommodating the intraluminal growth without impeding deglutition. Dysphagia sets in when the tumor encroaches on 90 percent of the esophageal circumference (52). Dysphagia is characteristically steadily progressive, affecting solids initially and then proceeding to total obstruction. Although most patients can localize the site of obstruction to the food bolus, this does not always correlate with the actual location of the tumor. Odynophagia occurs in about 20 percent of patients and on occasion may be the only presenting symptom. About half of the patients will report some degree of weight loss. Severe weight loss and cachexia are now rarely seen but are indications of advanced and widespread disease.

A variety of symptoms show extraesophageal extension with mediastinal invasion. Tracheoesophageal fistula is present in 5 percent of patients when they are first seen. Fistulae into the airway may occur with any lesion but are more common in tumors of the cervical and proximal esophagus because of the close apposition of the trachea and left mainstem bronchus to the organ in the neck and upper mediastinum (Fig. 1.15). Hoarseness of voice indicates recurrent laryngeal nerve invasion, either from the primary tumor or from metastatic deposits in the lymph nodes. Approximately 50 percent of patients will have clinical or radiologic evidence of metastatic disease at the time of diagnosis.

Physical examination of patients with esophageal cancer is often unremarkable, and diagnosis of cancer of the esophagus often relies on radiographic or endoscopic means.

Diagnosis

Contrast Studies

This is usually the initial study obtained in symptomatic patients. A complete radiographic study of the esophagus should include examination of the cervical, thoracic, and abdominal esophagus as well as the stomach and the duodenum. Single-contrast studies reveal gross structural abnormalities such as luminal masses (Fig. 1.16A), ulcerations, or strictures (Fig. 1.16B). Although various criteria are used to differentiate between malignant and benign strictures, these criteria are uniformly unreliable and the final determination lies with endoscopic biopsies. Double-contrast studies of the esophagus provide a clear definition of the

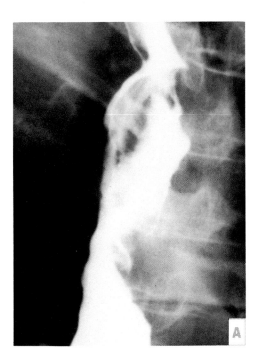
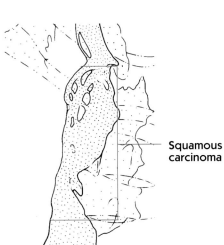

Squamous carcinoma

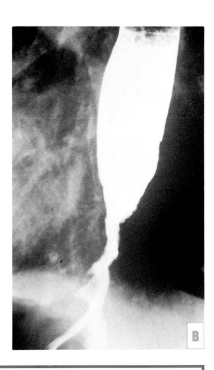

FIGURE 1.16 (A) A large, fungating squamous cell carcinoma. (B) The Barrett's adenocarcinoma shown is presented as a stricture but could be mistaken for a peptic stricture. (From Mitros, 1988.)

mucosal pattern, thereby permitting detection of early lesions (Fig. 1.17). Esophagograms have also been used as an aid to tumor staging by determining the esophageal axis, as proposed by Akiyama (53). Axis views are obtained with the esophagus full of barium in the posteroanterior, right anterior oblique, and left anterior oblique projections. The esophagus normally follows a relatively straight course, apart from a slight rightward deviation in the region of the aortic arch and a slight anterolateral indentation where the left mainstem bronchus crosses the viscus. Abnormalities from

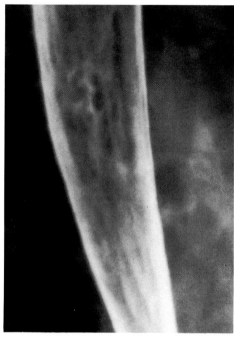

FIGURE 1.17 An early ulcerative squamous cell cancer is best shown by double contrast esophagogram. (From Mitros, 1988.)

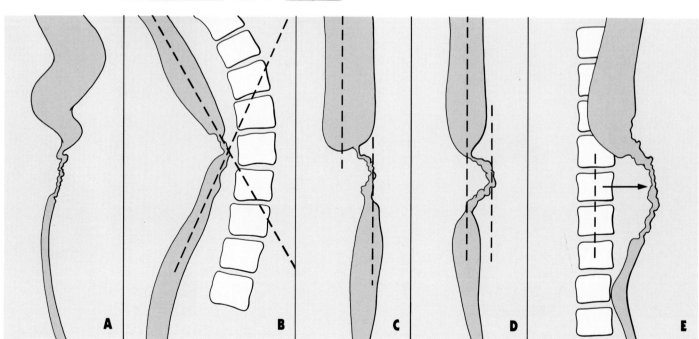

FIGURE 1.18 Axis views of abnormalities in the esophagograms of nonresectable tumors of the esophagus. (A) Tortuosity of the esophageal axis proximal to the tumor. (B) Angulation of the esophageal axis. (C) Deviation of the axis above and below the tumor. (D) Axis deviation of the tumor itself. (E) Abnormality of distance from the spine. (Adapted from Akiyama H. *Surgery for carcinoma of the esophagus*. Chicago: Year Book Medical Publishing, 1980.)

the normal axis, including angulation, tortuosity, or deviation, indicate extension of the tumor beyond the esophageal wall (Fig. 1.18). The test is relatively simple to perform but requires experience to interpret and is associated with a 20 percent false negative rate.

ESOPHAGOSCOPY

Endoscopy is an essential diagnostic modality, since it not only allows for tissue diagnosis but also maps the extent of the lesion for the surgeon, thus indicating the most effective operative approach. A normal radiographic study in the presence of symptoms should not preclude endoscopy. The flexible esophagoscope has now largely re-

placed the rigid instrument for this procedure. The morbidity of diagnostic endoscopy is less than 0.1 percent. The entire length of the esophagus, including the cervical esophagus, is examined carefully, regardless of the location of the lesion. The endoscopist should note the distance of distinctive markings from the patient's incisors, as well as the beginning and end of suspicious lesions. In the presence of Barrett's esophagus, the abnormality is documented by multiple biopsies and its proximal extent is carefully noted. One should be familiar with benign abnormalities such as glycogen acanthosis (Fig. 1.19A) and be able to differentiate these from areas suspected of being early carcinoma or satellite nodules (Fig. 1.19B,C,D). The

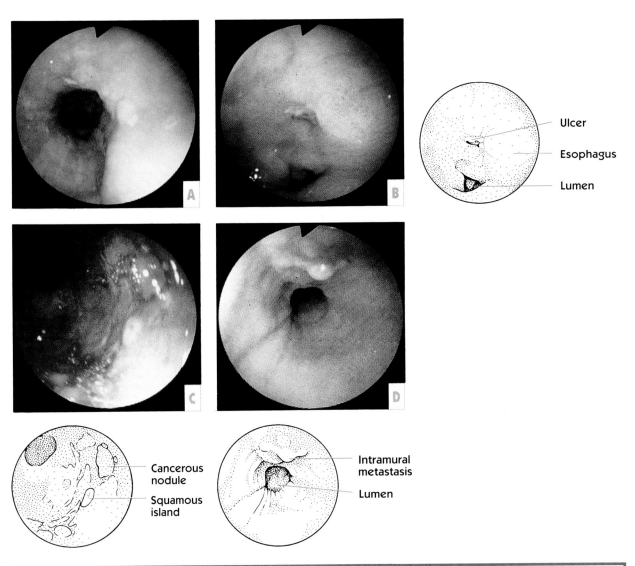

FIGURE 1.19 (A) Glycogen acanthosis: typical appearance. (B) The tiny ulcer shown proved to be squamous cell carcinoma on biopsy. **(C)** A small nodule in Barrett's esophagus proved to be a carcinoma. **(D)** Intramural metastasis from squamous cell carcinoma. (From Silverstein and Tytgat, 1987.)

appearance of early malignant lesions has been described; features include mild erythema, congestion, and small ulcerations. The use of vital stains such as toluidine blue or Lugol's iodine to guide endoscopic biopsies is occasionally quite valuable and is more widely practiced in Japan and western Europe than in North America. The esophagus is initially washed with 1 percent acetic acid, then stained with Lugol's iodine or toluidine blue, and finally decolorized with a second application of acetic acid. Malignant lesions retain the dye and permit direct biopsies and brushings. Strictures, when encountered, are dilated if necessary to permit passage of the endoscope. Direct brush cytologies are routinely performed and in 10 percent to 15 percent of patients have yielded a positive result in spite of negative biopsies. Multiple biopsies are obtained, preferably avoiding clearly necrotic areas of the tumor. The positive yield increases with the number of biopsies obtained; we usually perform three or four biopsies from the primary. The combination of both biopsy and cytology maximizes the accuracy of endoscopic diagnosis. Rarely, a stricture is undilatable and a diagnosis of malignancy is hard to establish. Rigid esophagoscopy under general anesthesia may be attempted in such situations, with another attempt at dilatation and four-quadrant biopsies. In the absence of a diagnosis, the patient is managed with a presumptive diagnosis of cancer of the esophagus, while the final answer rests in the resected specimen.

Staging

The concept of staging stems from the need to evaluate the anatomic extent of the disease in order to decide therapeutic strategy and to estimate prognosis. Previous staging systems for esophageal cancer proposed by the American Joint Committee on Cancer (AJCC) relied on tumor size, circumferential involvement, and clinical obstruction as discriminating staging criteria. A larger-size tumor was permissible in the T1 category than ordinarily allowed for in other organs. Furthermore, subjective clinical evaluation of esophageal obstruction separated stage 1 from stage 2 tumors. In 1981, a staging system was proposed that stressed wall penetration (W), nodal involvement (N), and distant metastases (M) as important determinants of survival (Fig. 1.20) (54). This resulted from a multivariate analysis for six prognostic factors in 58 patients after esophagectomy. Two-year survival with no evidence of renewed disease was compared with tumor location, cell type, degree of differentiation, tumor size, depth of wall penetration, and nodal involvement. Degree of wall penetration and nodal involvement emerged as the only independent prognostic factors. The validity of

---

FIGURE 1.20:
WNM CLASSIFICATION SYSTEM FOR ESOPHAGEAL TUMORS

STAGE	FEATURES
W0	Mucosal involvement
W1	Partial wall penetration
W2	Full wall penetration
N0	No nodal involvement
N1	1–4 positive nodes
N2	5 or more positive nodes
M0	No distant metastases
M1	Metastases present

the WNM staging system in predicting survival was later verified in a prospective series of 52 patients undergoing surgery from 1981 to 1984. The two studies combined resulted in 110 patients available for analysis. Patients with stages W1N1 and W2N0 had three-year survival rates of 55 percent and 44 percent, respectively (55). The concepts proposed by the WNM staging system have been reproduced in several studies and have recently been adopted by the AJCC and the UICC (International Union Against Cancer). Figures 1.21 and 1.22 show the most recent modification of the TNM staging system, in which the T has been modified to reflect wall penetration.

When the diagnosis of cancer of the esophagus is

FIGURE 1.21:
UICC TNM CLASSIFICATION OF ESOPHAGEAL TUMORS

STAGE	FEATURES
T: Primary tumor	
TX	Primary tumor cannot be assessed
T0	No evidence of primary tumor
Tis	Carcinoma in situ
T1	Tumor invades lamina propria or submucosa
T2	Tumor invades muscularis propria
T3	Tumor invades adventitia
T4	Tumor invades adjacent structures
N: Regional lymph nodes	
NX	Regional lymph nodes cannot be assessed
N0	No regional lymph node metastasis
N1	Regional lymph node metastasis
M: Distant metastasis	
MX	Presence of distant metastasis cannot be assessed
M0	No distant metastasis
M1	Distant metastasis (including celiac nodes)

From Speissl B, Beahrs OH, Hermanek P, et al. *UICC TNM atlas: illustrated guide to the TNM/pTNM classification of malignant tumours*, 3rd ed. Berlin and New York: Springer-Verlag, 1989.

established, further evaluation is aimed at defining the clinical stage of the disease, and a complete physiologic evaluation is done to determine the patient's ability to tolerate therapy. Obtaining a careful history during the initial visit is an essential component of the staging process. Patients are queried about symptoms suggestive of extraesophageal extension, such as new-onset cough associated with eating (suggesting tracheoesophageal fistula), hoarseness (suggesting recurrent nerve invasion), or, rarely, constant boring back pain (implying tumor penetration into the mediastinum). Bone or joint pains, or the more subtle features that indicate spread to the central nervous system, such as behavioral changes, somnolence, and head-

aches, should also be carefully sought. An evaluation of the degree of dysphagia, although not pertinent to the current staging system, may well dictate the speed of further evaluation and the urgency of intervention. Weight loss is a feature common to all patients with cancer of the esophagus except those with early lesions; therefore, most patients should be encouraged to consume several cans of high-caloric nutritional supplement per day for nutritional support as further workup continues on an outpatient basis. Patients with total dysphagia should be hospitalized and fed either enterally or parenterally. A careful history should also include evaluation of underlying cardiopulmonary disease. Patients with anginal symptoms, orthopnea, or

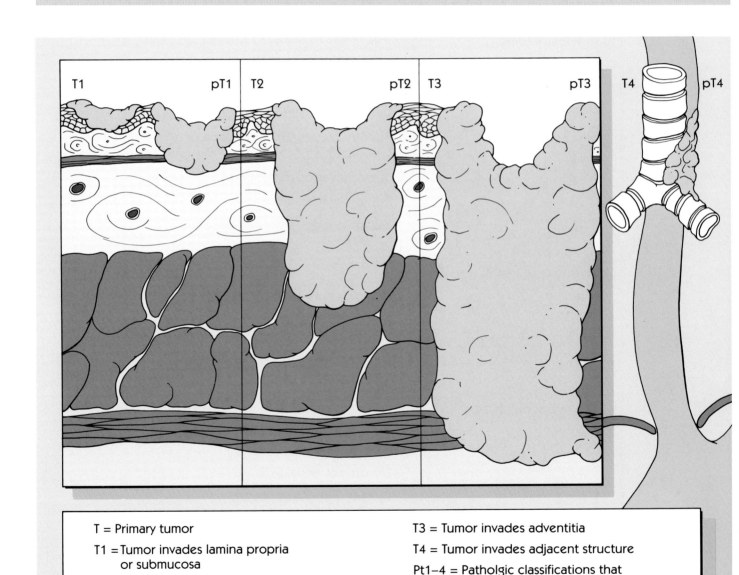

T = Primary tumor

T1 = Tumor invades lamina propria or submucosa

T2 = Tumor invades muscularis propria

T3 = Tumor invades adventitia

T4 = Tumor invades adjacent structure

Pt1–4 = Patholgic classifications that correspond to the T category

FIGURE 1.22 UICC staging, TNM clinical classification.

exertional dyspnea should receive a full cardiologic evaluation, up to and including coronary arteriography if necessary. Pulmonary function tests are also routinely obtained, and patients with an FEV_1 of less than 2 l are generally not considered candidates for transthoracic esophagectomy. As previously indicated, physical examination of patients with esophageal cancer is usually unremarkable; however, stigmata of widespread disease such as cervical adenopathy, hepatomegaly, ascites, and local bone tenderness should be carefully sought.

A barium swallow, as noted previously, is usually the first study obtained and determines the location of the tumor. Axis views, when available, may predict the likelihood of full wall penetration by the tumor. Bronchoscopy is a standard procedure for tumors of the cervical, upper, and middle thoracic esophagus. Bronchoscopy should be performed by physicians experienced in evaluating the subtle signs of airway invasion. A mere bulge into the membranous trachea or mainstem bronchi does not necessarily indicate malignant invasion, particularly if the membranous trachea moves readily with respiration. Erythema and edema, however, are ominous signs; biopsies of suspicious areas as well as material for cytology should be obtained. When an established tracheoesophageal fistula is identified, emergency intervention is usually indicated.

Computed tomography (CT) of the chest and upper abdomen is also routinely employed. The

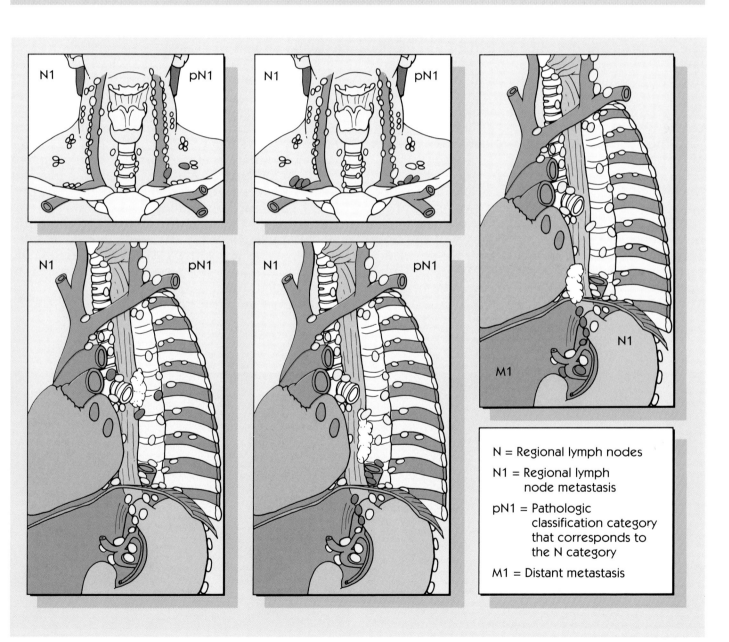

N = Regional lymph nodes

N1 = Regional lymph node metastasis

pN1 = Pathologic classification category that corresponds to the N category

M1 = Distant metastasis

FIGURE 1.22 (Continued).

primary tumor is usually marked by thickening of the esophageal wall. A blurring of the contour of the esophagus in the region of the tumor usually indicates full-thickness wall penetration (Fig. 1.23). Employing this criterion for the T descriptor, we were able to predict wall penetration with a 75 percent accuracy. Prediction of nodal involvement, however, is less reliable, with only a 50 percent diagnostic accuracy due to high false-negative rates with small nodes (56). The criteria determining invasion of adjacent structures are not well defined. Aortic invasion is predictable when the tumor encroaches on more than 90 degrees of the aortic circumference, but the diagnostic accuracy of this sign is poor with lesser degrees of encroachment (Fig. 1.24). CT criteria for airway invasion are similarly not well established, and computed tomography should not by itself prevent exploration based on presumed involvement of the trachea or bronchi. Evidence of hepatic or adrenal metastases should be diligently sought. Computed tomography has basically supplanted liver scintigraphy for detection of liver metastases; however, metastatic lesions from adenocarcinoma of the cardia or esophagus may on occasion be isodense with the liver parenchyma, and hence only detectable by radionuclide scintigraphy.

Endoscopic ultrasonography (EUS) has been developed over the last decade and has a clear application in the clinical staging of esophageal cancer. High-frequency ultrasound transducers have been incorporated into the distal tip of the fiberscope. Most experience has been with mechanical sector-scan instruments, using high-frequency transducers of 7.5 and 12 mHz (GF-UM3, Olympus Corp). The instruments provide a 360° view of a sector perpendicular to the insertion tube. Unique and detailed images of the esophageal wall can be produced, usually five wall layers thick, alternately hyperechoic and hypoechoic. Histologic correlates based on in vitro studies indicate that the first two layers represent the superficial and deep mucosa; the middle layer, the submucosa; the fourth layer, the muscularis propria; and the fifth layer, the adventitia (or serosa at the cardia) (Fig. 1.25).

Esophageal cancer is imaged as a relatively hypoechoic disruption of the normal wall layers (Fig. 1.26). According to the 1988 AJCC staging classification, T1 involves the first three layers, T2 the fourth layer, T3 disrupts the fifth, and T4 shows invasion of adjacent organs and structures. The accumulating data show that EUS is highly accurate for T staging. The accuracy of EUS ranges from 89 percent to 92 percent compared with 65 percent accuracy for CT (57).

EUS can also provide excellent images of the mediastinum and perigastric areas and can detect lymph nodes 2 to 3 mm in size. Lymph nodes that are sharply demarcated, rounded, and hypoechoic are more likely to be malignant, as are larger nodes above 10 mm in size. The accuracy of nodal involvement by EUS approaches 85 percent compared with 50 percent by CT alone. (57)

A major limitation of the current EUS instrument is its 13-mm diameter. Inability to pass a malignant stenosis has been reported in 26 percent to 62 percent of patients. Most cancers can be staged correctly in terms of T and N from the proximal portion, but staging of celiac axis nodes, considered distant metastases if positive (M1), is not possible unless the instrument can pass into the stomach. In general, high-frequency ultrasound has a more limited depth of field for staging M than for T and N.

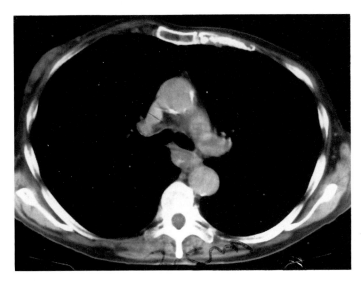

FIGURE 1.23 Thickening and blurring of the esophageal outline in this patient suggests tumor penetration through the wall of the organ.

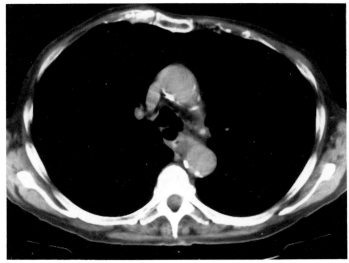

FIGURE 1.24 Tumor encroachment on 90° or more of the aortic circumference is predictable of tumor invasion in our experience.

EUS has also been shown to be sensitive (95 percent) and reasonably specific (80 percent) in diagnosing remnant esophageal cancer at the surgical anastomosis, where CT has not been effective (58).

Invasive measures such as mediastinoscopy, cervical node biopsy, laparoscopy, and occasionally laparotomy should be liberally employed when suggested by abnormal CT findings. Histologic documentation of metastatic disease should be obtained whenever possible, specifically in cases of isolated metastatic lesions.

Approach to the Patient

PHILOSOPHY OF THERAPY

An aura of pessimism has surrounded all therapeutic endeavors for patients with esophageal carcinoma. Survival after surgical extirpation is generally about 10 percent to 15 percent. When radiation therapy is used as a definitive therapeutic modality, survival rates at five years are generally 5 percent to 10 percent. Regardless of the method of local control, most failures occur at distant sites, prompting some investigators to suggest that esophageal cancer is a metastatic disease at the time of diagnosis. This latter view is challenged, however, by the excellent long-term disease-free survival obtained after surgery in Chinese patients diagnosed with early esophageal cancer or locoregional disease. Long-term disease-free survival has also been reported in the West for a small group of patients with early cancer of the esophagus, thus refuting the concept that

esophageal cancer in the Western hemisphere is an inherently more aggressive disease (56).

Furthermore, while staging systems have been established for most other solid tumors, the staging of esophageal cancer has lacked therapeutic or prognostic relevance. A staging system that is based on careful analysis of prognostic variables has only recently been adopted by the AJCC and UICC. Several issues remain to be resolved and are currently under evaluation by a staging committee of the International Society of the Diseases of the Esophagus. Concurrent with the re-evaluation of the staging system, the concept of combination chemotherapy was introduced, with several groups reporting response rates in the region of 60 percent to 70 percent. Finally, the surgical treatment of esophageal cancer has undergone significant developments in the last decade. Earlham in 1980 reported an operative mortality of 25 percent in an analysis of 81,000 esophagectomies (59). By the end of that decade, however, these figures no longer represented the state of the art. The mortality of esophagectomy is now generally under 10 percent. Unresolved, however, is the debate regarding the magnitude of the operation. Proponents of palliative operations such as the limited transthoracic esophagectomy or transhiatal esophagectomy believe that cure of the disease is a chance phenomenon. An alternate view is that survival is largely stage-related, with a cure possible in a small group of patients with either full wall penetration or limited nodal involvement (56). This

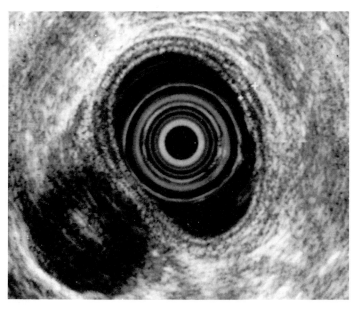

FIGURE 1.25 Normal distal esophagus at 35 cm from the incisors. The descending aorta is in the 7 o'clock position. The normal esophageal wall is seen as a five-layered structure in the 9 o'clock to 3 o'clock area.

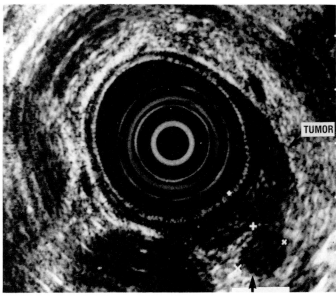

FIGURE 1.26 In the distal esophagus, a hypoechoic tumor is present at the 3 o'clock area to 6 o'clock position, and a round hypoechoic malignant lymph node is seen adjacent to the tumor. The descending aorta is at 6 o'clock.

could be accomplished by applying to the esophagus the same sound principles of surgical oncology that have been applied elsewhere in the gastrointestinal tract, with moderate improvement in survival rates. An esophagectomy with a thorough mediastinal and upper abdominal lymphadenectomy, together with resection of the posterior mesoesophagus and a wide margin of normal tissue around the tumor, was described for tumors of the lower thoracic esophagus and cardia as early as 1962 (60). The principle was extended to tumors of the midthoracic and cervical esophagus in 1969 (61). An operation of this magnitude is employed only if preoperative and intraoperative staging indicates that the tumor is potentially curable. We define potentially curable cancer of the esophagus as that in which the disease is limited to the wall of the esophagus with locoregional involvement within the limits of the proposed resection, without celiac nodal involvement and without evidence of hematogenous spread. Refinements in the staging systems and the variety of operative procedures now available should allow us to offer curative resections to patients with potentially curable disease, and also to select patients with less favorable tumors for neoadjuvant or adjuvant protocols. When palliation is the only reasonable goal of therapy, palliative modalities include surgical resection, radiotherapy, laser therapy, bougienage, and esophageal prosthesis. Feeding enterostomies, however, are not appropriate palliative measures, since they unnecessarily extend the suffering of a patient terminal with disease and fail to palliate the constant dysphagia to liquids and saliva.

SURGERY FOR ESOPHAGEAL CANCER

HISTORY Franz Torek performed the first successful transthoracic esophagectomy in 1913. The operation used the then novel technique of intratracheal ether insufflation rather than the standard negative-pressure Sauerbruch chamber. The hazards of an intrathoracic esophagogastric anastomosis were circumvented by a cervical esophagostomy and a gastrostomy. Torek's patient lived for 13 years, taking oral alimentation by connecting his cervical stoma and his gastrostomy via a red rubber tube. Successful intrathoracic esophagogastric reconstruction was first reported by Oshawa in the Japanese literature. Adams and Phemister from the University of Chicago are credited with the first successful transthoracic esophagectomy with intrathoracic reconstruction. Their report to the American Association for Thoracic Surgery in 1938 is a landmark in the history of esophageal surgery (62). Several surgeons contributed to refinements in transthoracic esophagectomy, including Sweet, Garlock, Belsey (63), and others. In 1962, Logan described his technique for en bloc resection of carcinoma of the cardia and

lower esophagus. The survival reported after this operation was 16 percent at five years, but wide adoption of the procedure was curtailed by a high operative mortality (60). More recently, the en bloc technique was reintroduced and extended to include carcinoma of the midthoracic and cervical esophagus, with acceptable mortality rates (56).

The transhiatal approach, or the esophagectomy without thoracotomy, was initially described by Turner in 1932. Akiyama reported the use of this technique for removal of the normal intrathoracic esophagus after resection of malignant tumors of the hypopharynx and cervical esophagus. Orringer popularized the technique for tumors of the cardia and lower esophagus. Although he advocates its use for cancer of the remainder of the thoracic esophagus, most surgeons (ourselves included) believe that these tumors are more appropriately treated by a transthoracic approach. Controversy continues in the literature as to which operation is best suited for patients with esophageal cancer. Our view is that the armamentarium of an esophageal surgeon should include different surgical approaches, since the operation is usually tailored to the individual patient based on the extent of disease and the ability to withstand major thoracotomy.

TUMOR LOCATION AND SURGICAL APPROACH The location of the tumor within the esophagus, as well as the tumor cell type, determines the surgical approach to a large extent. Tumors of the cervical esophagus are generally approached through a cervical incision with a simultaneous laparotomy. The cervical incision is used to mobilize the cervical esophagus and perform a neck node dissection, while through a laparotomy, the esophageal substitute (usually the stomach) is mobilized. In a cervical esophagogastrotomy, the intrathoracic esophagus is bluntly dissected and removed, and the stomach is advanced through the posterior mediastinum (Fig. 1.27). If the tumor straddles the thoracic inlet, a partial or complete sternotomy is occasionally required to complete the dissection around the great vessels under direct vision.

Tumors of the cardia or the lower esophagus are generally approached through a left thoracotomy, with access to the abdomen through a diaphragmatic incision, thus sparing the patient a separate abdominal incision or the increased morbidity of an extended thoracoabdominal approach (Fig. 1.28). The incision in the diaphragm is performed peripherally, about 1 inch from the chest wall from the back of the sternum anteriorly, to the tip of the spleen posteriorly. Thus performed, the diaphragmatic incision denervates the least amount of diaphragmatic muscle.

Tumors of the middle or upper third of the thoracic esophagus are best approached through a right tho-

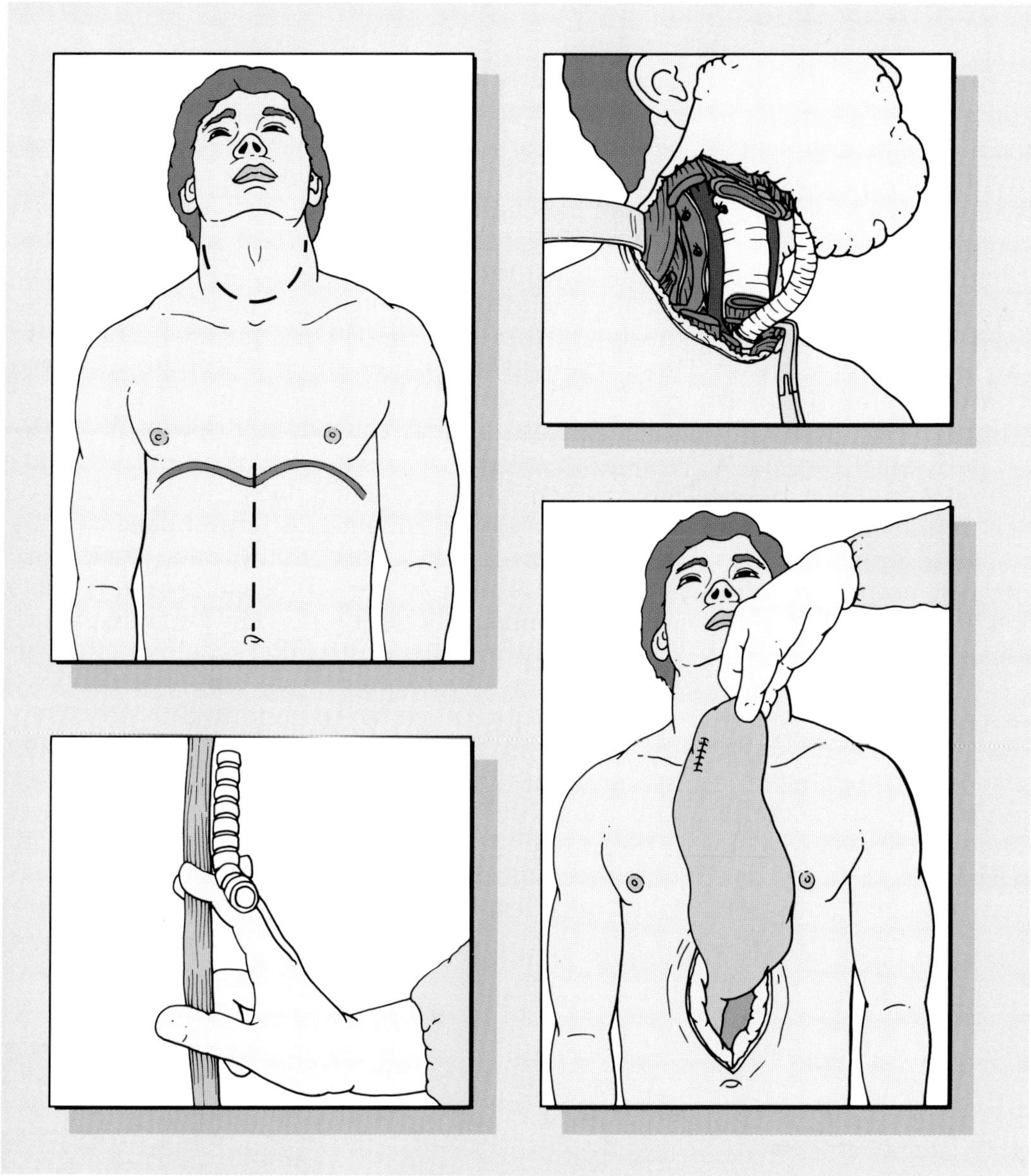

FIGURE 1.27 Resection of carcinoma of the cervical esophagus.

FIGURE 1.28 Left thoracotomy for resection. (Adapted from reference 25.)

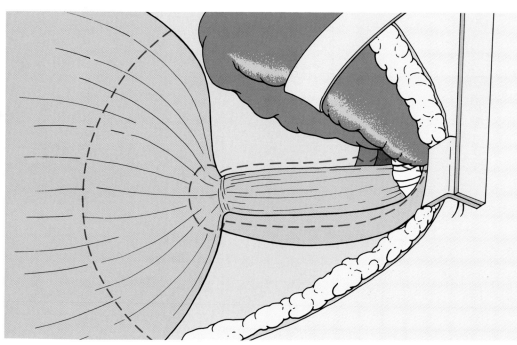

racotomy (Fig. 1.29). This provides the safest approach to tumors abutting the trachea, carina, or arch of the aorta. The thoracic duct is more vulnerable through this approach and must be carefully sought and ligated in the event of an en bloc resection. An abdominal incision is necessary to prepare the esophageal substitute. Hiebert and Belsey (63) describe mobilization of the stomach through the hiatus with a right thoracotomy, and we have occasionally performed this maneuver in patients without previous abdominal surgery in whom the tumor is located 10 cm proximal to the hiatus.

The transhiatal approach is performed through a cervical and abdominal incision with a blunt esophagectomy. This approach is primarily used for carcinomas of the cardia or lower esophagus or, as previously described, for removing a normal intrathoracic esophagus after resection of a carcinoma of the hypopharynx or cervical esophagus.

RECONSTRUCTION Several organs present themselves as esophageal substitutes. Since Sweet demonstrated that division of the left gastric artery does not impair gastric viability (64), surgeons have used the stomach for establishing esophagogastric continuity. The organ generally has a constant and reliable blood supply. Division of the left gastric, left gastroepiploic, and short

gastric vessels leaves the stomach with an adequate blood supply from the right gastric and right gastroepiploic arteries, with its arcade along the greater curvature. As such, the stomach could be advanced to the apex of the chest and even into the neck. The addition of a Kocher maneuver allows advancement of the stomach all the way to the hypopharynx, permitting its use for extended resections (Fig. 1.30). A single anastomosis is all that is required, thus reducing the operative time. The addition of a drainage procedure such as a pyloroplasty or a pyloromyotomy after the bilateral vagectomy incurred by esophageal resection is controversial. A recent, well-controlled, randomized study indicates that postprandial fullness, regurgitation, or vomiting develops in about one-third of patients without a drainage procedure. Symptoms were more severe, and were more likely to be multiple, in patients without drainage. Fourteen percent had clinical evidence of gastric outlet obstruction requiring total parenteral feeding or reoperation (65). Surgeons who have had occasion to reoperate to perform a pyloromyotomy will appreciate the need to perform this procedure at the primary operation. Regardless of whether the drainage procedure is done, most patients complain of a postprandial fullness that gradually improves with time. Occasional episodes of regurgitation occur, especially after high cervical esophagogastric or pharyn-

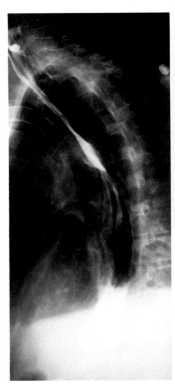

FIGURE 1.30 Complete gastric mobilization permits its advancement to the hypopharynx if necessary.

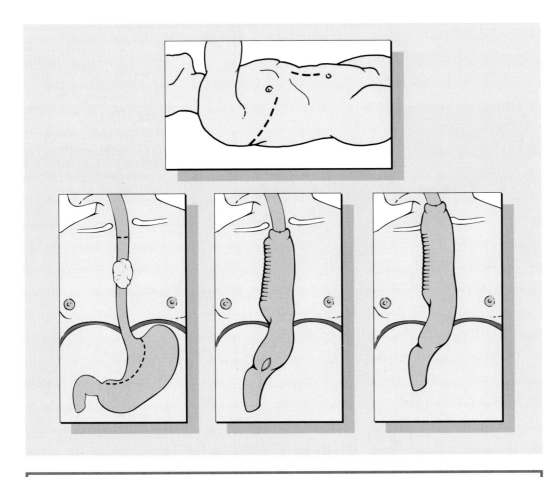

FIGURE 1.29 Right thoracotomy and laparotomy.

gogastric reconstruction. Patients are generally advised to divide their diet into six small meals daily and to avoid lying flat for two to three hours postprandially. We also place most patients on an H$_2$-blocker regimen to ameliorate the manifestations of gastroesophageal reflux that predictably follow intrathoracic esophagogastrostomy. When an esophagogastric anastomosis is performed in the neck rather than the mediastinum, the incidence of reflux esophagitis and strictures is decreased but not eliminated. In a report on the incidence of dysphagia and the need for postoperative dilatation after cervical esophagogastrostomy, Orringer found that 50 percent of patients required dilatation for a temporary period of time, and 15 percent required permanent home dilatations (66). Some believe that the occurrence of dysphagia after cervical esophagogastrostomy is a function of follow-up duration, since reflux in this circumstance has a more insidious and gradual onset than after intrathoracic reconstruction.

The sequelae of long-term reflux after esophagogastrostomy prompted us to use the colon for esophageal reconstruction after resection of favorable lesions, with expectations of long-term survival. The left colon is the conduit of choice because of the reliability of its blood supply. The transplant is used as a pedicled graft, based on the upper left colic branch of the inferior mesenteric artery, and is transposed to the required location in the posterior mediastinum or neck in an isoperistaltic manner (Fig. 1.31). A sufficient length of the viscus can usually be obtained to allow a cervical anastomosis. The operative procedure is prolonged by the need to construct three anastomoses—an esophagocolostomy, a cologastrostostomy, and a colocolostomy—to re-establish colonic continuity. The colon graft retains its peristaltic function, as compared with the transposed and denervated stomach, which contributes little to the transit of the food bolus. Dysphagia following colon interposition is related mainly to recurrent tumor or, on rare occasions, to redundancy of the colon within the chest. One may avoid the latter

problem by placing the graft under a moderate degree of tension throughout its intrathoracic course and fixing it to the edges of the diaphragmatic hiatus where it enters the abdomen. Although gastrocolic reflux is often seen, ulcerations or strictures are rare and are further minimized by constructing the cologastric anastomosis to the posterior wall of the stomach, leaving a sufficient length of colon within the abdomen subjected to the positive-pressure intra-abdominal environment, so that it acts as an antireflux mechanism. The retention of the stomach in its normal intra-abdominal location preserves its reservoir function, and dietary habits are not as deranged as after esophagogastrostomy.

Another option for reconstruction is the jejunum, which is used as either a pedicled or free graft. The jejunum, like the colon, retains its peristaltic function but has an unpredictable vascular pattern that may preclude its use for long-segment interpositions. The fairly thin, non-fat-laden mesentery of Oriental patients has allowed some in the Far East to use the jejunum as a conduit of choice. The use of a jejunum as a free graft is an exciting option, but one requiring microvascular techniques that add more time to an already lengthy and difficult operation.

RADIATION THERAPY

The results of irradiation delivered with curative intent to patients with esophageal carcinoma have been disappointing. Survival at five years has generally been reported to be in the region of 5 percent. A single report published in 1966 claimed a 20 percent survival at five years among a highly select group of patients (67). That result has not been duplicated by the original reporter or by others in the same institution in more than a decade since the first claim. Furthermore, 50 percent of the patients in the series could not complete the treatment protocol. Advocates of primary radiation therapy argue that poor survival rates in patients treated with that modality are a result of patient selection: patients with more advanced disease

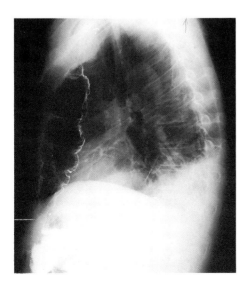

FIGURE 1.31 This patient was reconstructed by an isoperistaltic segment of left colon with a cervical esophagocolostomy.

are relegated to radiation and those with more favorable lesions are selected for surgical resection. Whether primary radiation therapy or surgical resection is the treatment of choice for locoregional esophageal carcinoma remains to be resolved by an adequately performed randomized trial. The argument that primary radiation therapy carries a lower mortality than surgical resection has not been validated by our own experience. Doses of radiation considered adequate to elicit a positive response with curative intent are generally in the region of 6000 rads and can cause permanent lung damage and necrosis of the esophagus along with tumor perforation and mediastinal abscesses. Furthermore, radiation may result in strictures that are difficult or even dangerous to dilate. The development of a tracheoesophageal fistula is accelerated by radiation of tumors invading the major airways. Of patients thus treated in our institution, 25 percent developed a tracheoesophageal fistula during therapy. The cumulative mortality of radiotherapy with curative intent approaches 10 percent and occurs primarily as a result of hemorrhage, abscess, fistula, or pneumonia (56). These figures are not significantly different from the mortality after esophageal resections.

Preoperative radiation to obtain the benefits of both kinds of treatment has long attracted interest. For many years Nakayama's group advocated brief, intense preoperative irradiation, employing 2000 rads over four consecutive days, followed on the next day by surgical resection (68). They estimated a 10 percent improvement in five-year survival, as compared with results achieved in patients not receiving radiotherapy. This outcome has been difficult to assess. A recent report from these authors, in fact, described no significant benefit from preoperative radiation (69). In the Western world, efforts at preoperative radiation have not produced improved results. Parker and associates found no significant improvement in long-term survival in their large experience (70). Two recent randomized studies have failed to show any benefit from preoperative radiation (71,72). The large trial coordinated by the European Organization for Research on Treatment of Cancer evaluated 200 patients with operable squamous cell esophageal carcinoma. The patients were randomized to a control arm treated by surgery alone or to an experimental arm receiving 3000 rads preoperatively. The study failed to show any advantage for preoperative radiation therapy in resectability or long-term survival.

PALLIATIVE MEASURES

RADIATION The role of radiation therapy for palliation of esophageal carcinoma is generally well accepted. The usual dose is in the range of 4500 rads delivered over a four-week period. An initial response is achieved in about two-thirds of patients and generally occurs toward the end of treatment. Unfortunately, however, only about one-third will have durable palliation

throughout the course of their disease, since recurrent dysphagia secondary to tumor occurs in most cases. Radiation therapy is contraindicated in patients with visible tumor invading the airway or in those with an established tracheoesophageal fistula, unless an esophageal exclusion procedure is initially performed.

LASER THERAPY The direct delivery of laser energy and subsequent vaporization of malignant tissue is an important addition to the available methods of palliating carcinoma of the esophagus. Among the various lasers, the neodymium:yttrium aluminum garnet (Nd:YAG) laser is the most commonly used for treating obstructing esophageal tumors. The procedure is appropriate for the relief of dysphagia in patients with disseminated disease or patients in whom surgical resection is contraindicated for medical reasons. The procedure results in adequate palliation in about 80 percent of patients and is accomplished with a reasonably low mortality during the procedure (73). Patients with odynophagia or chest pain have less effective symptom relief, since those symptoms probably represent evidence of mediastinal penetration. Patients having tumors with a large submucosal component, or with bleeding from large, ulcerating tumors of the cardia, are also less likely to derive significant benefit from laser treatment. The procedure is particularly attractive since it averts the mortality and major morbidity associated with esophagectomy and since it has no dose limitation (unlike radiation therapy) and hence can usually be repeated as often as required. Its application through the flexible esophagoscope permits its performance as an outpatient procedure using only mild intravenous sedation. The most feared complication, early or late perforation, is reported to occur in 10 percent to 30 percent of patients; if only early perforations directly related to laser therapy are considered, the rate is about 5 percent.

Treatment is performed under mild topical anesthesia and intravenous sedation with diazepam and/or meperidine. The flexible esophagoscope is advanced beyond the distal margin of the tumor. When the tumor does not permit passage of the endoscope, an initial bougienage over a guidewire may be attempted; usually Savary dilators are used for that purpose. Immediately following bougienage, or by the next day, a pediatric or adult-type esophagoscope is passed through the distal margin of the tumor. The wave guide carrying the laser beam is advanced through the biopsy channel to 1 cm beyond the edge of the lens. This permits all lasing to be done under direct vision (Fig. 1.32). The usual power setting is 80 to 100 watts for two-second intervals. As the scope is withdrawn, the tumor comes into view and the laser beam is aimed a 1-cm distance from the lesion, which is then treated circumferentially. Constant cognizance of the esophageal lumen is essential to reduce the risk of perforation. The initial reaction is blanching of the tissues. Endoscopy is done 48 hours later, and sloughed tumor tissue is either aspirated, removed with a biopsy forceps, or simply pushed downstream by the scope. Treatments are then continued until the desired effect is obtained. The mean number of sessions required is two to three per patient, with an increase in luminal diameter from 3 mm to 11 or 12 mm, allowing most patients a normal diet. When no lumen is identified, antegrade treatment is employed. The beam is aimed at the tumor tissue closest to the lumen and moved in a circular fashion around the tumor (Fig. 1.33). The laser beam is never directed at the esophageal wall. Fleischer reported relief of dysphagia in approximately 90 percent of patients so treated (73). Most patients develop a low-grade fever and a mild leukocytosis after treatment, but these eventually resolve. Major bleeding is rare in most series.

BOUGIENAGE AND ENDOPROSTHESIS Simple bougienage is an effective way of increasing esophageal luminal diameter in patients with malignant strictures. Restoration of the luminal diameter to 12 mm allows intake of a soft diet in most patients. Although Maloney mercury-weighted dilators are safe and easy to use, we prefer guidewire dilators under endoscopic control for most malignant strictures. Savary dilators are best suited for this purpose. The procedure is performed under light sedation and preferably, but not necessarily, under fluoroscopic guidance. A guidewire is passed through the biopsy channel of a flexible esophagoscope and is directed through the stricture into the distal esophagus and stomach. The scope is then removed, and the dilator of choice is passed over the wire and through the stricture. Resistance is generally felt with the first bougie, but

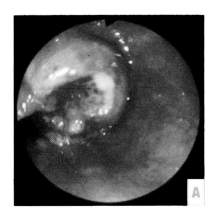 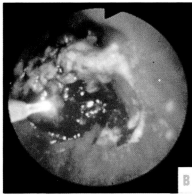 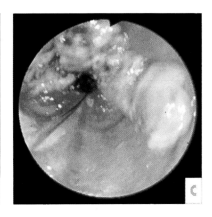

FIGURE 1.32 A fungating esophageal tumor (A) is lased under direct vision **(B)**. Bleeding is minimal and self-limiting. **(C)** The tumor bulk is reduced, and white coagulum is seen. (From

Waye JD, Geenen JE, Fleischer D, Venu RP. *Techniques in therapeutic endoscopy.* New York: Gower Medical Publishing, 1987.)

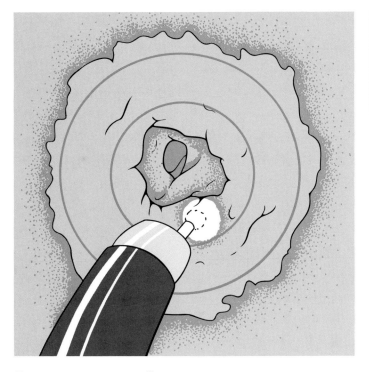

FIGURE 1.33 Antegrade therapy is "delivered" initially to tumor tissue closest to the lumen with the laser beam perpendicular to the tumor surface. Further treatments are done in concentric circles, avoiding aiming the beam perpendicular to the esophageal wall. (Adapted from Waye et al., 1987.)

dilation is easier beyond that. The tendency of malignant strictures to fracture rather than stretch accounts for the higher risk of perforation associated with bougienage reported in some series. It is essential when encountering resistance to apply gentle but firm pressure rather than forcible advancement of the dilator. One is usually able to dilate strictures gradually to accept a 46–50 French dilator. Cassidy reported a 2 percent mortality after bougienage in 154 patients, mainly due to perforation (74). The relief of dysphagia by simple bougienage, however, is short-lived. The desire to avoid repeated dilation prompted the introduction of the endoesophageal prosthesis. The development of the Nottingham introducer in 1977 greatly facilitated this approach. Several types are commercially available including the Proctor Livingstone, the Atkinson Key Med prosthesis, and the Celestin tube. All have a proximal flange to rest on the mucosal shelf of the tumor and to prevent distal migration. Some also have distal flanges that prevent proximal dislodgement. Recently introduced is a polyvinyl cuffed tube that is particularly adaptable to patients with tracheoesophageal fistula.

The procedure is performed under either intravenous sedation or general anesthesia. The stricture is initially dilated as described above, to 46–52 French. This could be done in one or several sessions. The exact distance of the proximal and distal ends of the tumor from the incisors is endoscopically measured. The prosthesis, together with the introducer mounted on the endoscope, is lubricated with silicone spray, and the whole assembly is advanced to the desired location in the esophagus, as based on previous measurements (Fig. 1.34). The introducer is disengaged and removed, and the position of the tube is confirmed endoscopically. Successful insertion of the prosthesis is possible in over 90 percent of patients. Insertion is contraindicated for tumors located within 2 cm of the cricopharyngeus due to the danger of tracheal compression and pharyngeal irritation. Tumors of the cardia can be intubated if appropriate measures are taken to prevent reflux (namely, avoiding recumbency at all times). Occasionally, malignant angulation at the cardia prevents insertion. The mortality of the procedure varies between zero and 16 percent, with most recent series reporting a 3 percent to 5 percent mortality. Tytgat, in a large survey, reported perforation in 7 percent, obstruction in 5 percent, and dislodgement in 7 percent. The incidence of major hemorrhage from pressure

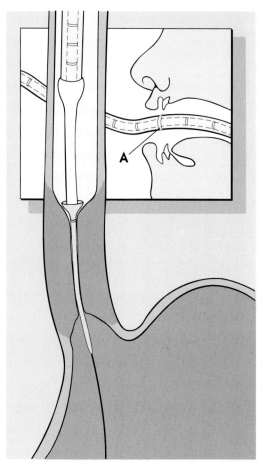
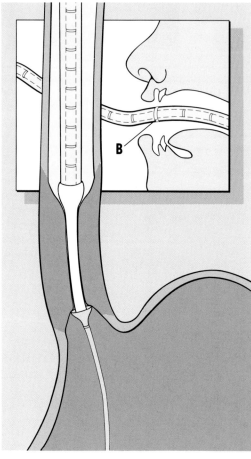

FIGURE 1.34 The peroral or "push" technique of insertion of endoesophageal prosthesis. Point (**A**) marked on the pusher tube indicates the start is at the proximal tumor edge, and (**B**) marks the seating of the flange at the proximal tumor shelf. (Adapted from Waye et al., 1987.)

necrosis into the mediastinum is about 1 percent (75). Perforation is treated, when recognized immediately, by prosthetic placement to seal the perforation. Delayed perforation is necessarily treated conservatively by antibiotics and by withholding oral feedings. Prosthetic obstruction results from food impaction, which can be prevented by frequent intake of fluids with meals and treated, once it occurs, by displacing the impacted food material downstream with either an endoscope or a nasogastric tube. Obstruction of the prosthesis can also result from tumor overgrowth, requiring removal and reinsertion (Fig. 1.35). The advent of laser therapy has limited the use of esophageal prostheses, which are now used only in selected patients with malignant tracheoesophageal fistulae (Fig. 1.36) who are not otherwise candidates for alternative palliative measures.

BIPOLAR ELECTROCOAGULATION Bipolar electrocoagulating probes have been developed which can be used to achieve thermal destruction of esophageal cancer. The tumor probe is similar in appearance to the Eder–Puestow dilator. The electrically active area corresponds to the dilating olive (15 mm, maximum size), and electric energy is delivered to a 360° area. An initial endoscopy and dilatation is performed, if necessary. Tumor margins are carefully measured. The procedure is carried out under fluo-

roscopic guidance, since there can be no direct visualization of probe-tissue interaction. The palpating sensation of tumor resistance is also used to guide therapy as the probe is passed beyond the cancer and then pulled retrograde in steps corresponding to the length of the electrically active area (Fig. 1.37). Decreased expense and increased portability are major advantages of this method as compared to laser therapy. A problem is that in noncircumferential cancer, normal tissue may be damaged, leading to stricture and perforation.

ALCOHOL INJECTION The least expensive and technically easiest method of nonoperative palliation of esophageal cancer is alcohol injection into the tumor via flexible endoscope (76). The technique is based on the freehand method for injection sclerosis of esophageal varices. The method involves passing an endoscope beyond the tumor and injecting 0.5-ml or 1-ml aliquots of absolute alcohol directly into the macroscopic tumor. Immediate blanching of the injection site is frequently observed. All visible tumor is injected, and injection into normal tissue is avoided. In a recent small series, ten of 11 patients so treated had improvement, with a mean period of 32 days between treatments (76).

PHOTODYNAMIC THERAPY In an effort to provide more selectivity in laser treatment of esophageal cancer,

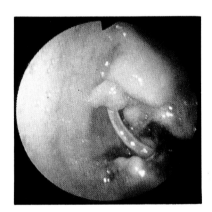

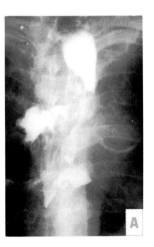

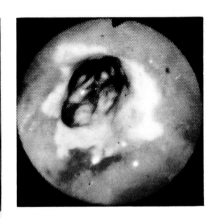

FIGURE 1.37 Tumor treated by bipolar electrocoagulation showing a circumferential white burn. (From Waye et al., 1987.)

FIGURE 1.36 Tracheoesophageal fistula complicating esophageal cancer (A) is effectively sealed by an endoesophageal prosthesis (B). (From Waye et al., 1987.)

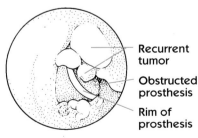

Recurrent tumor

Obstructed prosthesis

Rim of prosthesis

FIGURE 1.35 Tumor outgrowth obstructed this prosthesis. (From Silverstein and Tytgat, 1987.)

photodynamic therapy (PDT) is emerging as another high-technology approach (77). This involves injecting a photosensitizing chemical that is more selectively retained in malignant tissue than in normal tissue. A low-power laser is used to activate a photochemical reaction, which destroys the cancer but not the normal tissue. PDT has been mostly carried out with hematoporphyrin derivatives, and a major drawback has been skin sensitivity and the need to avoid bright light for prolonged periods. In one series of 40 patients, the lumen through the tumor increased from an average of 6 mm to 9 mm one month after treatment (77), and food intake improved from a liquid to a soft diet in 35 patients. Over an average survival time of 7.7 months, however, there were five sunburns, six pleural effusions, three tracheoesophageal fistulas, one chylothorax, and an endoscopic perforation. This type of therapy may be most effective in superficial cancers.

CHEMOTHERAPY

The last decade has witnessed an interest in the use of chemotherapy for treating patients with advanced esophageal cancer or with limited locoregional disease. Responses, mostly partial in degree, have been observed with both single-agent and combination chemotherapy (78). Most combinations are cisplatin-based. Although improvement in dysphagia may be achieved, it is usually short-lived. There are as yet insufficient data regarding the ultimate survival benefit of combination chemotherapy, either alone or in the neoadjuvant setting combined with surgical resection.

BENIGN TUMORS

Benign tumors of the esophagus are rare. Smooth muscle tumors are the most common, accounting for 80 percent of all benign tumors of the esophagus.

Leiomyoma

INCIDENCE

The actual incidence of esophageal leiomyoma is difficult to determine. Most small clinical series are not reported, and small tumors are likely to be missed except in the most thorough autopsies. In autopsy series the incidence of leiomyoma varies between one in 63 to one in 18,000, with an average of one leiomyoma reported for every 1000 autopsies (79). Oberhelman reported on 1105 leiomyomas of the gastrointestinal tract, of which 6 percent were located in the esophagus (80). In spite of the increasing number of reported cases in the last two decades, the incidence of esophageal carcinoma remains 50-fold higher than that of leiomyoma.

PATHOLOGY

Almost 90 percent of cases are found in the middle and distal esophagus. Tumors of the upper thoracic esophagus are seen in only 10 percent of patients, while those in the cervical region are very rare. The tumor originates in the muscularis mucosa and is located intramurally in 97 percent of cases. Pedunculated lesions or tumors extending mainly extramurally account for 3 percent of cases. The lesions vary between 2 to 5 cm in diameter, with rare reports of giant tumors. Some tumors measure only a few millimeters in size. Postlethwait and Musser reported on 51 leiomyomas, of which 30 measured less than 2 mm in diameter (81). The majority of the tumors are single, with multiple lesions noted in less than 3 percent of most series. The histologic features of leiomyomas have changed little since Virchow's initial description in 1863. The tumors are encapsulated and have no tendency toward invasion of the mucosa. Muscle fibers assume a whorly pattern characteristic of smooth muscle tumors with interspersed fibrous tissue. Malignant degeneration is rare; only two possible cases have been reported. Pathologically, the main issue is differentiating leiomyomas from leiomyosarcoma. The number of mitotic figures is no longer relied on to differentiate between malignant and benign smooth muscle tumors. The absence or poor development of intracellular organelles, normally seen in smooth muscles, is perhaps a more reliable indicator of malignancy. On occasion, the biologic behavior of the tumor is the only determinant of its malignant nature.

CLINICAL PRESENTATION AND COURSE

Over 90 percent of patients are between 20 and 60 years of age. The tumor is over twice as common in men as in women. Almost half the patients are asymptomatic, with the tumor discovered when radiographic examination is performed for other reasons. Dysphagia is present in 48 percent of patients, and is typically gradual in onset and occasionally intermittent. Chest pain, mainly in the form of substernal discomfort or epigastric fullness, is noted in half the patients. The pathogenesis of pain associated with leiomyoma is unclear, but may be related to an associated motor disorder. Various other symptoms such as pyrosis, belching, anorexia, and weight loss are also noted.

DIAGNOSIS

Chest radiography may reveal a retrocardiac posterior mediastinal mass. The diagnosis is usually made, however, by the esophagogram, where the tumor appears as a intraluminal bulge without mucosal ulceration. The acute angle between the tumor mass and the esophageal wall helps to differentiate leiomyomas from esophageal or mediastinal cysts. Hiatal hernias—or, less commonly, epiphrenic diverticulum—may be seen on the barium esophagogram. In fact, symptoms of gastroesophageal reflux or symptoms related to an epiphrenic diverticulum may have prompted clinical evaluation, with the leiomyoma being an incidental finding. Esophagoscopy is indicated in all cases to confirm the diagnosis and to evaluate associated lesions. The intact musosa overlying the tumor should not be breached by attempts at biopsy, which would complicate surgical removal (Fig. 1.38). A differential diagnosis includes mediastinal or esophageal cysts, mediastinal adenopathy, or esophageal compression by large aortic aneurysms. CT and occasionally aortography are essential to confirm the diagnosis.

MANAGEMENT

Surgical removal is usually indicated to confirm the benign nature of the tumor and to relieve dysphagia. The approach is determined by the location of the tumor and by the need to perform associated procedures such as an antireflux repair or excision of an epiphrenic diverticulum. Middle-third lesions are approached through a right thoracotomy, whereas leiomyomas of the lower esophagus or cardia are approached through a left thoracotomy. When operation is indicated for complications of gastroesophageal reflux, the operation is performed through a left thoracotomy. The esophagus is usually sufficiently mobilized to allow for removal of a middle-third leiomyoma. Enucleation is the procedure of choice, since the tumor peels easily off the mucosa. It is usually unnecessary to reapproximate the muscle layers after enucleation is complete. Resection is indicated only if malignancy is suspected or if tumors are extensive. An associated antireflux repair is performed after enucleation of tumors of the gastroesophageal junction, since the extent of dissection required disrupts the antireflux mechanisms. The mortality following enucleation is usually less than 2 percent.

Esophageal Polyps

Fibrovascular polyps are rare. They occur primarily in the cervical esophagus and may acquire a long pedicle as a result of swallowing and peristalsis, allowing occasional regurgitation of the tumor into the pharynx. Regurgitation of large polyps may have catastrophic consequences, with death secondary to asphyxiation. Microscopically, these lesions consist of a core of fibrovascular and adipose tissue (hence the name fibrolipoma) covered with normal mucosa.

Squamous papilloma is another polypoid lesion of the esophagus that may be sessile or pedunculated. It is more frequently recognized with the liberal use of esophagoscopy. The tumor consists of a fibrovascular connective-tissue core thrown into a papillary pattern and covered with hyperplastic squamous mucosa. The lesion is probably inflammatory rather than truly neoplastic.

Clinically, most cases of esophageal polyps are asymptomatic, except when large tumors result in dysphagia and weight loss. Lesions prolapsing into the lower esophageal sphincter may result in esophageal dilation and a radiographic appearance similar to that of achalasia.

Esophagoscopy is necessary to rule out pedunculated carcinoma and to determine the exact site of the pedicle, should surgical removal be necessary. Endoscopic removal is possible for small lesions with narrow pedicles. Larger lesions, however, are preferably excised by an esophagotomy sited opposite the origin of the pedicle.

Miscellaneous Tumors

A variety of other benign tumors of the esophagus have been reported, but they are exceedingly rare. These include hemangiomas, granular cell myoblastomas, lymphangiomas, neurofibromas, rhabdomyomas, osteochondromas, lipomas, and fibromas. Their management is essentially guided by ruling out malignancy and relieving symptoms.

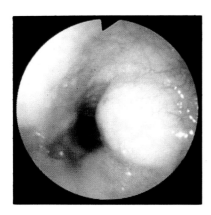

FIGURE 1.38 At endoscopy leiomyomas are seen as localized bulges covered by intact mucosa. (From Silverstein and Tytgat, 1987.)

References

1. Lu JB, Yang WX, Lui JM, et al. Trends in morbidity and mortality for esophageal cancer in Linxian county 1959–83. *Int J Cancer* 36:643–645, 1985.

2. Blot WJ, Fraumeni JF. Geographic epidemiology of cancer in the United States. In: Schotterfeld D, Fraumeni J, eds. *Cancer Epidemiology and Prevention*. Philadelphia: W.B. Saunders, 1982:179.

3. Fraumeni JF, Blot WJ. Geographic variation in esophageal cancer mortality in the United States. *J Chron Dis* 30:759–767, 1977.

4. Blot WJ, Fraumeni JF Jr. Trends in esophageal cancer mortality among U.S. blacks and whites. *Am J Public Health* 77: 296–298, 1987.

5. Bartsch J, Montesano R. Relevance of nitrosamines to human cancer. *Carcinogenesis* 5:1381–1391, 1984.

6. Hammond EC. Smoking in relation to death rates of one million men and women. *NCI Monogr* 19:127–204, 1966.

7. Rogot E, Murray JL. Smoking and causes of death among U.S. veterans: 16 years of observation. *Public Health Rep* 95: 213–222, 1980.

8. Doll R, Peto R. Mortality in relation to smoking: 20 years observation on male British doctors. *Br Med J* 2:1525–1536, 1976.

9. Mimic Y, Garabrant DH, Peters JM, et al. Tobacco, alcohol, diet, occupation and cancer of the esophagus. *Cancer Res* 48:3843–3848, 1988.

10. Chadirian P, Stein GF, Gorodetsky C, et al. Oesophageal cancer studies in the Caspian littoral of Iran: some residual results, including opium as a risk factor. *Int J Cancer* 35:593–597, 1985.

11. Pottern LM, Morris LE, Blot WJ, et al. Esophageal cancer among black men in Washington, D.C. I. Alcohol, tobacco and other risk factors. *J Natl Cancer Inst* 67:777–783, 1981.

12. Wynder EL, Bross IJ. A study of etiological factors in cancer of the esophagus. *Cancer* 14:389–413, 1961.

13. Tuyns AJ, Pequignot G, Jensen OM: Le cancer de l'oesophage en Ille-et-Vilaine en fonction des niveaux de consommation d'alcohol et de tabac: des risques qui se multiplient. *Bull Cancer* 64:63–65, 1977.

14. Tuyns AJ. Oesophageal cancer in non-smoking drinkers and non-drinking smokers. *Int J Cancer* 32:443–444, 1983.

15. Department of Chemical Etiology of CICAMS and LRTPTEC. Preliminary investigation on the carcinogenicity of extracts of pickles in Linxian. *Res Cancer Prev Treatment* 2:46–49, 1977.

16. Lu SH, Ohshima H, Fu HM, et al. Urinary excretion of N-nitrosamino acids and nitrate by high and low esophageal risk populations in northern China: endogenous formation of N-nitrosoproline and its inhibition by vitamin C. *Cancer Res* 46: 1485–1491, 1986.

17. O'Neill C, Pan Q, Clarke G, et al. Silica fragments from millet bran in mucosa surrounding oesophageal tumors in patients in northern China. *Lancet* 1:1202–1206, 1982.

18. Smith PG. Late effects of x-ray treatment of ankylosing spondylitis. In: Boice J, Fraumeni J, eds. *Radiation Carcinogenesis*. New York: Raven Press, 1984:107.

19. Norell S, Ahblom A, Lipping H, et al. Oesophageal cancer and vulcanization work. *Lancet* 1:462–463, 1983.

20. Selikoff IJ, Hammond EC, Seidman H. Mortality experience of insulation workers in the United States and Canada, 1943–76. *Ann N Y Acad Sci* 330:91–116, 1979.

21. Hille JJ, Markowitz S, Margoliusk A, et al. Human papillomavirus and carcinoma of the esophagus. *N Engl J Med* 213: 1707, 1985.

22. Crum CP, Ikenberg H, Richart R, et al. Human papillomavirus type 16 and early cervical neoplasia. *N Engl J Med* 310:880–883, 1984.

23. Shine J, Allison PR. Carcinoma of oesophagus with tylosis. *Lancet* 1:951–953, 1966.

24. Ellis FH, Gibb SP, Watkins E. Esophagogastrectomy: a safe, widely applicable and expeditious form of palliation for patients with carcinoma of the esophagus and cardia. *Ann Surg* 198:531, 1983.

25. Skinner DB. En bloc resection for neoplasms of the esophagus and cardia. *J Thorac Cardiovasc Surg* 85:59–70, 1983.

26. Hamilton S, Smith R, Cameron J, et al. Prevalence and characteristics of Barrett's esophagus in patients with adenocarcinoma of the esophagus or the esophagogastric junction. *Hum Pathol* 19:942–948, 1988.

27. Kalish RJ, Clancy PE, Orringer MB, et al. Clinical, epidemiological and morphologic comparison between adenocarcinomas arising in Barrett's esophageal mucosa and in the gastric cardia. *Gastroenterology* 86:461–467, 1984.

28. Spechler JS, Robbins AH, Rubbins HB, et al. Adenocarcinoma and Barrett's esophagus: an overrated risk? *Gastroenterology* 87:927–933, 1984.

29. Cameron AJ, Ott BJ, Payne WS. The incidence of adenocarcinoma in columnar-lined (Barrett's) esophagus. *N Engl J Med* 313:857–859, 1985.

30. Sprung DJ, Ellis FH, Gibb P. Incidence of adenocarcinoma in Barrett's esophagus. *Gastroenterology* 79:817, 1984.

31. Robertson CS, Mayberry JF, Nicholson DA. Value of endoscopic surveillance in the detection of neoplastic changes in Barrett's esophagus. *Br J Surg* 75:760–763, 1988.

32. Altorki N, Skinner DB, Ferguson MR, et al. Barrett's adenocarcinoma: long term survival and recurrence patterns. In: *Proceedings of the Fourth World Congress of the International Society for Diseases of the Esophagus*. 1989:132.

33. Sprung DJ, Ellis FH, Gibb SP. Regression of Barrett's epithelium after anti-reflux surgery. *Gastroenterology* 79:817, 1984.

34. Hamilton SR, Hutcheon DF, Ravich WJ, et al. Adenocarcinoma in Barrett's esophagus after elimination of gastroesophageal reflux. *Gastroenterology* 86:356–360, 1984.

35. Dowlatshahi K, Daneshbod A, Mobarhan S. Early detection of cancer of the oesophagus along the Caspian littoral. *Lancet* 1:125, 1978.

36. Shu YJ. Cytopathology of the esophagus: an overview of esophageal cytopathology in China. *Acta Cytol* 27:7–16, 1983.

37. Shu YJ, Yang SG, Gin SP. Further studies on the relationship between epithelial dysplasia and carcinoma of the esophagus. *Natl Med J China* 60:39–41, 1980.

38. Mandard AM, Marnay J, Gignoux M, et al. Cancer of the esophagus and associated lesions: detailed pathologic study of 100 esophagectomy specimens. *Hum Pathol* 15:660–669, 1984.

39. Schmidt HG, Riddell RH, Walther B, et al. Dysplasia in Barrett's esophagus. *Cancer Res Clin Oncol* 110:145–152, 1985.

40. Reid BJ, Weinstein WM, Lewin KJ, et al. Endoscopic biopsy can detect high grade dysplasia or early adenocarcinoma in Barrett's esophagus without grossly recognizable neoplastic lesions. *Gastroenterology* 94:81–90, 1988.

41. Lee RG. Dysplasia in Barrett's esophagus. *Am J Surg Pathol* 9:845–852, 1985.

42. Altorki N, Sunagawa M, Little AG, Skinner DB. High grade dysplasia in the columnar-lined esophagus: to resect or not? *Am J Surg* (in press).

43. Tateishi R, Taniguchi H, Wada A, et al. Argyrophil cells and melanocytes in esophageal mucosa. *Arch Pathol* 98:87–89, 1974.

44. Bosman FT, Louwerens JWK. APUD cells in teratoma. *Am J Pathol* 104:174–180, 1981.

45. Takubo K, Kanada Y, Ishii M, et al. Primary malignant melanoma of the esophagus. *Hum Pathol* 14:727–730, 1983.

46. Gaede JT, Postlethwait RW, Shelburne JD, et al. Leiomyocarcoma of the esophagus. Report of two cases, one with associated squamous cell carcinoma. *J Thorac Cardiovasc Surg* 75:74–746, 1978.

47. Shao LF, Hunag GJ, Zhang DW, et al. Detection and surgical treatment of early esophageal carcinoma. In: *Proceedings of the Beijing Symposium on Cardiothoracic Surgery, Beijing, 1981.* New York: John Wiley & Sons, 1981:168.

48. Huang GJ. Recognition and treatment of the early lesion. In: Delarue N, Wilkins E, Wong J, eds. *International Trends in General Thoracic Surgery*, Vol. 4. St. Louis: CV Mosby Inc., 1988:144.

49. Nabeya K, Hanoaka T, Onozawa K, Ri S, et al. New measures for early detection of carcinoma of the esophagus. In: Siewert Jr, Holscher AH, eds. *Diseases of the Esophagus*. Berlin: Springer-Verlag, 1988:105.

50. Dowlatshahi K, Skinner DB, DeMeester TR, et al. Evaluation of brush cytology as an independent technique for detection of esophageal carcinoma. *J Thorac Cardiovasc Surg* 89:848–851, 1985.

51. Yangin M, Gangyi L, Xianchi G, et al. Detection and natural progression of early oesophageal carcinoma: preliminary communication. *J R Soc Med* 74:864, 1981.

52. Skinner DB. Esophageal malignancies: experience with 110 cases. *Surg Clin North Am* 56:137–147, 1976.

53. Akiyama H, Kogure T, Itai Y. The esophageal axis and its relationship to the resectability of carcinoma of the esophagus. *Ann Surg* 176:30–36, 1972.

54. Skinner DB, Dowalatshahi KD, DeMeester TR. Potentially curable cancer of the esophagus. *Cancer* 50:2571–2575, 1982.

55. Altorki N, Skinner DB. En bloc esophagectomy: the first 100 patients. *Hepato-Gastroenterology* (in press, 1990).

56. Skinner DB, Ferguson MK, Soriano A, et al. Selection of operation for esophageal cancer based on staging. *Ann Surg* 204:391–401, 1986.

57. Lightdale CJ, Botet JF, Zauber AG, Brennan MF. Endoscopic ultrasonography in the staging of esophageal cancer: comparison with dynamic CT and surgical pathology. *Gastrointest Endosc* (in press, 1990).

58. Lightdale CJ, Botet JF, Kelsen DP, et al. Diagnosis of recurrent upper gastrointestinal cancer at the surgical anastomosis by endoscopic ultrasound. *Gastrointest Endosc* 35:407–412, 1989.

59. Earlam R, Cunha-Melo JR. Oesophageal squamous cell carcinoma. I. A critical review of surgery. *Br J Surg* 67:381, 1980.

60. Logan A. The surgical treatment of carcinoma of the esophagus and cardia. *J Thorac Cardiovasc Surg* 46:150–161, 1963.

61. Skinner DB. En-bloc resection for neoplasms of the esophagus and cardia. *J Thorac Cardiovasc Surg* 85:59–69, 1983.

62. Adams WE, Phemister DB. Carcinoma of the lower thoracic esophagus: report of a successful resection and esophagogastrostomy. *J Thorac Surg* 7:621–632, 1938.

63. Belsey R, Hiebert CA. An exclusive right thoracic approach for cancer of the middle third of the esophagus. *Ann Thorac Surg* 18:1–5, 1974.

64. Sweet RH. Surgical managment of cancer of the mid esophagus. Preliminary report. *N Engl J Med* 233:1–7, 1945.

65. Fok M, Wong J. Pyloroplasty in esophageal replacement by stomach: a prospective, randomized controlled study. In: *Proceedings of the Fourth World Congress of the I.S.D.E.*. Chicago: I.S.D.E., 1989:91.

66. Orringer MB, Sterling MC. Cervical esophagogastric anastomosis for benign disease: functional results. *J Thorac Cardiovasc Surg* 96:887–883, 1988.

67. Pearson JG. The present status and future potential of radiotherapy in the management of esophageal cancer. *Cancer* 39:882, 1977.

68. Nakayama K. Pre-operative irradiation in the treatment of patients with carcinoma of the oesophagus and of some other sites. *Clin Radiol* 15:232, 1964.

69. Endo M, Kinoshita Y, Yamada A, et al. Surgical treatment of thoracic esophageal cancer, including clinical evaluation of early esophageal cancer. In: Pfeiffer CJ, ed. *Cancer of the Esophagus*, Vol. 2. Boca Raton: CRC Press, 1982:57.

70. Parker EF, Gregorie HB. Carcinoma of the esophagus: long-term results. *JAMA* 235:1018, 1976.

71. European Organization for Research Treatment of Cancer, Gastrointestinal Cooperative Group. Preoperative radiotherapy for carcinoma of the esophagus: results of a prospective multicentric study. In: DeMesster TR, Skinner DB, eds. *Esophageal Disorders, Pathophysiology and Therapy*. New York: Raven Press, 1985:367.

72. Huang GJ, Xian-Zhi G, Liang JW, et al. Combined preoperative irradiation and surgery for esophageal carcinoma. In: Delarue NC, Wilkins EW, Wong E, eds. *International Trends in General Thoracic Surgery*, Vol. 4. St. Louis: CV Mosby Co., 1988: 315.

73. Fleischer D. Endoscopic laser therapy for gastrointestinal neoplasms. *Surg Clin North Am* 64:947–953, 1984.

74. Cassidy DC, Nord HJ, Boyce HW Jr. Management of malignant esophagus strictures: role of esophageal dilatation and peroral prostheses. *Am J Gastroenterol* 76:173–176, 1981.

75. Tytgat GN. Endoscopic methods of treatment of gastrointestinal stenoses. *Endoscopy* (suppl): 57–63, 1980.

76. Payne-James JJ, Spiller RC, Misiewicz JJ, Silk DBA. Use of ethanol-induced tumor necrosis to palliate dysphagia in patients with esophagogastric cancer. *Gastrointest Endosc* 36:42–43, 1990.

77. McCaughan JS, Nima TA, Guy GT, et al. Photodynamic therapy for esophageal tumors. *Arch Surg* 124:74–80, 1989.

78. Kelsen DP. Chemotherapy of esophageal cancer. *Semin Oncol* 11:159–168, 1984.

79. Postlethwait RW. Benign tumors and cysts of the esophagus. *Surg Clin North Am* 63:925–931, 1983.

80. Oberheim HA, Gordon JB, Guzanskas AC. Leiomyoma of the gastrointestinal tract. *Surg Clin North Am* 32:111, 1958.

81. Postlethwait RW, Musser AW. Changes in the esophagus in 1000 autopsy specimens. *J Thorac Cardiovsc Surg* 68:953,1974.

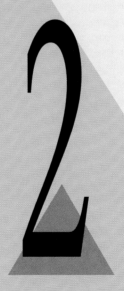

Tumors of the Stomach

Man-Hei Shiu, Charles J. Lightdale, and Robert C. Kurtz

chapter two

ADENOCARCINOMA

Almost all malignant tumors of the stomach—more than 90 percent—are adenocarcinomas. The remaining malignancies are made up of lymphomas, leiomyosarcomas, malignant carcinoid tumors, and metastatic tumors from other sites such as melanoma, breast cancer, and lung cancer.

Epidemiology

Gastric adenocarcinoma ranks third in incidence among gastrointestinal cancers in the United States. An estimated 20,000 new cases occurred in 1989 (1), with a slightly male predominance. The disease is relatively uncommon in people under 50 years old. Most important, the death rate of gastric adenocarcinoma has been decreasing continually over the last several decades. The reason for this decline remains unknown.

Gastric cancer rates vary markedly worldwide. For example, in Japan gastric cancer represents a leading cause of cancer death. Chile, Iceland, Finland, and adjoining parts of Russia also have high rates. There is a high prevalence of gastric cancer in the mountainous regions of Colombia, South America, but not in its coastal regions. This variability suggests that environmental factors are at least partially responsible for gastric cancer development. Japanese who have emigrated to the United States show a 25 percent reduction in the incidence of gastric cancer. Second generation Japanese living in the United States have over a 50 percent reduction in the incidence of gastric cancer when compared to their relatives on mainland Japan (2).

Pathophysiology

Numerous dietary factors have been suggested as the putative agents in the promotion of gastric adenocarcinoma. Nitrosamines and polycyclic hydrocarbons are two such agents. Nitrosamines, chemical compounds with well-documented carcinogenic potential in laboratory animals, are ubiquitous in nature and may also be formed in vivo in the human stomach. In patients with high intragastric pH and intestinal metaplasia of the stomach, bacteria present in the stomach can produce nitroso compounds from dietary nitrogen and endogenous nitrate (3). Nitrate is found in high concentration in foods that use it as a preservative. Processed meats and vegetables account for much of the daily nitrate intake; the remainder comes from drinking water. Correa and colleagues (4) have correlated the high water nitrate concentration with the high gastric cancer incidence in Narino, Colombia. Hill made similar observations for the English town of Worksop (3). Soil nitrate levels also appear to correlate with gastric cancer incidence, and they have been implicated in the high rate of cancer in the mountainous areas of Colombia, when compared to

coastal areas. Chile's high gastric cancer rate may be related to nitrate fertilizer exposure.

Polycyclic hydrocarbons such as benzopyrene have been associated with smoked foods in countries such as Iceland. Other dietary studies have demonstrated that patients without gastric cancer ate substantially more fresh vegetables than those with gastric cancer. These vegetables included lettuce, tomatoes, carrots, green cabbage, and red cabbage. The high vitamin C content of fresh vegetables may be responsible for their apparent protective effect. Vitamin C has been shown to interfere with in vivo nitrosation (5). The popularity of vitamin C and the widespread use of refrigeration, which has eliminated the need for salting foods with sodium chloride and nitrate for preservation, may be in part responsible for the falling gastric cancer incidence in the United States.

There have been familial aggregations in gastric cancer, but the influence of heredity in the development of the disease is not well understood. Cregan and Fraumeni (6) reported one family with 12 members in four generations who had developed gastric cancer. They attempted to associate this cancer aggregation with abnormalities in T-lymphocyte function and showed impaired in vitro lymphocyte transformation, skin test anergy, and lymphopenia. Many family members also had antiparietal cell antibodies. There have been a number of instances in which gastric cancer has occurred in twins (7,8).

In a large population-based study in Shandong, China (9), the risk of developing gastric cancer was influenced not only by dietary factors and cigarette use but by heredity. This risk rose by 80 percent among those who had a family member with gastric cancer.

Studies of the ABO blood groups show that blood type A is most commonly associated with gastric cancer. Correa and colleagues (10) showed that 49 percent of patients with the diffuse type of gastric cancer had type A blood, whereas only 38.3 percent of the general population had this blood type. The reason for this difference is not known, but it has been noted in other studies dating back to 1953 (11).

Premalignant Conditions

ATROPHIC GASTRITIS

Chronic gastritis is a common finding in older adults. Hypochlorhydria or achlorhydria is frequently seen when the chronic gastritis is severe. There have been several classifications of chronic gastritis (13,14). Cell kinetic studies have demonstrated that atrophic gastritis represents a hyperproliferative state in which the rapidly replicating proliferative compartment of the gastric gland has moved up to the luminal surface from its usual location in the gland neck (15). While early such changes may be reversible, decrease in acid production, colonization by bacteria, and endogenous formation of nitroso compounds with potential mutagenicity may eventually lead to the development of cancer. Although all patients with gastric cancer have underlying atrophic gastritis, the vast majority of people with atrophic gastritis never develop gastric cancer.

Recent studies have suggested that the previously observed higher risk of gastric cancer in pernicious anemia is no longer seen. Eriksson and colleagues [16] evaluated all patients with autopsy-documented gastric cancer in Malmö, Sweden, from 1958–1976. Pernicious anemia was present in 2.0 percent of the cancer patients which was not significantly different from the control group in which only patients who had a known history of pernicious anemia for more than five years were included.

IMMUNODEFICIENCY DISORDERS

Atrophic gastritis and a pernicious anemia-like syndrome have been identified in a number of patients with immunoglobulin deficiency. A group of these patients have gone on to develop gastric cancer [17]. They differ from patients with classic pernicious anemia in that they are younger, have antral involvement with atrophic gastritis, and have concomitant low serum gastrin levels [18]. They also lack parietal cell and intrinsic factor antibodies [19].

It is likely that the association of gastric cancer and pernicious anemia initially observed was a reflection of the high incidence of gastric cancer at that time. Gastric mucosal damage can also occur in patients with common-variable immunodeficiency and is thought to be related to a cell-mediated immune mechanism.

SUBTOTAL GASTRECTOMY

Carcinoma occurring in gastric remnant following surgery for benign disease was described initially in 1922 [20]. Several studies demonstrated that the frequency of gastric cancer increases substantially with time, up to sixfold in one series, when compared to age-matched controls operated on 25 years earlier [21]. The overall estimated risk of developing cancer in the gastric remnant was observed to be about 3 percent [22]. The initial finding that the majority of cancer cases occurred after Billroth II anastomosis probably reflected the greater number of Billroth II anastomoses performed. Cancer occurred in patients with Billroth II anastomosis with a frequency of 5 percent to 6 percent [23] (Fig. 2.1).

Other studies have demonstrated no increased cancer risk after subtotal gastrectomy. It appears that the risk for gastric cancer after subtotal resection is high only in countries at high risk for gastric cancer.

GASTRIC POLYPS

Gastric polyps are most often hyperplastic (75 percent to 95 percent) (Fig. 2.2) and less commonly adenomatous (5 percent to 10 percent) [26]. Adenomatous gastric polyps may be associated with gastric cancer. Hyperplastic gastric polyps are not.

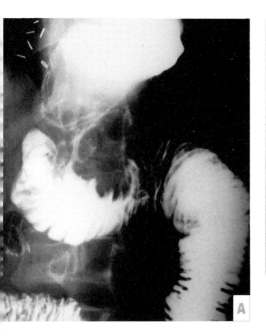
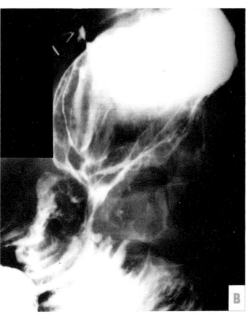
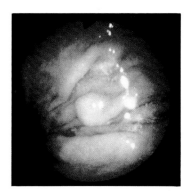

FIGURE 2.2 The small, sessile hyperplastic polyp has a smooth, dome-shaped surface. The background gastric mucosa shows atrophic gastritis. (From reference 2.)

FIGURE 2.1 Carcinoma of gastric remnant in a Billroth II partial gastrectomy. **(A,B)** These two spot films of an upper GI series demonstrate thickened folds in the distal portion of the gastric remnant, coarse nodularity of the mucosal folds in the efferent loop, and narrowing of the stoma. There is a mass effect on the superior aspect of the efferent loop. (From reference 24.)

Tomasulo (26) found that in patients operated on for gastric cancer, 35 percent had gastric adenomatous polyps, and changes of carcinoma in situ were seen in five of 23 polyps (22 percent). Berg (27) noted that 13 percent of 106 adenomas in 45 patients had carcinomatous changes and concluded that these polyps are precancerous. Although adenomatous polyps of the stomach are premalignant, the majority of gastric adenomatous cancers seen in the United States do not have an identifiable pre-existing adenomatous polyp.

Pathology

Gastric adenocarcinoma has been divided by Lauren into diffuse (Fig. 2.3A and B) and intestinal types (Fig. 2.4) (29). The intestinal type resembles small bowel mucosa. Correa ascribes cell cohesion as the morphologic element that causes the neoplastic cells to attach to each other and form gland-like structures. When this cohesive element is absent, the malignant cells infiltrate the stomach walls, forming the so-called diffuse type of gastric adenocarcinoma (30). In high-risk areas of the world, the intestinal type of gastric cancer accounts for the additional incidence. The diffuse cancer has a poorer prognosis, is more common in women and younger patients, and generally is not associated with the premalignant conditions noted above.

Clinical Presentation

Unfortunately, most gastric cancers in the United States present at an advanced stage. Symptoms such as dysphagia, weight loss, and abdominal pain often herald advanced disease. There is often a substantial lag time between onset of symptoms

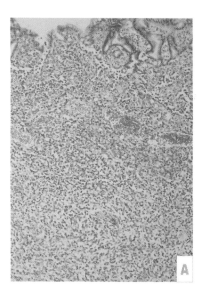
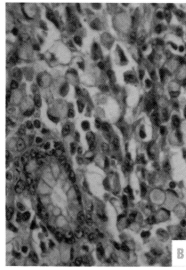
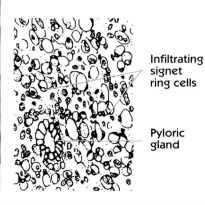

FIGURE 2.3 A diffuse pattern gastric carcinoma. (A) A low-power view (H&E stain, x50). (B) In the high-power view (H&E stain, x320), the discrete nature of the mucin-laden tumor cells (signet ring cells) is apparent in contrast to the surviving pyloric gland. (From reference 28.)

Infiltrating signet ring cells

Pyloric gland

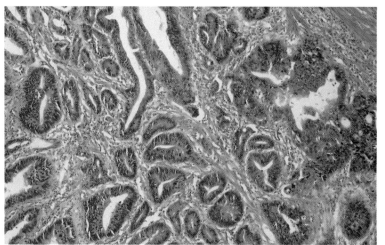

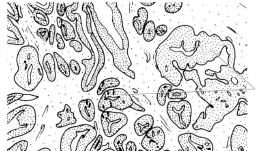

FIGURE 2.4 Histologic appearance of an intestinal type of carcinoma, showing well-formed malignant glandular elements (H&E stain, x75). (From reference 28.)

Malignant glandular elements

and appropriate diagnostic evaluation, related in part to patient denial and in part to treatment without investigation of the source of symptoms.

Diagnosis

The most important aspect in the diagnosing of gastric cancer is a high physician index of suspicion. Early evaluation of patients for gastric cancer should be undertaken whenever there is a strong family history of gastric cancer or a personal history of gastric polyps or immunodeficiency. New and persistent dyspeptic symptoms should be evaluated with upper gastrointestinal radiography or endoscopy (Fig. 2.5).

The initial evaluation of patients with carcinoma of the stomach includes a physical examination with particular attention to sites of possible nodal metastases in the supraclavicular areas and the liver. Chest x-ray will allow assessment of possible pulmonary metastases. Computed tomographic (CT) scanning of the abdomen is reasonably accurate for detecting metastases to the liver and other intra-abdominal organs. Magnetic resonance imaging (MRI) is still being evaluated in gastric cancer staging, but it seems to add little information to that obtainable by CT scans (Fig. 2.6A–C).

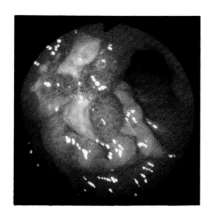

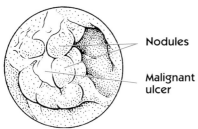

Nodules

Malignant ulcer

FIGURE 2.5 Malignant gastric ulcer in the antrum. The nodular heaped-up margins are particularly suggestive of malignancy. (From reference 12.)

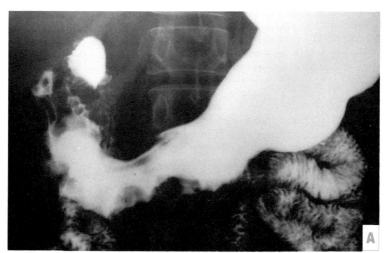

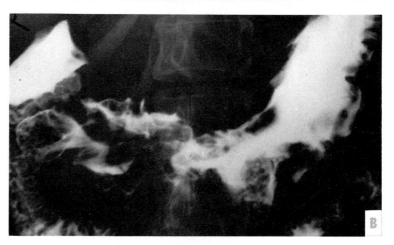

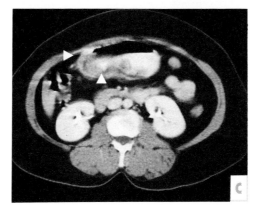

FIGURE 2.6 An upper GI series (A,B) shows a nodular, ulcerating mass measuring about 10 cm in length. **(C)** CT shows the circumferential tumor (*arrows*) encroaching on the antral lumen. (From reference 24.)

BARIUM X-RAY EXAMINATION

Traditionally, the first diagnostic technique for patients with upper gastrointestinal symptoms has been the barium upper gastrointestinal series. Under optimal conditions, an accuracy of about 90 percent has been established for this procedure (31). The x-ray appearance of gastric cancer is variable, depending on the nature of the tumor and its location in the stomach. Abnormalities seen on x-ray include a lack of distensibility of the stomach (Fig. 2.7A), an obstructing mass (Fig. 2.7B), enlarged gastric folds, or a mass effect surrounding an ulceration. One major difficulty with contrast radiography, however, is in differentiating benign from malignant gastric ulcers. Another problem is that early gastric cancer may not be seen on a barium upper gastrointestinal series without carefully performed air-contrast techniques.

The radiographic differentiation of a benign and malignant gastric ulcer may be extremely difficult. Healing of the ulcer, as assessed by radiologic methods, used to be considered a good indicator of its benign state; this, however, is no longer true. With potent H_2-receptor antagonists, malignant gastric ulcers have been shown to heal on barium x-ray examinations. A strong case can therefore be made for early endoscopy and biopsy in all patients with gastric ulcers before placing them on medical management (Fig. 2.8).

Barium and air-contrast radiologic examination of the upper gastrointestinal tract can be employed to find the small mucosal lesions of early cancer. A thin layer of barium coats the gastric mucosal surface as the stomach is distended with air or gas (CO_2). Multiple views are obtained, which evaluate the entire stomach in great detail (32). Many of the lesions identified by this procedure would no doubt be overlooked using conventional radiologic techniques (Fig. 2.9).

ENDOSCOPY, BIOPSY, AND CYTOLOGY

Upper gastrointestinal endoscopy provides the best overall method of diagnosing gastric cancer. Substantial technical advances have made this procedure much less difficult for both the patient and physician. Fiberoptic endoscopy has been widely utilized in Japan in detecting early gastric cancer (Fig. 2.10). This type of cancer is found in 0.88 percent of all upper endoscopies in Japan, but only 0.37 percent of endoscopies in Western Europe and 0.1 percent in the United States (33).

The accuracy of endoscopy in diagnosing gastric cancer has been well established. Winawer, Sherlock, and Hajdu (34) studied 63 patients with gastric adenocarcinoma. A correct endoscopic diagnosis was made visually in 57 (90 percent) of these patients. In patients in whom the cancer was classi-

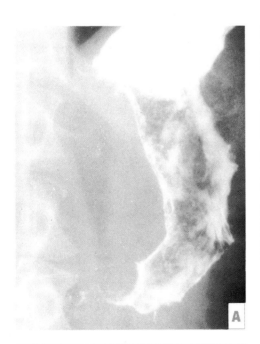

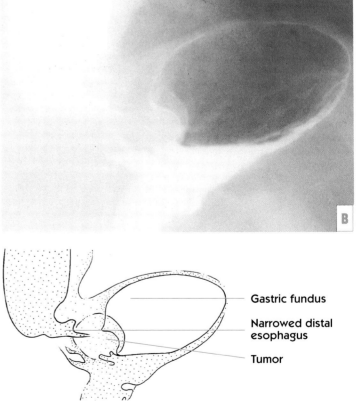

Gastric fundus

Narrowed distal esophagus

Tumor

FIGURE 2.7 (A) The characteristic rigidity, irregular contour, and narrowed lumen of linitis plastica are seen affecting the entire stomach. **(B)** This fungating mass of the gastric cardia is extending into the distal end of the esophagus, causing high-grade obstruction. (From reference 2.)

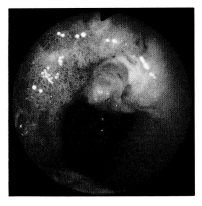

FIGURE 2.8 This benign-looking gastric ulcer proved to be malignant after multiple biopsies. (From reference 12.)

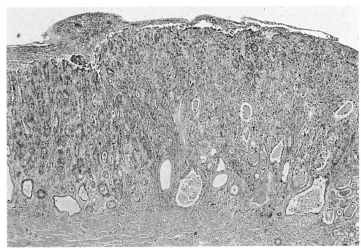

FIGURE 2.9 The entire mucosa is replaced by malignant glandular structures in this early gastric carcinoma. Some surface erosions are present (x16). (From reference 2.)

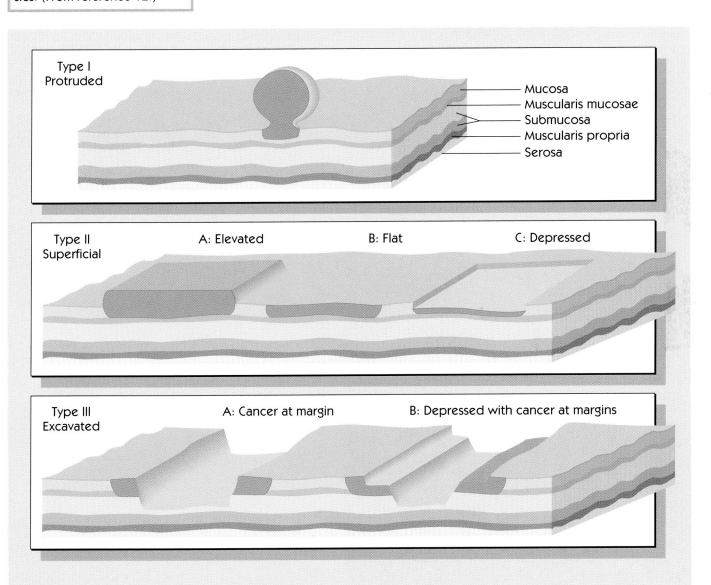

Type I
Protruded

— Mucosa
— Muscularis mucosae
— Submucosa
— Muscularis propria
— Serosa

Type II
Superficial

A: Elevated   B: Flat   C: Depressed

Type III
Excavated

A: Cancer at margin   B: Depressed with cancer at margins

FIGURE 2.10 Schematic diagram of early gastric carcinoma. (Adapted from reference 2.)

fied as exophytic, a combination of brush cytology (Fig. 2.11) and biopsy studies was accurate histologically in 92 percent of patients. This accuracy was replicated in only 50 percent of the patients with infiltrative cancers. A minimum of four biopsies was obtained from each exophytic lesion. Up to 12 biopsies were required for diagnosis in the infiltrating lesions. Brush cytology did better than biopsy in making the correct diagnosis.

Early gastric cancer can be quite difficult to differentiate from benign gastric ulcer disease even with endoscopy. Kobayashi and associates (35) from Nagoya, Japan, noted that in 42 (11 percent) of 381 patients with early gastric cancer seen at the Aichi Cancer Center Hospital, endoscopic observation alone failed to make the correct diagnosis. The early cancer that presented as an excavated lesion similar to a benign peptic ulcer was most commonly mistaken for a benign ulcer (Fig. 2.12). These authors stress the important point that endoscopic biopsy of benign-appearing gastric ulcers must be carefully done. Twelve biopsies should be taken from the inside edge of the ulcer. If the ulcer is an early gastric cancer, at least one biopsy will be positive. In their experience, biopsy of these lesions is accurate in 95 percent of cases (Fig. 2.13).

Staging

The International Union Against Cancer (UICC) and the American Joint Committee on Cancer (AJCC) published essentially identical classifications for staging adenocarcinoma of the stomach in 1987 and 1988 (Fig. 2.14) (36,37). The Japanese Committee on Cancer (JCC) endorsed the same staging classification for stomach cancer in 1987 (38).

These classifications are based on the TNM staging system:

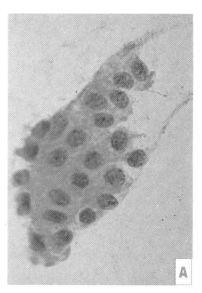

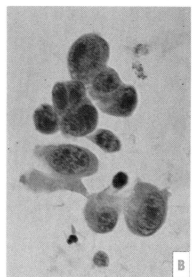

FIGURE 2.11 Brush cytologic preparations contrasting benign gastric epithelial cells (**A**) with obviously malignant cells (**B**). The latter have an increased nuclear cytoplasmic ratio and hyperchromatic nuclei with coarsely clumped chromatin (Papanicolaou stain, x500). (From reference 28.)

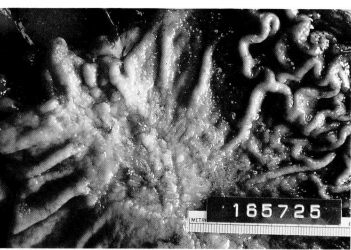

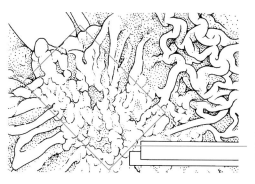

Approximate extent of carcinoma

FIGURE 2.12 A small, shallow ulcer and the irregular, distorted mucosa with an effacement of rugal folds mark the extensive involvement by this superficial spreading gastric carcinoma. (From reference 2.)

T—Indicates the depth of primary tumor invasion, recognizing that gastric adenocarcinomas originate in the mucosa and invade progressively deeper layers of the stomach wall as they advance.

N—Indicates the spread of cancer to specified regional lymph nodes. For the stomach, there are two positive lymph node designations, depending on the location of the nodes and their distance from the primary tumor.

M—Indicates distant metastases to lymph nodes outside specified regional nodes, or to the peritoneum or organs such as liver and lung, not involved by direct extension from the primary cancer.

It is important to note that these classifications do not recognize symptoms, or whether the primary cancer is circumferential, or the length or size of the primary cancer as stage determinants. Clinical and pathologic stages are identical. Imaging methods of potential value for clinical staging are computerized tomography (CT), magnetic resonance imaging (MRI), ultrasonography (US), and endoscopic ultrasonography (EUS) (39). Only high-frequency EUS can produce detailed images of the stomach wall, allowing an accurate assessment of depth of tumor invasion (T) (40,41). CT and MRI produce only a measurement of total wall thickness and contour to estimate T.

The accumulating data indicate that EUS represents a significant advance in the clinical staging of gastric cancer. Because of its limited depth of field, EUS cannot replace CT for detection of distant metastases. However, EUS is more accurate in assessing depth of cancer invasion, and it also appears to be more accurate in determining cancer spread to regional lymph nodes.

CT, MRI, and EUS can judge nodal metastases by the size of imaged structures consistent with lymph nodes. Lymph nodes greater than 10 mm are more likely to be malignant. EUS can image much smaller nodes (2–3 mm), and in addition can provide diagnostically helpful echo patterns. Malignancy is suggested if imaged lymph nodes are round, sharply demarcated, and hypoechoic (42,43). EUS has a limited depth of field. Distant lymph nodes, the entire liver, and the lungs cannot be imaged, as they can with CT or MRI.

Most clinical EUS has been performed with mechanical sector scan ultrasound endoscopes using frequencies of 7.5 and 12 MHz (Olympus Corp., Tokyo). With this system, a 360° gray scale image is produced, which routinely shows five layers of the stomach wall. The five alternating hyperechoic (bright) and hypoechoic (dark) layers are best seen after filling the gastric lumen with water for acoustical contact. The histologic correlates of the five layers for clinical staging are shown

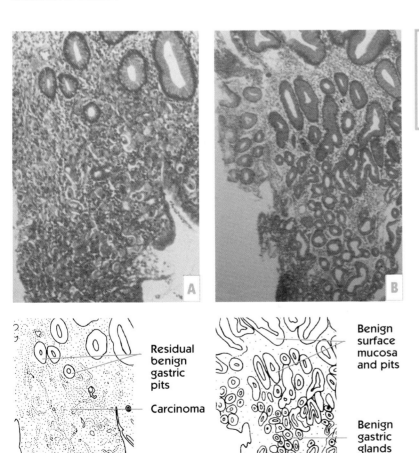

Residual benign gastric pits

Carcinoma

Benign surface mucosa and pits

Benign gastric glands

FIGURE 2.13 Two biopsies from an ulcer, part of an endoscopic series of ten. Only one of the ten (**A**) showed an infiltrating adenocarcinoma; the others were benign (**B**). This demonstrates the sampling error inherent in endoscopic biopsies (H&E stain, x75). (From reference 28.)

FIGURE 2.14:
AJCC/UICC STAGING OF GASTRIC CANCER

PRIMARY TUMOR (T)

TX	Primary tumor cannot be assessed
T0	No evidence of primary tumor
Tis	Carcinoma in situ: intraepithelial tumor without invasion of the lamina propria
T1	Tumor invades lamina propria or submucosa
T2	Tumor invades the muscularis propria or the subserosa
T3	Tumor penetrates the serosa (visceral peritoneum) without invasion of adjacent structures[1]
T4	Tumor invades adjacent structures[2]

REGIONAL LYMPH NODES (N)

NX	Regional lymph nodes cannot be assessed
N0	No regional lymph node metastasis
N1	Metastasis in perigastric lymph node(s) within 3 cm of the edge of the primary tumor
N2	Metastasis in perigastric lymph node(s) more than 3 cm from the edge of the primary tumor, or in lymph nodes along the left gastric, common hepatic, splenic, or celiac arteries[3]

DISTANT METASTASIS (M)

MX	Presence of distant metastasis cannot be assessed
M0	No distant metastasis
M1	Distant metastasis[4]

STAGE GROUPING

Stage 0	Tis	N0	M0
Stage IA	T1	N0	M0
Stage IB	T1	N1	M0
	T2	N0	M0
Stage II	T1	N2	M0
	T2	N1	M0
	T3	N0	M0
Stage IIIA	T2	N2	M0
	T3	N1	M0
	T4	N0	M0
Stage IIIB	T3	N2	M0
	T4	N1	M0
Stage IV	T4	N2	M0
	Any T	Any N	M1

1. Tumor invasion of muscularis propria without serosal penetration, but with spread to gastrohepatic or gastrocolic ligaments or to lesser or greater omentum is still considered T2.
2. Adjacent structures are spleen, transverse colon, liver, diaphragm, pancreas, abdominal wall, adrenal gland, kidney, small intestine, and retroperitoneum.
3. Regional lymph nodes include perigastric lymph nodes, not otherwise specified and those along the inferior (right) gastric, splenic, superior (left) gastric, celiac, and hepatic arteries. All other lymph nodes are considered distant, including retropancreatic, hepatoduodenal, aortic, portal, retroperitoneal, and mesenteric.
4. Most common metastatic sites include liver, lungs, supraclavicular lymph nodes, and widespread intraperitoneal sites.

in Figure 2.15. The fourth hypoechoic layer corresponding to the muscularis propria can serve as a boundary for separating early from advanced cancer. Resectability may also be assessed according to the presence or absence of local tumor extension and the pattern of lymph node metastases. In 36 patients with gastric cancer, Tio and Tytgat judged local resectability correctly in nine of 11 patients, palliative resectability in 13 of 15, and local nonresectability in eight of ten (44). Aibe reported EUS staging in 34 patients with gastric cancer, of which 22 had early stage disease on pathology. EUS had an accuracy of 88 percent in differentiating between early and advanced cancer (45).

In a group of 34 patients with gastric cancer reported by Grimm and associates, EUS was accurate in 28. Metastatic lymph nodes were detected in 21 out of 22 patients by EUS, and in only three out of 22 by CT (46). Tio and colleagues studied 74 patients preoperatively with EUS and found the accuracy for T to be 84 percent and for N, 81 percent (47).

In a study from Memorial Sloan-Kettering Cancer Center, EUS and CT were compared to surgical pathology for staging gastric cancer preoperatively in 50 patients according to the UICC/AJCC staging system. For clinical staging with EUS, invasion of the first three wall layers was Tl (cancer involving mucosa/submucosa); invasion of the fourth layer, T2 (cancer involving muscularis propria); invasion through the fifth layer, T3 (cancer penetrating the serosa); and direct invasion of adjacent organs or structures, T4 (Figs. 2.16–2.19). Results showed that EUS agreed with surgical pathology in 92 percent vs. 42 percent for CT in staging T (p < 0.00042), and in 78 percent vs. 48 percent in staging N (p < 0.038) (48).

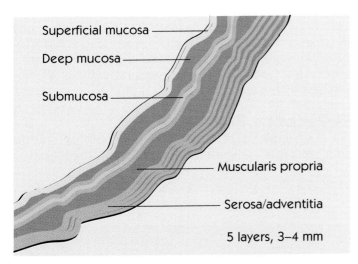

FIGURE 2.15 Histologic correlates for clinical staging of five-layer gastric wall structure imaged with high-frequency EUS.

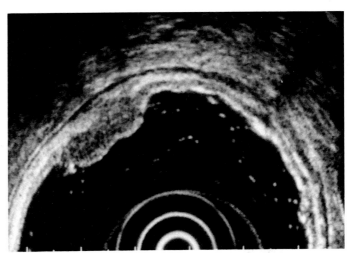

FIGURE 2.16 A T1 cancer of the stomach involving mucosa and submucosa is imaged as a hypoechoic disruption of the first three wall layers in the 11 o'clock position.

FIGURE 2.17 A T2 cancer of the gastric cardia is imaged from 2 to 5 o'clock as a nodular disruption of the wall extending into but not through the fourth hypoechoic layer, the muscularis propria.

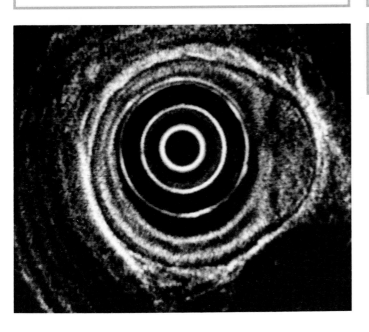

Treatment of Gastric Adenocarcinoma

SELECTION OF PATIENTS WITH POTENTIALLY CURABLE CANCERS

The first consideration in treatment is to determine which patients have localized disease suitable for potential cure, and which patients have disseminated or incurable disease who would benefit from a program of palliative treatment (Fig. 2.20). Careful physical examination and a few selected diagnostic tests will often separate these two categories. Supraclavicular lymph node enlargement, jaundice, hepatomegaly, or ascites are signs of advanced disseminated cancer. When corroborated by biopsy or cytologic confirmation, these signs preclude consideration of curative surgical treatment for gastric carcinoma. Chest roentgenographs and blood chemistry determinations should be routinely performed. As noted above, computed tomography (CT) of the abdomen and endoscopic ultrasound can be helpful in staging the patient's tumor according to the TNM schema. It is important to note that the CT scans may reveal benign hepatic cysts or hemangiomas, which can be confused with metastatic gastric cancer. In the absence of obvious distant metastases, most patients should undergo surgical exploration to determine whether the gastric tumor is suitable for resection and potential cure. Even patients who have a large palpable tumor or radiologic evidence of contiguous involvement of an adjacent organ, such as the spleen, colon, or pancreas, need not be denied surgical treatment based on this consideration alone. Such tumors may be resectable and potentially curable.

At the time of surgical exploration, the surgeon looks for metastases in the liver and on the peritoneal surfaces, particularly under the diaphragm, in the pelvis, and on the serosal surfaces of the small and large intestine, omentum, and mesentery. Sometimes metastases are quite small and not detectable by CT or endoscopic ultrasound examination. Once biopsy confirmation of metastatic gastric carcinoma in the liver or peritoneum is obtained, the patient is no longer a candidate for curative surgical resection, although resection can still be considered for palliation. A tumor with enlarged perigastric lymph nodes can be resected with prospects of cure, but bulky lymph nodes fixed to the retroperitoneum usually indicate incurability, because of fixation to the celiac axis or hepatic artery. On the other hand, a tumor intimately attached to or actually invading an adjacent organ can often be managed with curative intent by gastrectomy en bloc, with, for example, splenectomy, distal pancreatectomy, or partial colectomy, provided that complete tumor excision can be accomplished with a clear resection margin.

PREOPERATIVE PREPARATION

An overnight fast, preoperative intravenous hydration, and mechanical cleansing of the large intestine

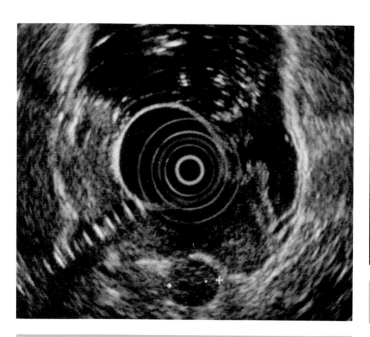

FIGURE 2.18 A T3 cancer of the fundus seen from 5 to 9 o'clock invades through the entire stomach wall. Outside the primary cancer is a round, sharply demarcated, hypoechoic 1.4-cm diameter lymph node metastasis (N1).

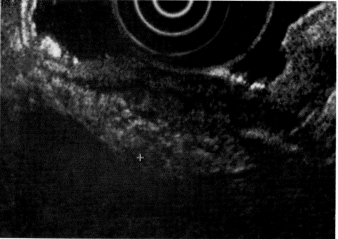

FIGURE 2.19 A T4 cancer of the body of the stomach is imaged invading posteriorly into the pancreas.

are standard preoperative measures. If the stomach is obstructed or distended, it should be completely drained by nasogastric suction to prevent intraoperative contamination. Because coexisting hypochlorhydria is common, the stomach tends to harbor many bacterial organisms. Oral antibiotics, such as those with a neomycin and erythromycin base, can be given for gut sterilization and are important when the adjacent colon must be resected. Intravenous antibiotics such as a newer generation cephalosporin, or metronidazol, can also be given immediately before laparotomy, to decrease the risk of intra-abdominal and wound infection.

PRINCIPLES OF CURATIVE SURGICAL TREATMENT
To satisfy the intent of cure, a gastric resection must completely remove the cancer in its entire visible and palpable extent, including also all

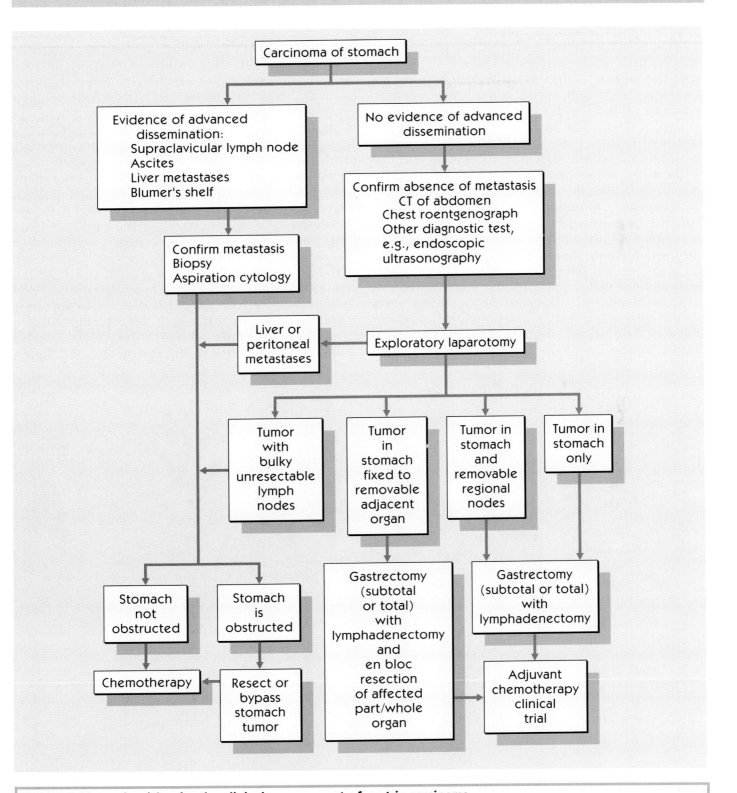

FIGURE 2.20 An algorithm for the clinical management of gastric carcinoma.

deposits of tumor in lymph nodes that are suspected or known to be present. The extent of gastric resection and the scope of lymphadenectomy constitute the two main considerations in the concept and technical execution of a curative gastrectomy for carcinoma. Methods of reconstruction and the indications for surgical resection of organs adjacent to the stomach must also be considered.

Radical gastric resection performed with intent of cure for gastric carcinoma differs considerably from gastrectomy performed for peptic ulcer disease. In performing gastrectomy for ulcer disease, the surgeon removes the affected part of the stomach with minimal margins. In performing gastrectomy for carcinoma, the surgeon strives to dissect as far away from the stomach and the carcinoma as possible, removing the greater omentum and lesser omentum which are attached to the two curvatures.

EXTENT OF GASTRECTOMY   Lateral spread of carcinoma within the gastric wall is very common and may not be easily appreciated by palpation or naked-eye examination. With the exception of small "early" gastric cancers, a minimal resection margin of 5 cm from the grossly appreciated edge of the tumor is recommended; for poorly differentiated tumors an even wider margin is required. Most tumors located in the pyloric antrum of the stomach can be resected by a high distal subtotal gastrectomy with an adequate margin at both ends. Larger tumors of the pyloric antrum may reach high up on the lesser curvature of the stomach, requiring resection up to the cardia. Tumors of the mid-stomach and fundus can

be resected by distal or proximal subtotal gastrectomy if the tumor is small; unfortunately many of these carcinomas are bulky and require total gastrectomy to achieve complete excision with adequate margins. On the other hand, deliberate use of total gastrectomy, when subtotal gastrectomy is adequate, has not shown any advantage in a prospective randomized clinical study (49). Carcinomas of the gastric cardia often involve the distal esophagus; esophagogastrectomy with thoracotomy is therefore indicated for many of these tumors.

SCOPE OF LYMPHADENECTOMY   In 50 percent to 90 percent of gastric carcinomas, metastases are present in the lymph nodes draining the stomach; their frequency depends on the particular patient population. Even in early gastric cancers lymph node metastases develop in up to 15 percent of patients. These metastatic deposits may be large and easily recognized on CT, endoscopic ultrasonography, or during surgery. More often they escape recognition because of their small or microscopic size, and are found lodged within otherwise normal-appearing lymph nodes. Many pathoanatomic studies have been performed to document the frequency of metastases in the various lymph node groups around the stomach (50–53). The pattern of lymphatic metastasis depends on the location of the primary tumor. Thus cancers of the pyloric region tend to metastasize first to lymph nodes along the lesser and greater curvature and those of the subpyloric and supra-

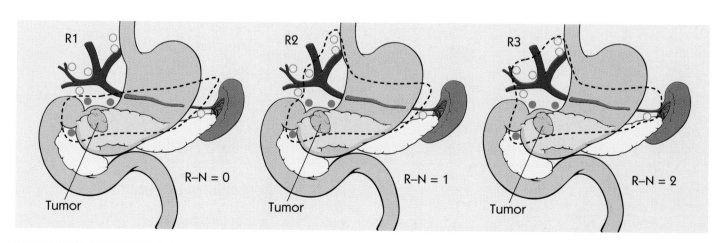

FIGURE 2.21 Extent of radical lymphadenectomy with removal of two echelons of draining lymph nodes (R2 lymphadenectomy) according to the pattern of lymphatic drainage of the tumor in the curative resection of gastric carcinoma.

pyloric groups (N1) and, second, to nodes along the left gastric, celiac, and hepatic arteries (N2). The staging notations N1 and N2 refer to metastases in these nodal echelons. Cancers of the fundus and cardia tend first to metastasize to the nodes on the lesser and greater curvature and those in the right and left cardiac groups (N1) and, second, to the nodes along the left gastric, celiac, and splenic artery, as well as those in suprapyloric and subpyloric groups (N2). Radical gastric lymphadenectomy requires dissection and removal of these two echelons according to the anatomic site of the primary tumor (Fig. 2.21).

Numerous retrospective studies have confirmed that many but not all patients with such lymph node metastases, who underwent gastrectomy and radical lymphadenectomy, have been cured of their disease (50–55). Because many of these metastases are not clinically obvious, a wide scope of lymphadenectomy must be performed to encompass fully any visible disease, if cure is the intent (54–57). A retrospective study of a series of patients treated at the Memorial Sloan–Kettering Cancer Center (Fig. 2.22) has shown a survival advantage when the scope of lymphadenectomy widely encompassed any lymph node metastasis (58). Recent experience in this and other centers has also shown that wide lymphadenectomy does not significantly increase the risk of operative morbidity or mortality.

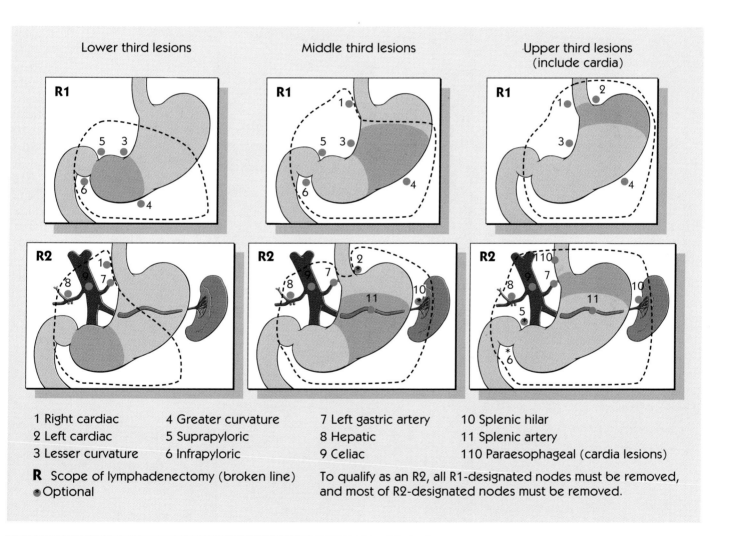

1 Right cardiac	4 Greater curvature	7 Left gastric artery	10 Splenic hilar
2 Left cardiac	5 Suprapyloric	8 Hepatic	11 Splenic artery
3 Lesser curvature	6 Infrapyloric	9 Celiac	110 Paraesophageal (cardia lesions)

R Scope of lymphadenectomy (broken line)
● Optional

To qualify as an R2, all R1-designated nodes must be removed, and most of R2-designated nodes must be removed.

FIGURE 2.22 The upper, middle, and lower third lesions show increasingly wide lymphadenectomy (R) for a gastric carcinoma with metastatic deposits in the perigastric lymph nodes (N1). Patients who underwent wider scope lymphadenectomy *relative* to the nodal stage, $(R - N) > 1$, had a significantly higher survival rate. (From reference 58.)

RECONSTRUCTION OF FOOD PASSAGE   Reconstruction after distal subtotal gastrectomy (Fig. 2.23) is usually performed with a gastrojejunal anastomosis, by manual suturing, or by stapling. Reconstruction by gastroduodenal anastomosis, though sometimes used for ulcer disease, is less commonly employed for the treatment of cancer, because the gastric stump is often too short to reach the duodenum and any recurrence in the stomach bed is more likely to cause gastric outlet obstruction. After esophagogastrectomy, or proximal partial gastrectomy (Fig. 2.24), the remaining lower segment of the stomach is brought up to be anastomosed to the esophagus; most surgeons also perform a pyloroplasty or pyloromyotomy, to prevent gastric stasis which may occur in 10 per-cent to 20 percent of

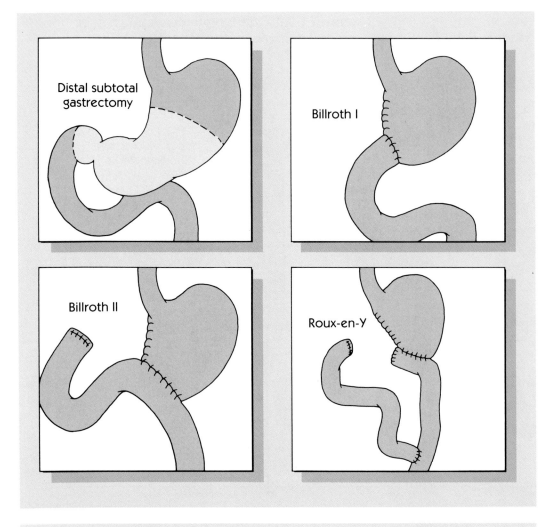

FIGURE 2.23 Reconstruction after distal subtotal gastrectomy.

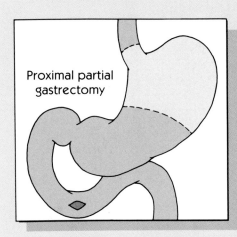
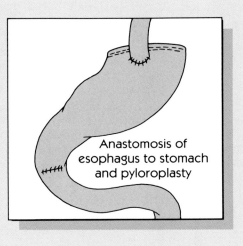

FIGURE 2.24 Reconstruction after proximal partial gastrectomy.

these patients. After total gastrectomy (Fig. 2.25), reconstruction utilizes the jejunum, either by a variety of anastomoses using the Roux-en-Y configuration to prevent bile reflux, or by direct reconnection of the esophagus to the duodenum using an interposed segment of jejunum. A pouch of jejunum can also be made to serve as a food reservoir below the esophageal anastomosis. It takes three to six months before patients can comfortably ingest a meal of moderate size; most need to take six or more small meals a day to maintain nutrition. All patients after total gastrectomy require iron and vitamin B_{12} supplements because iron absorption is poor and the gastric fundus that synthesizes B_{12} has been removed.

RESECTION OF ADJACENT ORGANS Advanced carcinomas may encroach upon or directly invade an adjacent organ, such as the left lobe of the liver, the spleen, body and tail of the pancreas, and the transverse colon. If cure is the intent of surgical treatment, it is important to consider resecting the affected portion of the involved organ with the stomach, to avoid violation and spilling of tumor.

The risk of morbidity and mortality from an extended organ resection is greater than that of radical gastrectomy alone. Serious and potentially lethal complications may occur, such as pancreatic or enteric fistula with attendant intra-abdominal abscess formation. However, even for patients whose tumor showed pathologically confirmed direct invasion of an adjacent organ, a five-year survival rate of 7 percent may be achieved by such resection, with even higher survival rates when lymph node metastasis was absent or minimal (59,60). Concern has been raised about the negative effect of splenectomy on survival (61). An analysis of patients treated from 1960 to 1984 at the Memorial Sloan—Kettering Cancer Center showed that while splenectomy did increase the risk of septic com-plications after gastrectomy, any effect it had on sur-vival was due to that of other coexisting factors (62).

RESULTS OF CURATIVE SURGICAL TREATMENT
Figure 2.26 shows the five-year survival rates after surgical treatment of two large collected series of patients with different TNM stages of gastric cancer in Japan (63) and the United States (64). It can be

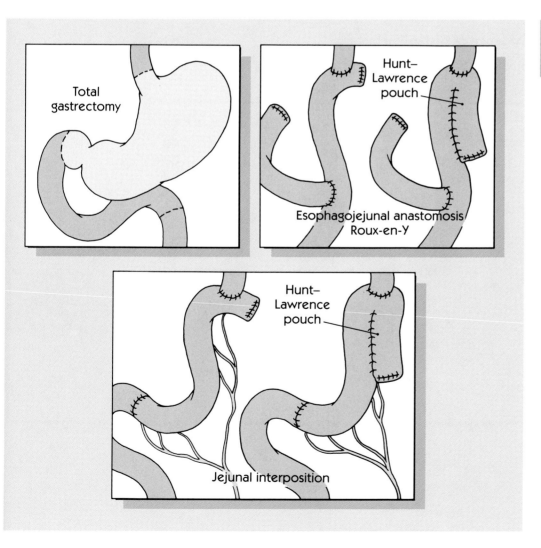

FIGURE 2.25 Reconstruction after total gastrectomy.

Total gastrectomy

Hunt–Lawrence pouch

Esophagojejunal anastomosis Roux-en-Y

Hunt–Lawrence pouch

Jejunal interposition

FIGURE 2.26:
NEW INTERNATIONAL TNM STAGING OF GASTRIC CANCER (1985): FIVE-YEAR SURVIVAL RATES IN JAPAN AND UNITED STATES

				% OF FIVE-YEAR SURVIVAL	
PRIMARY TUMOR (T)				IN JAPAN*	IN U.S.A.**
T1	Tumor limited to mucosa or mucosa and submucosa			98	76
T2	Tumor involves the muscularis propria/subserosa			70	34
T3	Tumor penetrates the serosa			34	15
T4	Tumor involves contiguous structures			16	—
REGIONAL LYMPH NODES (N)					
N0	No metastases to regional lymph nodes			87	54
N1	Involvement of perigastric lymph nodes within 3 cm of the primary tumor			45	20
N2	Involvement of regional lymph nodes more than 3 cm from the primary tumor, including those located along left gastric, common hepatic, splenic, and celiac arteries			24	—
	Note: Involvement of other intra-abdominal lymph nodes is regarded as distant metastasis.				
DISTANT METASTASIS (M)					
M0	No evidence of distant metastasis			63	—
M1	Evidence of distant metastasis			6	—

STAGE GROUPING

Stage I	Ia:	T1	N0	M0	99	—
	Ib:	T1	N1	M0	90	—
		T2	N0	M0	88	—
Stage II		T1	N2	M0	79	—
		T2	N1	M0	71	—
		T3	N0	M0	69	—
Stage III	IIIa:	T2	N2	M0	52	—
		T3	N1	M0	46	—
		T4	N0	M0	52	—
	IIIa:	T3	N2	M0	23	—
		T4	N1	M0	26	—
Stage IV		T4	N2	M0	16	—
		Any	Any	M1	10	—

* Adapted from reference 63.
** Adapted from reference 64.

seen that, stage for stage, the survival figures are much lower for patients in North America. However, the surgical treatment, pathologic examination, and hence the staging methods applied to the two patient populations were quite different. Some of the patients in the American series would probably have been classified as palliative resections according to the reporting format used by the Japanese investigators. Extensive lymphadenectomy and detailed pathologic processing techniques were seldom performed in the American patients, so that many must have been assigned a TNM stage lower than the actual stage, due, for example, to metastatic deposits in lymph nodes that were not removed or, if removed, to microscopic deposits that could have been re-

vealed only by detailed step-section examination of the lymph nodes.

Some of the difference in survival rates may be attributable to the more aggressive surgical resections offered in the Japanese centers. More limited experience of radical resections in the United States (58) and Europe (65) has also shown improved survival rates compared with those after less extensive resections.

PROGNOSTIC FACTORS AFFECTING SURVIVAL AFTER CURATIVE RESECTION

Age and sex have only a minimal influence on prognosis (Figs. 2.27 and 2.28). Antral carcinomas in general have a better prognosis than carcinomas

FIGURE 2.27:
UNIVARIATE ANALYSIS OF CLINICAL AND PATHOLOGIC FACTORS*
IN CURATIVE RESECTION OF GASTRIC CARCINOMA
AT THE MEMORIAL SLOAN–KETTERING CANCER CENTER (1960–1984)

| PROGNOSTIC VARIABLE | FAVORABLE | | UNFAVORABLE | | |
	FEATURE	% OF 5-YEAR SURVIVAL**	FEATURE	% OF 5-YEAR SURVIVAL**	$p^\dagger$
Sex	Male	45	Female	37	NS
Age	Over 65	49	65 or less	35	< 0.1
Site of tumor	Antrum or body	47	Fundus or diffuse	18	< 0.001
Tumor diameter	10 cm or less	44	Over 10 cm	23	< 0.1
TMN stage	IB or II	62	III or higher	23	< 0.0001
N stage	N0	67	N1	32	< 0.001
	N1	32	N2	9	< 0.001
No. of lymph nodes involved by metastases	0–3	55	4 or more	17	< 0.0001
Histologic grade of malignancy	1 or 2	58	3	32	< 0.001
Serosa involved	T1 or T2	56	T3	32	< 0.005

* Analysis excluded T1N0 cases.
** 5-year survival according to the method of Kaplan and Meier.
† Log-rank test, NS indicates not statistically significant.

Adapted from Shiu MH, et al. Adenocarcinoma of the stomach: a multivariate analysis of clinical, pathologic and treatment factors. *Hepato-Gastroenterology* 36:7–12, 1989.

arising from the fundus and cardia. The histopathologic features of the tumor also carry prognostic significance: the prognosis is better when the tumor is well differentiated, with the intestinal type of tumor having a more favorable prognosis than the diffuse type. Recently, studies by flow cytometry have shown that aneuploid tumors have significantly worse prognosis compared to diploid tumors (66). DNA ploidy is closely linked to tumor invasion, lymph node metastasis, and prognosis in gastric cancer. It has also been found that most tumors of the cardia and gastroesophageal junction are aneuploid as compared with about half of those in the body and antrum of the stomach. In the absence of flow cytometry, the factors of prognostic importance are the depth of tumor invasion in the gastric wall and the extent of involvement of the regional gastric lymph nodes. Multivariate statistical analyses (Fig. 2.29) have shown that the anatomic site, the TNM stage, the number of lymph nodes involved by metastases, and the histologic differentiation (grade) are important predictors of survival (58,63). Such analyses have also shown the beneficial effect of wide-scope lymphadenectomy.

PATTERNS OF RECURRENCE

Autopsy studies showed that the main sites of disease were the stomach remnant or stomach-bed, the liver, the peritoneum, and—less commonly—distant organs such as the lung. Gunderson and Sosin at the University of Minnesota studied the pattern of recurrence after curative gastric resection by single or multiple reoperations (67). Of 107 patients studied, 86 developed failure, with complete documentation

FIGURE 2.28:
UNIVARIATE ANALYSIS OF SURGICAL TREATMENT FACTORS*
IN CURATIVE RESECTION OF GASTRIC CARCINOMA
AT THE MEMORIAL SLOAN–KETTERING CANCER CENTER (1960–1984)

PROGNOSTIC VARIABLE	FAVORABLE		UNFAVORABLE		
	FEATURE	% OF 5-YEAR SURVIVAL**	FEATURE	% OF 5-YEAR SURVIVAL**	P†
Type of gastrectomy	Distal	50	Total or proximal subtotal	27	< 0.0001
Margin of resection	No tumor	44	Showed tumor	19	< 0.05
Splenectomy	Not done	48	Done	32	< 0.005
Scope of lymphadenectomy	R ≥ 1.5	40	R < 1.5	45	NS
Scope of lymphadenectomy relative to nodal state (R minus N)	(R – N) ≥ 1.5	72	(R – N) < 1.5	32	< 0.0001
Adjuvant chemotherapy	Not given	43	Given	32	NS

* Analysis excluded T1N0 cases.
** 5-year survival according to the method of Kaplan and Meier.
† Log-rank test, NS indicates not statistically significant.

Adapted from Shiu MH, et al., 1989.

in 82. Local or regional (stomach-bed or nodes) relapse was the only failure in 29 percent, local/regional plus localized peritoneal relapse in 53 percent, diffuse peritoneal disease in 4 percent, and distant metastases, mostly liver, in 5 percent. When occurring as a component of any pattern of relapse, local or regional disease accounted for 88 percent, peritoneal disease for 54 percent, and distant metastases for 29 percent. In a series of 77 patients who had documentation of recurrence after curative gastric resection at the Memorial Sloan–Kettering Cancer Center (58), the peritoneal surfaces showed disease in 49, the liver in 36, the lung in 11, and the stomach remnant or stomach-bed in nine. Many patients had multiple sites of recurrence, but the peritoneum was the only site of relapse in 36 percent of the patients.

ADJUVANT THERAPY

A number of chemotherapeutic agents, including mitomycin-C, fluorouracil (5-FU), doxorubicin, and the nitrosoureas, have been used in trials of adjuvant therapy after potentially curative resection of gastric cancer (Fig. 2.30). The Japanese centers have conducted a large number of clinical trials using mitomycin-C and derivatives of 5-FU. Most of these trials were not randomized in design. Recently, the Cooperative Study Group of Surgical Adjuvant Chemotherapy for Gastric Cancer in Japan reported on the experience in 2064 patients treated according to two protocols in a randomized, prospective, controlled trial (68), comparing mitomycin-C given alone vs. mitomycin-C given with Futraful, a derivative of 5-FU. No enhancement of survival was observed in either arm of the study although subset analysis suggested

---

FIGURE 2.29:
INDEPENDENT VARIABLES IN CURATIVE RESECTION OF GASTRIC CARCINOMA, IDENTIFIED BY COX PROPORTIONAL HAZARDS MODEL,* AT THE MEMORIAL SLOAN–KETTERING CANCER CENTER (1960–1984)

PROGNOSTIC VARIABLE	ADVERSE FEATURE	LOG-HAZARD RATIO**	RELATIVE RISK OF DEATH**
CLINICOPATHOLOGIC VARIABLES			
Number of lymph nodes involved by metastases	4 or more nodes	0.6828	1.9790
Histologic grade of malignancy	High grade (3)	0.5874	1.7993
TNM stage	IIIA or IIIB	0.5517	1.7362
TREATMENT VARIABLES			
Scope of lymphadenectomy relative to nodal stage (R minus N)	(R − N) < 1.5	0.4930	1.6372
Splenectomy	Performed	0.4524	1.5721[†]

* Cox model analyses using the covariates listed in Figures 2.26 and 2.27.

** The log-hazard ratios are the natural logarithms of the relative risk of death; they permit evaluation of the additive influence of one or more of the above-listed prognostic factors on the risk of death (last column) in a given patient with some or all of the adverse features.

[†] Borderline significance. Subsequent analysis of a larger number of patients failed to show a significant effect of splenectomy on survival (see reference 68).

Adapted from Shiu MH, et al., 1989.

an improvement of survival in patients whose tumor had serosal invasion and lymph node metastasis, after combined treatment of mitomycin-C and Futraful. In North America, the Gastrointestinal Tumor Study Group (GITSG) investigated the benefit of adjuvant chemotherapy using 5-FU plus methyl lomustine given postoperatively for two years, compared with no postoperative therapy in a randomized prospective trial (69). An improvement of survival was noted with adjuvant therapy. However, three similar trials failed to confirm the positive results of the GITSG study (70). A large multi-institutional trial of 5-FU, doxorubicin, and mitomycin-C (FAM) also showed no benefit (71).

New approaches to adjuvant treatment include regional chemotherapy by direct instillation of drugs into the peritoneal cavity (72) which is the most common site of recurrence, and the application of hyperthermia with drugs (73). Kim and his associates in Korea have reported encouraging results on the use of adjuvant chemotherapy combined with immunotherapy using a *Streptococcus pyogenes* preparation (74).

Abe and associates studied tumor-bed irradiation by intraoperative radiation therapy (IORT) after curative and palliative gastric resection for carcinoma, and have observed some benefit in a small series of patients (75). Because of lack of generally

FIGURE 2.30:
ADJUVANT CHEMOTHERAPY OF GASTRIC CARCINOMA

GROUP	TREATMENT	SIGNIFICANT SURVIVAL BENEFIT	COMMENTS
Gastrointestinal Tumor Study Group U.S.A. (1982)	5-FU + methyl-CCNU vs. control	Significant	Survival rate of control patients unusually low; results have not been corroborated
Eastern Cooperative Oncology Group U.S.A. (Engstrom, 1985)	5-FU + methyl-CCNU vs. control	Not significant	Surgical and chemotherapy treatments seem to lack uniformity
British Stomach Cancer Group (Fielding, 1983)	5-FU + mitomycin-C vs. 5-FU + mitomycin-C with initial multidrug induction vs. control placebo	Not significant	Survival improved at 1 year for 5-FU + mitomycin-C if started within 1 month of surgery, but benefit was lost at 3 years
Cooperative Study Group of Surgical Adjuvant Chemotherapy for Gastric Cancer in Japan (Inokuchi, 1984)	Mitomycin-C in two schedules randomized to with or without Futraful, a 5-FU derivative	Not significant	Subset analysis showed survival benefit in node positive, serosa positive patients who received bolus mitomycin-C plus Futraful. Drugs were started on day of surgery
European Organization for Research and Treatment of Cancer (EORTC, 1988)	5-FU, doxorubicin, and mitomycin-C	Not significant	
Korea (Kim, 1987)	Chemotherapy + immunotherapy vs. control Drugs: mitomycin-C, 5-FU, cytosine arabioside, or 5-FU, methyl CCNU + *Streptococcus pyogenes* preparation	Significant	

proven efficacy, and the potential toxicity of these treatments, adjuvant chemotherapy with or without other treatment modalities for gastric carcinoma remains investigational.

Palliative Treatment of Incurable Gastric Carcinoma

Relief of distressing symptoms constitutes the main aim of palliative treatment of gastric cancer. While a few patients treated palliatively may live for several years, most die within one year. In deciding on how best to offer palliative treatment, the clinician needs to consider the risk of the treatment, and the quality of life it may provide.

SURGICAL TREATMENT

If obstruction of the food passage is the main symptom, there is no doubt that partial gastrectomy with removal of the obstructing tumor gives the best results. The risk is relatively low, relief of obstruction is effective, and the patient enjoys rapid recovery with return to normal or near normal alimentation. Numerous studies have shown that such palliative resection yielded more satisfactory results than a bypass procedure such as gastrojejunostomy. Lawrence and McNeer (76) reported from their experience at the Memorial Sloan–Kettering Cancer Center that bypass gastrojejunostomy rarely relieved symptoms or prolonged life expectancy. Similar observations have been made by Remine and associates from the Mayo Clinic (77), Dupont and Cohn at Tulane University (78), Stern and colleagues at the Roswell Park Memorial Institute (79), Meifer and co-workers in the Netherlands (80), Hallissey and associates in the United Kingdom (81), and others. Patients who underwent palliative resection had an average survival time of nine to 19 months, as compared with three to seven months for patients who underwent bypass only.

When bleeding and pain are the main symptoms rather than obstruction, resection can provide equally worthwhile relief. However, if the patient's symptoms are mainly due to liver, peritoneal or bulky lymphatic metastases rather than the primary tumor, little benefit can be obtained by gastric resection.

Partial gastrectomy is preferred to total gastrectomy in a palliative resection for obvious reasons. The risk of complications from anastomotic leakage is significantly higher with a total gastrectomy. Also, patients resume eating and tend to achieve nutritional balance much more rapidly after a partial gastrectomy. While total gastrectomy should generally be avoided when palliation is the aim, special circumstances may justify its use (82). In some patients, it may be the only means to remove a bulky, obstructing tumor, or to control massive hemorrhage.

In other circumstances, the clinician can weigh the risks and benefits, and consider other options such as a near-total gastrectomy and nonsurgical modalities of treatment.

Surgical resection of liver metastases from gastric carcinoma is rarely performed, even though such resection is often done, with an added survival benefit, for liver metastases from colon and rectal cancer. In most patients, liver metastases from gastric carcinoma are multiple, with associated peritoneal and extensive lymphatic metastases. Very few reports of hepatic resection for metastatic gastric cancer have appeared in the literature; long-term survival is virtually unknown (83).

ENDOSCOPIC LASER THERAPY

As an alternative to resection or bypass, endoscopic laser therapy can offer relief of obstruction due to gastric cancer (84). Encouraging results have been reported, particularly when the obstructing lesion is short, such as in the cardia or prepyloric region. The neodymium aluminum garnet laser (Nd:YAG) is usually used. Fleischer and Sivak treated 15 patients with obstructing lesions of the gastric cardia who had a mean tumor length of 6.3 cm and narrowest lumen diameter of 3.3 mm. After an average of 2.8 treatments over six days, the mean diameter of the lumen increased to 12.1 mm. Increased food intake was noted in all patients, with no major complications. The scope of usefulness of laser therapy and its precise role in the palliative management of gastric cancer await further study in a larger number of patients. There is no doubt that certain subsets of patients, particularly those who are poor risks for surgery, will benefit from this treatment.

CHEMOTHERAPY AND RADIATION THERAPY

Most clinical studies of palliative chemotherapy and/ or radiation therapy performed from 1950 to 1980 failed to show significant benefit. However, recent advances have shown some encouraging results.

Radiation therapy has not been commonly used in the management of locally advanced, unresectable gastric cancer (67,85–87). Low tolerance of the normal stomach and adjacent intestines, and the nausea and vomiting that accompany treatment, generally preclude effective tumor control. Nevertheless, radiation therapy can sometimes control bleeding. Abe and his associates (88) have advocated the use of intraoperative radiation therapy as a method capable of giving a high radiation dose with sparing of adjacent sensitive organs. The efficacy of this technique requires further clinical study.

Chemotherapy combined with radiation therapy was studied by the Gastrointestinal Tumor Study Group in a prospective randomized trial. Considerable toxicity was experienced in this study, with many of the patients requiring intensive nutritional support. No significant improvement in survival was observed.

Numerous clinical trials of chemotherapy of advanced gastric carcinoma have appeared in the literature. The FAM regimen (5-FU, doxorubicin, and mitocycin-C) has received much attention during the last decade, since its first report by MacDonald and colleagues in 1979 (89). Initial experiences suggested an objective response rate of 37 percent to 63 percent with this regimen. In recent years, most centers have found that the response rate is about 20 percent, with complete response rates below 5 percent (90,91). Alopecia, nausea, vomiting, and myelosuppression are common and moderately severe. More recently two protocols have yielded significantly higher response rates (see Fig. 2.26). The first (92) consisted of 5-FU, doxorubicin (adriamycin), and methotrexate, with leucovorin rescue (FAMTX protocol); the second (93), of etoposide, doxorubicin, and cisplatin (EAP protocol). Kremer and associates (94) treated 42 patients with advanced, metastasized gastric carcinoma in the University of Hamburg using mostly the FAMTX protocol. Complete tumor regression documented by reoperation was achieved in six patients, four of whom continued to be alive at eight to 55 months. Moderately severe toxicity was also experienced. Studies are continuing at a number of centers to corroborate these improved results.

GASTRIC LYMPHOMA

Gastric lymphoma accounts for 1 percent to 5 percent of all gastric malignancies. There are indications that the incidence has increased in recent years (95). The stomach may be one of multiple anatomic sites involved by generalized lymphoma. Sometimes, however, lymphoma presents only in the stomach. Of all anatomic locations in which extranodal lymphoma can manifest, the stomach is the most common site (96). The term *primary gastric lymphoma* refers to this condition and is justifiable if diagnostic evaluation reveals no evidence of systemic disease.

Pathology

Although intra-abdominal Hodgkin's disease sometimes invades the stomach, primary gastric lymphomas are almost exclusively of the non-Hodgkin varieties. For many years, the Rappaport terminology was used for the histopathologic classification of the non-Hodgkin's lymphomas (97). Recently an expert international panel has recommended a Working Formulation that can be used in clinical trials and in international comparisons of reported results (98). In the Working Formulation, the lymphoma is assigned as high, low, or intermediate grade, with corresponding prognostic significance; the large-cell immuno blastic, lymphoblastic, and small-noncleaved-cell lesions have the worst prognosis. The most common

---

FIGURE 2.31:
HISTOPATHOLOGIC CLASSIFICATION OF THE NON-HODGKIN'S LYMPHOMAS: COMPARISON OF THE RAPPAPORT AND WORKING FORMULATION SCHEMES

WORKING FORMULATION	RAPPAPORT TERMINOLOGY
HIGH GRADE	
Large-cell immunoblastic	Diffuse, histiocytic
Lymphoblastic	Lymphoblastic
Small noncleaved cell	Diffuse, undifferentiated
INTERMEDIATE GRADE	
Follicular, predominantly large cell	Nodular histiocytic
Diffuse cleaved cell	Diffuse, poorly differentiated lymphocytic
Diffuse mixed large, small	Diffuse, mixed cell
Diffuse large cell	Diffuse, histiocytic
LOW GRADE	
Small lymphocytic, consistent with chronic lymphocytic leukemia	Diffuse, well-differentiated lymphocytic
Follicular, small cleaved cell	Nodular, poorly differentiated lymphocytic
Follicular, mixed small cleaved and large cell	Nodular, mixed lymphocytic histiocytic

types of gastric lymphoma are the diffuse histiocytic or diffuse poorly differentiated lymphocytic varieties according to the Rappaport scheme, or the diffuse large-cell and diffuse-cleaved-cell varieties according to the Working Formulation scheme (Fig. 2.31). Figures 2.32 and 2.33A and B show typical examples of the gross appearance and microscopic features of these tumors.

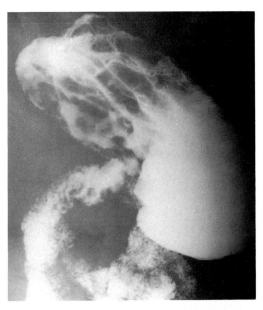

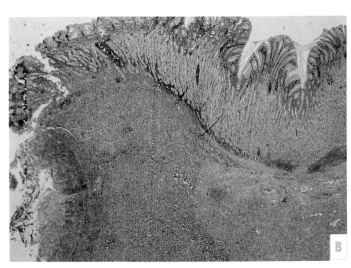

FIGURE 2.32 Gastric lymphoma. An upper GI series shows grossly enlarged thickened rugal folds in the body and fundus of the stomach. (From reference 24.)

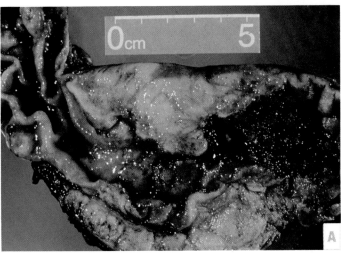

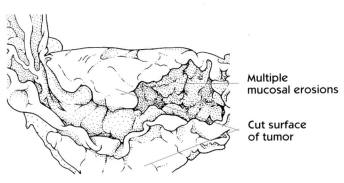

Multiple mucosal erosions

Cut surface of tumor

Mucosa

Lymphoma

Ulcer edge

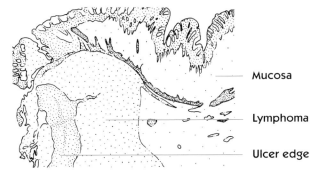

FIGURE 2.33 (A) This gastric lymphoma involves all layers of the stomach wall. Rugal folds are enlarged or effaced. The mucosa shows multifocal erosions and ulcers. (B) The lymphomatous infiltrate at the edge of this central ulcer shows no evidence of cohesiveness between the tumor cells in this gastric lymphoma (x4). (From reference 2.)

Clinical Presentation

Gastric lymphoma can cause dyspepsia, bleeding, obstruction, and perforation, closely mimicking the manifestations of peptic ulcer disease. A mass may be palpable on physical examination of the patient. Barium study of the stomach (Fig. 2.34) and gastroscopy (Fig. 2.35) reveal a variety of appearances, including polypoid, fungating, or ulcerated lesions. Large, thick rugal folds, often rigid due to mucosal and submucosal tumor infiltration, are characteristic. Single or multiple lesions may be seen. Unlike adenocarcinomas, a gastric lymphoma may extend across the pylorus to the duodenum. It may also involve an adjacent organ, and the gastric and extra-gastric lymph nodes.

Diagnosis

Before the advent of flexible fiberoptic endoscopy, biopsy was seldom possible. Many patients with gastric lymphoma underwent surgical treatment with a presumptive diagnosis of gastric carcinoma. Radical surgical resection by subtotal, total, or extended types of gastrectomy was performed based on this presumed diagnosis. While about 30 percent of patients so treated were cured (99), this treatment may not be optimal for most patients with gastric lymphoma. Chemotherapy and radiation therapy, used alone or in combination, have proven to be effective methods of treatment for lymphoma during the last two decades. It is, therefore, important to obtain a preoperative diagnosis of lymphoma, so that the role of surgery, radiation therapy, and chemotherapy can be appropriately planned by consultation among the treating physicians in these disciplines. Today endoscopic biopsy and cytologic examination permit an accurate diagnosis of gastric lymphoma in most patients.

Because the lymphoma often lies deep under the mucosa or submucosa, superficial biopsies may miss the diagnosis. Multiple biopsies and also cytologic brushings are recommended and may need to be repeated if they are not sufficiently diagnostic. The additional use of endoscopic ultrasound examination allows not only visualization of the mucosal aspect of the stomach but also an assessment of the depth of tumor penetration as well as involvement of adjacent lymph nodes and organs.

Staging

With an established diagnosis of gastric lymphoma, the patient should undergo a thorough diagnostic workup to determine the extent of the disease. In addition to a complete history and physical examination, standard blood count, blood chemistry, immunoglobulin analysis, chest roentgenographs, bone marrow biopsy, and computed tomography of the thorax and abdomen are performed. The CT may show enlargement or another abnormality in the spleen, liver, and the mediastinal, para-aortic, mesenteric, and iliac lymph nodes. Pedal lymphangiograms were formerly used to visualize the para-aortic and iliac nodes, but since the availability of CT, lymphangiography has seldom been necessary. CT-guided needle biopsy of the liver and other gross abnormalities within the abdomen can be carried out, if necessary, for staging purposes. The

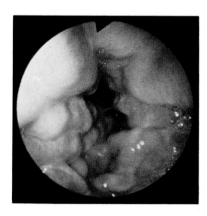

FIGURE 2.34 In this lymphoma the gastric rugae are infiltrated and may be confused with linitis plastica. (From reference 12.)

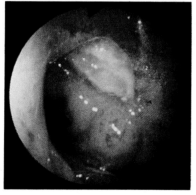

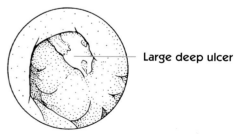

Large deep ulcer

FIGURE 2.35 A large deep ulcer associated with gastric lymphoma. (From reference 12.)

results of these diagnostic studies allow a tentative clinical staging of the disease, categorizing patients as having stomach involvement alone or stomach plus extragastric disease. This may suffice for the planning of treatment in many patients. If surgery is indicated, detailed, accurate, pathologic staging information can be obtained at laparotomy, including whether disease is present in the liver and the para-aortic, iliac, and mesenteric lymph nodes. If surgical resection is not indicated, the clinician will treat the patient by either chemotherapy or radiation therapy or both. Laparotomy for the purpose of staging alone, though sometimes recommended in the management of Hodgkin's disease, is rarely performed for patients with non-Hodgkin's lymphoma of the stomach.

The Ann Arbor Staging Classification (Fig. 2.36) is widely accepted in the stage designation of Hodgkin's disease as well as the non-Hodgkin's lymphomas (100). For gastric and other extranodal lymphomas, the qualifier "E" is added to denote extranodal origin according to a modification of the basic scheme by Musshoff (101).

Approach to the Patient

Because gastric lymphoma can be treated by surgical resection, radiation therapy, as well as chemo-therapy, it is important to appreciate what each of the three modalities can and cannot accomplish, and the risks attendant to each. Surgical resection can eradicate the lymphoma in the stomach and adjacent lymph nodes but offers no control of extragastric disease. In carefully selected patients, the risk of complications or death from the surgical operation is small (102,103). On the other hand, a serious complication, should it develop, may prevent initiation of needed chemotherapy or radiation therapy.

Radiation therapy can control not only local disease but can be extended to cover the para-aortic, iliac, and other nodal areas that may be involved. It cannot, however, effectively treat parenchymal organs such as the liver and lung. The radiation portals and dose must be carefully planned so as to avoid damage to the bowel and other sensitive organs.

Chemotherapy offers effective treatment of local as well as systemic lymphoma. Drug-induced myelosuppression often occurs with chemotherapy: the resulting leukopenia may lead to infectious complications, and thrombocytopenia to hemorrhage, particularly from the gastric lymphoma if not resected.

The extent and stage of the gastric lymphoma determine which modality or combination of modalities should best be used for the management of a

FIGURE 2.36:
ANN ARBOR STAGING CLASSIFICATION FOR HODGKIN'S AND NON-HODGKIN'S LYMPHOMAS

STAGE I   Involvement of a single lymph node region (I) or a single extralymphatic organ or site (IE)

STAGE II   Involvement of two or more lymph node regions on the same side of the diaphragm (II) or localized involvement of an extralymphatic organ or site with one or more lymph node regions on the same side of the diaphragm (IIE)

STAGE III   Involvement of lymph node regions on both sides of the diaphragm with (IIIE) or without (III) involvement of an extralymphatic organ or site, or spleen (IIIS), or both (IIIES)

STAGE IV   Diffuse or disseminated involvement of one or more extralymphatic organs with or without associated lymph node involvement given patient. Figure 2.37 shows an algorithm that summarizes the approach to management. In general, most patients need either surgical resection or radiation therapy for control of the local disease, and also chemotherapy for control of systemic lymphoma which is presumably present in at least 70 percent of cases. There have also been trials of treatment by chemotherapy alone. A spectrum of opinion exists regarding the exact indications for using the different modalities as well as combinations of them. Some centers favor surgery as an important part of treatment before chemotherapy (102–107), while others offer primary chemotherapy without preliminary resection of the gastric lymphoma (108). Many use an intermediate strategy, advising surgical resection before chemotherapy if the lesion involves the full thickness of the gastric wall or is deeply ulcerated and thus prone to hemorrhage and perforation (109).

PRIMARY SURGICAL RESECTION

Primary surgical resection followed by chemotherapy, radiation therapy, or both, is the standard method of management of most patients with gastric lymphoma at the Memorial Sloan–Kettering Cancer Center (102). Surgery is performed in patients who are judged to be good risks for surgery and whose tumor is considered resectable. There were no surgical deaths in a consecutive series of 48 patients treated from 1971 to 1982 (102). The resectability rate was 100 percent for stage IE, 66 percent for stage IIE, and 59 percent for stage IV, according to the complete staging information available after laparotomy. Subtotal gastrectomy was the preferred surgical method of resection; total gastrectomy was avoided. Patients received postsurgical abdominal radiation therapy with a boosting dose to the stomach-bed to 3700 cGy, and/or chemotherapy using mainly the CHOP (cyclophosphamide, doxorubicin, vincristine, prednisone) regimen. No patient developed known relapse in the abdomen after abdominal irradiation, and none developed relapse after adjuvant chemotherapy. The estimated survival rates at five years after treatment were 95 percent, 78 percent, and 25 percent, respectively, for stages IE, IIE, and IV.

Two other important observations were made with regard to surgical treatment. First, *total* gastrectomy can cause an immediate nutritional problem due to malabsorption and dumping, making chemotherapy or radiation therapy very difficult if not impossible to administer. This adverse effect of total gastrectomy has previously been reported (99,110). Second, observations in this study and elsewhere (111) indicate that it is unnecessary to perform total gastrectomy for no other reason than to gain a wide margin of resection. If all gross tumor can be removed, a partial gastrectomy will suffice even if microscopic or even minimal macroscopic tumor is left behind, provided that the patient receives adjuvant therapy. Three of four such patients in this study survived free of relapse.

A number of other centers also favor primary surgical resection with postoperative radiation therapy and/or chemotherapy in the management of gastric lymphoma. In adopting such an approach, the clinician needs to have a potentially resectable lesion in a patient who is medically fit to withstand the surgical operation. Other treatment options must be considered if these criteria cannot be met.

RADIATION THERAPY

Radiation therapy has been used for many years in the management of non-Hodgkin's lymphoma, and can achieve a high percentage of control of localized disease with substantial survival rates in stage I and stage II patients (112,113). The commonly used radiation dose is 3500 cGy over 3.5 weeks, with the exception of histiocytic lymphomas for which a higher dose of 4500 to 5000 cGy in 200 cGy fractions is used. In the treatment of localized lymphoma, radiation is generally given only to the involved anatomic region (involved field), with or without extension of the field to adjacent areas. For a gastric lymphoma, the stomach and stomach bed, including the celiac, perigastric, and splenic lymph nodes, are treated, as well as nodes in the hepatoduodenal ligament and porta hepatis. Optionally the field can be extended to cover the lower para-aortic and mediastinal nodes, or the entire abdomen with shielding of the kidneys.

Radiation therapy can be used successfully without surgical resection in the management of gastric lymphoma, but several reports have emphasized the risk of bleeding and perforation in 10 percent or more of patients treated. Bleeding and perforation have occurred mostly in patients who had bulky tumors. The risk of such complications in less advanced lesions has not been clearly documented.

Radiation therapy used as an adjunct after surgical resection has yielded a substantially higher rate of local control as well as survival in many reported series (99, 102–106). Most centers have used stomach-bed field radiation with extension of the treatment field to include adjacent upper abdominal nodes, and the hepatoduodenal and splenic regions. Total abdominal irradiation (2000 to 2500 cGy) with stomach and upper abdominal boost was used by some centers before the established use of multidrug chemotherapy (102,114). Although a lower rate of intra-abdominal relapse may have been achieved by total abdominal irradiation, treatment-related diarrhea and nutritional problems tended to be more severe.

Relapse, when it occurs, is often outside the treatment field. The addition of chemotherapy to radiation therapy has shown statistically significant

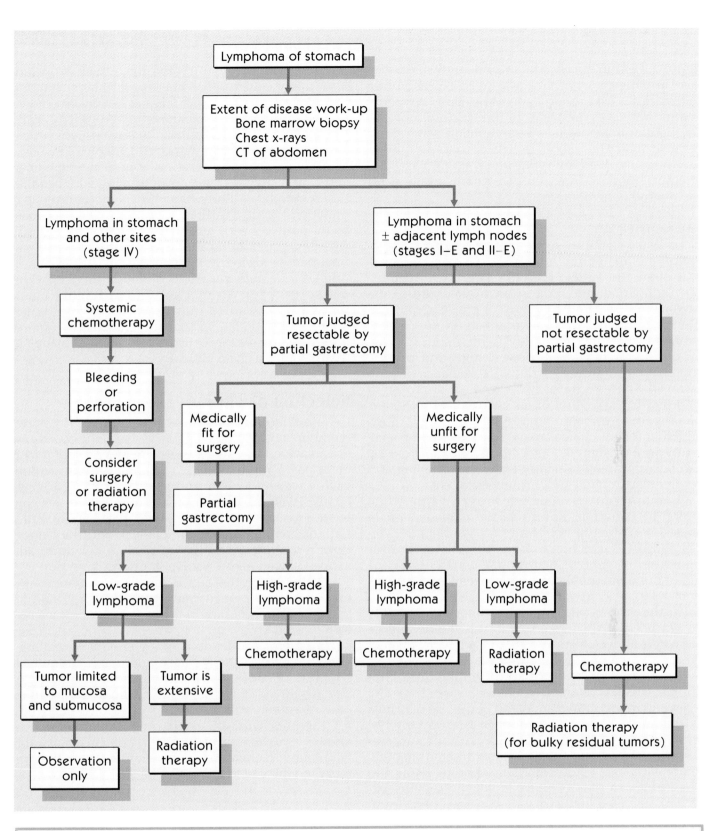

FIGURE 2.37 Algorithm for treatment of gastric lymphoma.

improvement in survival in several studies, particularly in patients who have advanced disease or an unfavorable histologic type (115–117). In recent years, therefore, the trend in the treatment of gastric lymphoma as well as lymphoma in general has been to limit the use of radiation therapy only to the area involved by lymphoma, using systemic chemotherapy as the main treatment method for the overall control of disease.

CHEMOTHERAPY

Increasingly effective chemotherapy of non-Hodgkin's lymphoma using multiple drugs has become available since the 1970s (118,119). The CHOP regimen (cyclophosphamide, doxorubicin, vincristine, and prednisone) is commonly used. It consists of cyclophosphamide 600–700 mg/m^2 given on day 1, doxorubicin 40–50 mg/m^2 on day 1, vincristine 1.4 mg/m^2 on day 1 (maximum dose 2 mg), and prednisone 60 mg/m^2 orally on days 1 through 5, in each cycle of 21 to 28 days, for a total of six to eight cycles (102,120). Other drugs such as methotrexate, bleomycin, etoposide, and cytarabine have been added in recent clinical trials. The treatment is generally well tolerated. However, myelosuppression can occur, leading to nadir sepsis and bleeding as a result of leukopenia and thrombocytopenia.

Chemotherapy has shown proven value when added to radiation therapy in the management of stage I and stage II non-Hodgkin's lymphoma (117, 121,122). It is also commonly administered after resection of gastric lymphoma, particularly for tumors of unfavorable histology, because of the risk of developing systemic disease. Stage I lesions limited to the gastric mucosa and submucosa probably do not need further treatment by chemotherapy, as indicated above. Also, the role of adjuvant chemotherapy is uncertain for low-grade lesions such as nodular, poorly differentiated lymphocytic lymphoma, which is often an indolent disease (123).

Several reports have appeared of the use of primary chemotherapy plus radiation therapy for the treatment of gastric lymphoma without surgical resection. Maor and his associates treated nine patients with four cycles of chemotherapy using the CHOP regimen plus bleomycin, which was alternated with involved field radiation therapy (108). Treatment was started after endoscopic biopsy in six patients, and after exploratory laparotomy which showed unresectable disease in three patients. Complications such as bleeding and perforation did not occur, and all nine patients were alive at the time of the report. Taal and his group similarly advocated primary chemotherapy with radiation therapy; however, they encountered serious hemorrhage and perforation in four patients and recommended that patients who had bleeding or deeply ulcerated tumors should first undergo resection (109). Bleeding and perforation following radiation or chemo-

therapy of gastric lymphoma have been reported from many centers (107,114,115,124). Most tumors that bleed or perforate are large or deeply ulcerated, involving the entire thickness of the gastric wall. Taal and others have proposed that endoscopic ultrasound examination can visualize the depth of involvement and extent of ulceration of gastric lymphoma, and that it may be used to determine whether the tumor can safely be treated by chemotherapy and radiation therapy without resection (109). Because many patients with gastric lymphoma are elderly and have coexisting medical disorders, surgical treatment is always risky. The efficacy and safety of primary chemotherapy and radiation therapy without surgery for various subsets of tumors must therefore be studied more extensively in a large number of patients, so that the clinician can more accurately weigh the benefits and risks in planning treatment for a given patient.

Selection of Therapy

Debate continues on the best treatment of gastric lymphoma; it will not be conclusive until questions are answered by clinical trials. For the present, most clinicians agree that stage I tumors localized to the gastric wall, of low- or intermediate-grade histology, can be treated by resection alone; radiation therapy is an equally effective alternative, particularly if the patient has increased surgical risk and the tumor does not show extensive ulceration. For more advanced stage I and for stage II lesions, resection followed by chemotherapy is usually recommended, especially for tumors of high-grade histology, but the value of chemotherapy has yet to be confirmed by randomized study. If chemotherapy is not used for such patients, radiation therapy should be administered to at least the stomach and upper abdominal lymph node areas. For patients who have unresectable disease, and for those have who had bulky disease resected, radiation therapy is also recommended, together with chemotherapy. In patients with known involvement of the liver, spleen, or distant lymph nodes, chemotherapy must constitute the primary modality of treatment.

Prognosis and Treatment Failure

Several clinicopathologic variables of gastrointestinal lymphoma have been found to be associated with prognosis according to multivariate statistical analyses (103,106,116,125). Favorable characteristics include low Ann Arbor stage (stage IE), low- or intermediate-grade histology in the Working Formulation scheme, and surgical resectability. Absence of deep penetration such as invasion of the serosa also correlated with a better prognosis (103,106,107,126).

Failures of treatment is due to either local or systemic disease or both. Systemic failure is more common after gastric resection, whereas local failure is more common when the gastric lesion is not resected. Multidrug chemotherapy improves the probability of survival in patients with high-grade non-Hodgkin's lymphoma, but no such effect has yet been demonstrated for patients with nodular, poorly differentiated lymphocytic lymphomas (follicular small-cleaved-cell type, according to the Working Formulation scheme), which tend to have an indolent clinical course. In patients who develop relapse after initial control of the disease, salvage treatment by chemotherapy or resection and radiation therapy can sometimes be attempted, with a successful outcome in carefully selected patients.

GASTRIC SARCOMA

Sarcomas of the stomach are almost exclusively myosarcomas. These tumors represent about 1 percent of the malignant neoplasms of the stomach. They occur in either sex and at all ages, though most commonly between 50 and 70. There is no known etiologic association.

Pathology

Histopathologically, they are either spindle-cell-type leiomyosarcomas (Figs. 2.38A and B; 2.39A and B) or malignant leiomyoblastomas with round or epithelioid cells (127–130). The malignant leio-

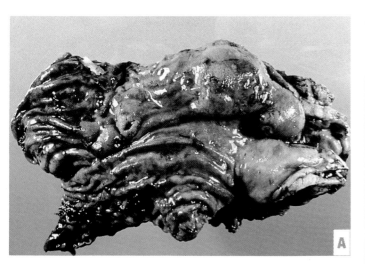

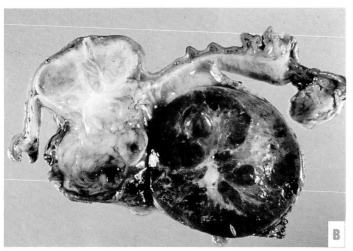

FIGURE 2.38 (A) This sizeable leiomyosarcoma was visible only as a large, smooth bulge underlying a largely intact mucosa. **(B)** The cut surface of the tumor revealed its intramural nature, with a prominent projection beyond the serosa. (From reference 2.)

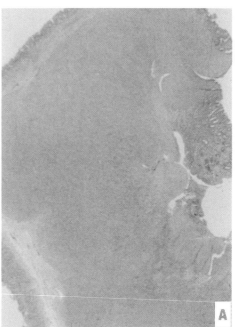

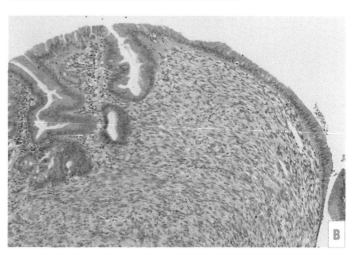

FIGURE 2.39 (A) The central ulcer in this densely cellular leiomyosarcoma shows mucosal invasion at its edge (x3.3). **(B)** In this same example of mucosal invasion by leiomyosarcoma, the mitotic rate was greater than 10 mitoses per 50 high-power fields. This tumor measured 12 cm (x25). (From reference 2.)

myoblastoma is also known as bizarre leiomyosarcoma or epithelioid leiomyosarcoma. An occasional gastric myosarcoma may show the presence of both cell types. Despite distinctly different microscopic appearances, the two types of myosarcomas show similar clinical behavior.

Gastric myosarcomas arise in the muscular wall of the stomach, presenting either as an intragastric or extragastric mass. In some patients it may be attached to the outer surface of the stomach wall by a long stalk. These sarcomas range from a few centimeters to over 30 cm in diameter. The larger ones often undergo cystic degeneration and hemorrhage. They may invade an adjacent organ such as the left lobe of the liver, transverse colon, spleen, or pancreas. Exophytic tumors may perforate, resulting in transperitoneal dissemination. Poorly differentiated tumors (high histopathologic grade of malignancy) often develop meta- stases, typically to the liver. Lymphatic metastases are rare and usually indicative of advanced disease (128,131). Well-differentiated (low-grade) tumors usually remain confined to the stomach, but may enlarge, invade adjacent organs, or perforate into the free peritoneal cavity, causing transabdominal metastases.

Determination of the histologic grade of malignancy is an important part of the pathologic diagnosis because it has a bearing on prognosis. The method for grading is similar to that for sarcoma of soft tissues (128,130,132,133). The pathologist assigns the grade according to the degree of cellularity, nuclear and cytoplasmic features, mitotic rate, and other microscopic features such as vascularity, amount of stroma, and necrosis. While all of these characteris-

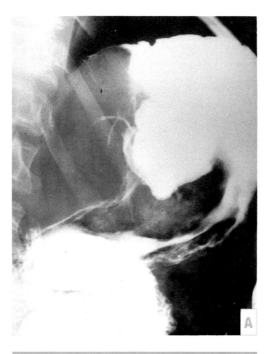

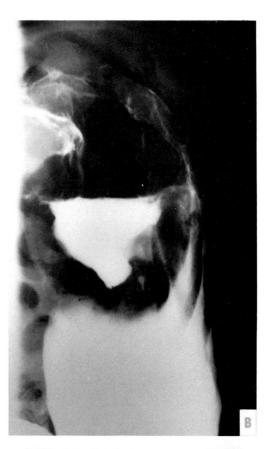

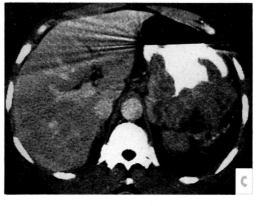

FIGURE 2.40 Leiomyosarcoma. This 69-year-old man complained of early satiety, epigastric fullness, increasing abdominal girth, and dark stools. Physical examination revealed an epigastric mass. **(A,B)** Recumbent and erect films of an upper GI series show a large ulcerating mass arising from the lesser curvature and posterior wall of the stomach. (In **B,** note the gas-fluid level in the ulcer on the erect film.) The tumor has both intra- and extraluminal components, with a blind tract extending from the intraluminal ulcer to the extraluminal mass. **(C)** CT scan demonstrates a bulky exophytic mass arising from the gastric wall. A portion of the sinus tract (*arrow*) is opacified by barium. The low-attenuation area represents necrosis. (From reference 24.)

tics of a given tumor must be taken into account in assigning the grade, the mitotic count is the most objective and reproducible. High-grade tumors generally show ten or more mitoses per ten high-power fields, with other corroborative features such as sparcity of stroma, pleomorphism of cells, and evidence of necrosis.

Clinical Presentation

The symptoms caused by gastric myosarcomas resemble those of peptic ulcer disease and gastric carcinoma. Some patients may have a very large tumor, discovered by either the patient or a physician. Hematemesis, melena, or anemia may be caused by hemorrhage from ulcerated tumors.

Diagnosis

Barium examination of the stomach shows the characteristic appearance of a space-occupying lesion often with a deep crater (Fig. 2.40A–C). When the tumor has an intragastric component, gastroscopy and biopsy can provide a preoperative diagnosis. CT or magnetic resonance imaging (MRI) gives an accurate image of these tumors as well as liver metastases when present.

Approach to the Patient

Surgical resection is the principal method of treatment of a primary gastric myosarcoma. The principles of resection for myosarcoma differ from those for gastric carcinoma (128,130). Because extensive intramucosal or submucosal spread seldom occurs with gastric myosarcomas, resection need not include as wide a margin of the normal stomach as is recom-

mended for gastric carcinoma. Excision of the tumor with a wedge or sleeve of the adjacent stomach will satisfactorily control most of the smaller lesions. A large tumor, or one located at the cardia or pylorus, may require resection by partial gastrectomy. Total gastrectomy is needed only for the very rare tumor involving the entire stomach from cardia to pylorus. For tumors that abut or invade an adjacent organ, en bloc excision of the particular organ such as the spleen, colon, or pancreas must be performed for local tumor control. Figure 2.41 shows the type and extent of surgical resection in a series of 32 gastric myosarcomas treated at the Memorial Sloan–Kettering Cancer Center. Nine patients underwent excision of their tumors which measured 5 cm or less in diameter; all nine patients survived free of disease for five or more years. The larger tumors needed partial gastrectomy or more extensive gastric resections.

During surgery, a question sometimes arises as to whether a tumor is benign or malignant. It is important to note that pathologic diagnosis by frozen-section examination of many of these tumors is unreliable, because differentiation from benign leiomyosarcoma cannot be made by this technique. In practice, the surgical treatment need not be much different, because only a limited resection margin of 2 to 3 cm of the stomach wall is needed for most lesions whether benign or malignant. The surgeon can decide at the time of surgery in such a way that the scope of resection would be adequate if the tumor proves to be a sarcoma, and would not be unjustifiably excessive if it proves to be a benign leiomyoma.

Adjunctive chemotherapy and radiation therapy are sometimes used to advantage in the management of patients with sarcoma of soft tissues in somatic sites. The effectiveness of adjuvant radia-

FIGURE 2.41:
EXTENT OF RESECTION AND FIVE-YEAR SURVIVAL OF GASTRIC MYOSARCOMAS: THE MEMORIAL SLOAN–KETTERING CANCER CENTER (1949–1973)

	TUMOR ≤ 5 cm	TUMOR invades adjacent organs	TOTAL
Wedge resection	6/6		7/9
Subtotal gastrectomy	1/1		6/7
Total gastrectomy	1/1		1/1
Extended resections (plus pancreas, liver, colon, etc.)	1/1	0/6	3/10
All cases	9/9	0/6	17/27

Numerator denotes number of patients alive; denominator, number of patients treated. (Adapted from reference 128.)

tion therapy in local control has been confirmed by randomized clinical trials. The role of adjuvant chemotherapy for sarcoma of soft somatic tissues is controversial, with survival advantage having been demonstrated in a few but not in most randomized studies. For gastric leiomyosarcomas, however, neither retrospective nor prospective randomized studies have shown any benefit of adjuvant radiation therapy or chemotherapy after resection.

The prognosis of gastric myosarcoma is governed by the size of the tumor, its histopathologic grade of malignancy, and whether it has invaded an adjacent organ structure (128). The overall survival rate at five years is approximately 50 percent, depending on the admixture of these prognostic factors in the patient population. Low-grade tumors smaller than 5 cm in diameter have a cure rate approaching 100 percent after simple excision by wedge gastrectomy. On the other hand, the cure rate is less than 10 percent with large, high-grade tumors that have invaded adjacent organs, despite radical extirpation by extensive multiorgan resection.

References

1. American Cancer Society. *Ca—A Cancer Journal for Clinicians* 39:12–13, 1989.

2. Buell P, Dunn JE Jr. Cancer mortality among Japanese Issei and Nisei of California. *Cancer* 18:656–664, 1965.

3. Hill MJ, Hawksworth G, Tattersall G. Bacteria, nitrosamines, and cancer of the stomach. *Br J Cancer* 28:562–567, 1973.

4. Correa P, Haenszel W, Cuello C, Tannenbaum S, Archer M. A model for gastric cancer epidemiology. *Lancet* 2:58–60, 1975.

5. Raineri R, Weisburger JH. Reduction of gastric carcinogens with ascorbic acid. *Ann NY Acad Sci* 258:181–189, 1975.

6. Creagan ET, Fraumeni JF. Familial gastric cancer and immunologic abnormalities. *Cancer* 32:1325–1331, 1973.

7. Lee FI. Carcinoma of the gastric antrum in identical twins. *Postgrad Med J* 47:622–623, 1971.

8. Cwern M, Garcia RL, Davidson MI, Friedman IH. Simultaneous occurrence of gastric carcinoma in identical twins. *Am J Gastroenterol* 75:41–47, 1981.

9. You W-C, Blot WJ, Chang Y-S, et al. Diet and high risk of stomach cancer in Shandong, China. *Cancer Res* 48:3518–3523, 1988.

10. Correa P, Sasano N, Stemmerman GN, Haenszel W. Pathology of gastric carcinoma in Japanese populations: comparisons between Miyagi Prefecture, Japan and Hawaii. *J Natl Cancer Inst* 51:1449–1459, 1973.

11. Aird I, Bentall HH, Roberts JAF. A relationship between cancer of the stomach and the ABO blood groups. *Br Med J* 1:799–801, 1953.

12. Silverstein FE, Tytgat GNJ. *Atlas of gastrointestinal endoscopy.* New York: Gower Medical Publishing, 1987.

13. Correa P. Epidemiology and pathogenesis of chronic gastritis: three etiologic entities. *Front Gastroenterol Res* 6:98–108, 1980.

14. Siurala M, Isokoski M, Varis K, Kekki M. Prevalence of gastritis in a rural population. *Scand J Gastroenterol* 3:211–223, 1968.

15. Deschner EE, Winawer SJ, Lipkin M. Patterns of nucleic acid and protein synthesis in normal human gastric mucosa and atrophic gastritis. *J Natl Cancer Inst* 48:1567–1574, 1972.

16. Eriksson S, Clase L, Moquist-Olsson I. Pernicious anemia as a risk factor in gastric cancer. The extent of the problem. *Acta Med Scand* 210:481–484, 1981.

17. Hermans PE, Huizenga KA. Association of gastric carcinoma with idiopathic late-onset immunoglobulin deficiency. *Ann Intern Med* 76:606–609, 1972.

18. Hughes WS, Brooks FP, Conn HO. Serum gastrin levels in primary hypogammaglobulinemia and pernicious anemia—studies in adults. *Ann Intern Med* 77:746–750, 1972.

19. Cowling DC, Strickland RG, Ungar B, Whillingham S, Rose W McI. Pernicious anemia-like syndrome with immunoglobulin deficiency. *Med J Aust* 1:15–17, 1974.

20. Balfour DC. Factors influencing the life expectancy of patients operated on for gastric ulcers. *Ann Surg* 75:405–408, 1922.

21. Stalsberg H, Taksdal S. Stomach cancer following gastric surgery for benign conditions. *Lancet* 2:1175–1177, 1971.

22. Eberlein TJ, Lorenzo FV, Webster MW. Gastric carcinoma following operation for peptic ulcer disease. *Ann Surg* 197:251–256, 1978.

23. Domellof L, Eriksson S, Janunger KG. Late precancerous changes and carcinoma of the gastric stump after Billroth I resection. *Am J Surg* 132:26–31, 1976.

24. Kassner EG. *Slide atlas of radiologic imaging.* New York: Gower Medical Publishing, 1988.

25. Mitros FA. *Atlas of gastrointestinal pathology.* New York: Gower Medical Publishing, 1988.

26. Tomasulo J. Gastric polyps—histologic types and their relationship to gastric carcinoma. *Cancer* 27:1346–1355, 1971.

27. Berg JW. Histologic aspects of the relation between gastric adenomatous polyps and gastric cancer. *Cancer* 11:1149–1155, 1958.

28. Misiewicz JJ, et al. *Atlas of clinical gastroenterology.* London: Gower Medical Publishing, 1985.

29. Lauren P. The histological main types of gastric cancer—diffuse and so-called intestinal-type carcinoma: an attempt at histological classification. *Acta Pathol Microbiol Scand* 64:31–49, 1965.

30. Correa P. Clinical implications of recent developments in gastric cancer, pathology, and epidemiology. *Semin Oncol* 12:2–10, 1985.

31. Mitty WF, Rousselot LM, Grace WJ. Carcinoma of the stomach. *Am J Dig Dis* 5:249–258, 1960.

32. Kreel L, Herlinger H, Glaville J. Techniques of double-contrast barium meal with examples of correlation with endoscopy. *Clin Radiol* 24:307–314, 1973.

33. Morrissey JF. The diagnosis of early gastric cancer. *Gastroinest Endosc* 23:14–15, 1976.

34. Winawer SJ, Sherlock P, Hajdu SI. The role of upper gastrointestinal endoscopy in patients with cancer. *Cancer* 37:440–448, 1976.

35. Kobayashi S, Kasugai T, Yamazaki H. Endoscopic differentiation of early gastric cancer from benign peptic ulcer. *Gastrointest Endosc* 25:55–57, 1979.

36. International Union Against Cancer. *TNM classification of malignant tumors,* 4th ed. Berlin: Springer-Verlag, 1987: 40–42.

37. American Joint Committee on Cancer. *Manual for staging of cancer,* 3rd ed. Philadelphia: J.B. Lippincott, 1988: 63–67.

38. Kennedy BJ. The unified international gastric cancer staging classification system. *Scand J Gastroenterol* 2(Suppl 133): 11–13, 1987.

39. Mauro MA, Lee JKT, Heiken JP, Balfe DM. Radiologic staging of gastrointestinal neoplasms. *Surg Clin North Am* 64:67–88, 1984.

40. Kimmey MB, Martin RW, Haggitt RC, Wang KY, Franklin DW, Silverstein FE. Histologic correlates of gastrointestinal ultrasound images. *Gastroenterology* 96:433–441, 1989.

41. Tio TL, Tytgat GNJ. Endoscopic ultrasonography in analyzing peri-intestinal lymph node abnormality. *Scand J Gastroenterol* 21(Suppl 123):158–163, 1986.

42. Aibe T, Ito T, Yoshida T, et al. Endoscopic ultrasonography of lymph nodes surrounding the upper GI tract. *Scand J Gastroenterol* 21(Suppl 123):164–169, 1986.

43. Yasuda K, Kiyota K, Mukai H, Cho E. Anatomical aspects of endoscopic ultrasonography. In: K Kawai, ed. *Endoscopic*

Ultrasonography in Gastroenterology. Tokyo: Igaku-Shoin, 1988:140–158.

44. Tio TL, den Hartog Jager FC, Tytgat GNJ. The role of endoscopic ultrasonography in assessing local resectability of oesophagogastric malignancies. Accuracy, pitfalls, and predictability. *Scand J Gastroenterol* 21(Suppl 123):78–86, 1986.

45. Aibe T, Takemoto T. Diagnosis of the infiltrating depth of gastric cancer by endoscopic ultrasonography. *Gan No Rinsho* 32(10):1173–1175, 1986.

46. Grimm H, Sollano J, Hamper K, Noar M, Soehendra N. Endoscopic ultrasound (EUS) of esophago-gastric cancer: a new requirement for preoperative staging? (Abstract) *Gastrointest Endosc* 34:176–177, 1988.

47. Tio TL, Schovwink MH, Likot RJLM, Tytgat GNJ. Preoperative TNM classification of gastric carcinoma by endosonography. *Gastroenterology* 96:A512, 1989.

48. Lightdale CJ, Botet JF, Brennan MF, Shiu MH, Coit DG. Endoscopic ultrasonography (EUS) compared to computerized tomography (CT) for pre-operative staging of gastric cancer. (Abstract) *Gastrointest Endosc* 35:154–155, 1989.

49. Gouzi JL, Hugier M, Fagniez PL, et al. Total versus subtotal gastrectomy for adenocarcinoma of the gastric antrum. *Ann Surg* 209:162–166, 1989.

50. Coller FA, Kay EB, McIntyre RS. Regional lympatic metastases of carcinoma of the stomach. *Arch Surg* 43:748–761, 1941.

51. Sunderland DA, McNeer G, Ortager LG, Pearce LS. The lymphatic spread of gastric cancer. *Cancer* 6:987–996, 1953.

52. McNeer G, Pack GT. *Neoplasms of the stomach.* Philadelphia: J.B. Lippincott, 1967.

53. Arhelger SW, Lober PH, Wangensteen OH. Dissection of the hepatic pedicle and retro-pancreaticoduodenal areas for cancer of the stomach. *Surgery* 38:675–678, 1955.

54. Remine WH, Gomes MMR, Dockerty MB. Long-term survival (10 to 56 years) after surgery for carcinoma of the stomach. *Am J Surg* 117:177–184, 1969.

55. McNeer G, Bowden L, Booher RJ, McPeak CJ. Elective total gastrectomy for cancer of the stomach. *Ann Surg*

56. Korenaga D, Tsujitani S, Haraguchi M, et al. Long-term survival in Japanese patients with far advanced carcinoma of the stomach. *World J Surg* 12:236–240, 1981.

57. Kodoma Y, Sugimachi K, Soejima K, et al. Evaluation of extensive lymph node dissection for carcinoma of the stomach. *World J Surg* 5:241–248, 1981.

58. Shiu MH, Moore E, Sanders M, et al. Influence of the extent of resection on survival after curative treatment of gastric carcinoma. *Arch Surg* 122:1347–1351, 1987.

59. Kajitani T, Miwa K (for Japanese Research Society for Gastric Cancer). *Treatment results of stomach carcinoma in Japan, 1963–1966.* WHO-UICC Mongraph No. 2. Tokyo: WHO Collaborating Center for Evaluation of Methods of Diagnosis and Treatment of Stomach Cancer, c/o National Cancer Center, 1979: 115–118.

60. Papachristou DN, Shiu MH. Management by en bloc multiple organ resection of carcinoma of the stomach invading adjacent organs. *Surg Gynecol Obstet* 152:483–487, 1981.

61. Suchiro S, Nagasue N, Ogawa Y. The negative effect of splenectomy on the prognosis of gastric cancer. *Am J Surg* 148:645–648, 1984.

62. Brady MS, Rogatko A, Dent L, Shiu MH. Effect of splenectomy on morbidity and survival after curative resection of gastric carcinoma. *Arch Surg* 126:359–364, 1991.

63. Miwa K, et al. Evaluation of the TNM classification of stomach cancer and a proposal for its rational stage-grouping. *Jpn J Clin Oncol* 14:385–410, 1984.

64. Kennedy BJ. TNM classification for stomach cancer. *Cancer* 26:971–983, 1970.

65. Diggory RT, Cuschieri A. R 2/3 gastrectomy for gastric carcinoma: an audited experience of a consecutive series. *Br J Surg* 72:146–148, 1985.

66. Nanus DM, Kelsen DP, Niedzwiecki D, et al. Flow cytometry as a predictive indicator in patients with operable gastric cancer. *J Clin Oncol* 8:1105–1112, 1989.

67. Gunderson LL, Sosin H. Adenocarcinoma of the stomach: areas of failure in a reoperation series (second or symptomatic looks); clinicopathologic correlation and implicaions for adjuvant therapy. *Int J Radiat Oncol Biol Phys* 8:1–11, 1982.

68. Inokuchi K, Hattori T, Taguchi T, Abe O, Ogawa N. Postoperative adjuvant chemotherapy for gastric carcinoma. *Cancer* 53:2393–2397, 1984.

69. The Gastrointestinal Tumor Study Group. Controlled trial of adjuvant chemotherapy following curative resection for gastric cancer. *Cancer* 49:1116–1122, 1982.

70. Schreml W, Schlag P, Herfarth C, et al. Adjuvant 5-FU/BCNU chemotherapy in gastric cancer. In: Jones SE, Salmon SE, eds. *Adjuvant Therapy of Cancer IV*. New York: Grune & Stratton, 1984:441.

71. Shein PS, Coombes RC, Chilvers C. A controlled trial of FAM (5-FU, doxorubicin, and mitomycin C) chemotherapy as adjuvant treatment for resected gastric carcinoma: an interim report. *Proc Am Soc Clin Oncol* 5:78, 1986.

72. Atiq O, Kelsen D, Shiu MH, et al. Postoperative adjuvant intraperitoneal (IP) and intravenous (IV) chemotherapy in poor-risk gastric cancer patients. (Abstract) *Proc Am Soc Cli Oncol*, 1991.

73. Koga S, Hamazue R, Maeter M, et al. Prophylactic therapy for peritoneal recurrence of gastric cancer by continuous hyperthermic peritoneal perfusion with mitomycin C. *Cancer* 61:232–237, 1988.

74. Kim JP. The concept of immunochemosurgery in gastric cancer. *World J Surg* 11:465–472, 1987.

75. Abe M, Shibamoto Y, Takahashi M, et al. Intraoperative radiotherapy in carcinoma of the stomach and pancreas. *World J Surg* 11:459–464, 1987.

76. Lawrence W Jr, McNeer G. The effectiveness of surgery for palliation of incurable gastric cancer. *Cancer* 11:28–32, 1958.

77. Remine WH, Priestley JT, Berkson J. *Cancer of the stomach.* Philadelphia: W.B. Saunders Co., 1964.

78. Dupont BJ, Cohn I Jr. Gastric adenocarcinoma. In: Hickey RC, ed. *Current Problems in Cancer*, Vol. 4 (No. 8). Chicago: Year Book Medical Publishers, Inc., 1980: 38–41.

79. Stern JF, Denman S, Elias EG, Didolkar M, Holyoke ED. Evaluation of palliative resection in advanced carcinoma of the stomach. *Surgery* 77:291–298, 1975.

80. Meijer S, De Bakker OJGB, Hoitsma HFW. Palliative resection in gastric cancer. *J Surg Oncol* 23:77–80, 1983.

81. Hallissey MT, Allum WH, Roginski C, Fielding JW. Palliative surgery for gastric cancer. *Cancer* 62:440–444, 1988.

82. Boddie AW Jr, McMuretry MJ, Giacco GG, et al. Palliative total gastrectomy and esophagogastrectomy: a re-evaluation. *Cancer* 51:1195–1200, 1983.

83. Hughes K, Sugarbaker PH. Resection of the liver for metastatic solid tumors. In: Rosenberg SA, ed. *Surgical Treatment of Metastatic Cancer*. Philadelphia: J.B. Lippincott, 1987: 143–144.

84. Fleischer D, Sivak MV. Endoscopic Nd:YAG laser therapy as palliative treatment for advanced adenocarcinoma of the gastric cardia. *Gastroenterology* 87:815–820, 1984.

85. Goldstein HM, Rogers LF, Fletcher GH, et al. Radiological manifestation of radiation induced injury to the normal upper gastrointestianl tract. *Radiology* 117:135, 1975.

86. Nodman E, Kauppinin C. The value of megavoltage therapy in carcinoma of the stomach. *Strahlentherapie* 144:635, 1972.

87. Wieland C, Hymmen U. Megavolttherapie maligner Neoplasien des Magens. *Strahlentherapie* 140:20–26, 1970.

88. Abe M, Takahashi T, Yabumoto E, et al. Clinical experiences with intra-operative radiotherapy of locally advanced cancers. *Cancer* 45:40–48, 1980.

89. MacDonald JS, Wooley PV, Smythe T, et al. 5-fluorouracil, adriamycin and mitomycin C (FAM) combination chemotherapy in the treatment of advanced gastric cancer. *Cancer* 44: 42–47, 1919.

90. Gastrointestinal Tumor Study Group. A comparative clinical assessment of combination chemotherapy in the management of advanced gastric carcinoma. *Cancer* 49:1362–1366, 1981.

91. Haim N, Epelbaum R, Cohen Y, Robinson E. Further studies on the treatment of advanced gastric cancer by 5-fluorouracil, adriamycin (doxorubicin) and mitomycin C (modified FAM). *Cancer* 54:1999–2002, 1984.

92. Klein HO, Wickramanayake PD, Schultz V, et al. 5-fluorouracil, adriamycin and methotrexate: a combination protocol (FAMeth) for the treatment of metastasized stomach cancer. In: Kimura K, Fuji S, Ogawa M, et al., eds. *Fluoropyrimidines in Cancer Therapy*. Amsterdam: Excerpta Medica, 1984: 280–287.

93. Preusser P, Wilke H, Achterrath W, et al. Phase II Studie mit Etoposi, Adriamycin, Cisplatin (EAP) beim primar inoperablen, metastasierenden Magenkarzinom. *Tumor Diagnostik & Therapie* 3:43–48, 1987.

94. Kremer B, Henne-Bruns D, Effenberger TH. Advanced gastric cancer: a new combined surgical and oncological approach. *Hepato-Gastroenterology* 36:23–26, 1989.

95. Hayes J, Dunn E. Has the incidence of primary gastric lymphoma increased? *Cancer* 63:2073–2076, 1989.

96. Freeman C, Berg JW, Cutler SJ. Occurrence and prognosis of extranodal lymphomas. *Cancer* 29:252–260, 1972.

97. Rappaport H. Tumors of the hematopoietic system. In: *Atlas of Tumor Pathology*, Section 3, Fascicle 8. Washington, DC: US Armed Forces Institute of Pathology, 1966.

98. The Non-Hodgkin's Lymphoma Pathologic Classification Project. National-Cancer-Institute-sponsored study of classification of non-Hodgkin's lymphomas. *Cancer* 49:2112–2135, 1982.

99. Shiu MH, Karas M, Nisce LZ, Lee BJ, Filippa DA, Lieberman PH. Management of primary gastric lymphoma. *Ann Surg* 195:196–202, 1982.

100. Carbone PP, Kaplan HS, Mussoff K, Smithers DW, Tubiana M. Report of the committee on Hodgkins's staging classification. *Cancer Res* 31:1860–1861, 1971.

101. Musshoff K. Klinische Stadieneinteilung der Nicht-Hodgkin-Lymphome. *Strahlentherapie* 153:218–221, 1977.

102. Shiu MH, Nisce LZ, Pinna A, et al. Recent results of multimodality therapy of gastric lymphoma. *Cancer* 58:1389–1399, 1986.

103. Rosen CB, Van Heerden JA, Martin JK, Wold LE, Ilstrup DM. Is an aggressive surgical approach to the patient with gastric lymphoma warranted? *Ann Surg* 205:634–640, 1988.

104. Shepherd FA, Evans WK, Yau JC, et al. Chemotherapy following surgery for stage IE and IIE non-Hodgkin's lymphoma of the gastrointestinal tract. *J Clin Oncol* 6:253–260, 1988.

105. Hockey MS, Powell J, Crocker J, Fielding JWL. Primary gastric lymphoma. *Br J Surg* 74:483–487, 1987.

106. Dragosics B, Bauer P, Radaszkiewics T. Primary gastrointestinal non-Hodgkin's lymphomas: a retrospective clinicopathologic study of 150 cases. *Cancer* 55:1060–1073, 1985.

107. Brooks JJ, Enterline HT. Primary gastric lymphomas: a clinicopathologic study of 58 cases with long-term follow-up and literature review. *Cancer* 51:701–711, 1983.

108. Maor MH, Maddux B, Osborne BM, et al. Stages IE and IIE non-Hodgkin's lymphomas of the stomach: comparison of treatment modalities. *Cancer* 54:2330–2337, 1984.

109. Taal BG, Den Hartog Jager FCA, Burgers JMV, Van Heerd P, Tio TL. Primary non-Hodgkin's lymphoma of the stomach: changing aspects and therapeutic choices. *Eur J Cancer Clin Oncol* 1989.

110. Lim FE, Hartman AS, Tan EGC, Cady B, Meissner WA. Factors in the prognosis of gastric lymphoma. *Cancer* 39:1715–1720, 1977.

111. Weingrad DN, DeCosse JJ, Sherlock P, Straus D, Lieberman PH, Filippa DA. Primary gastrointestinal lymphoma: a 30-year review. *Cancer* 49:1258–1265, 1982.

112. Jones SE, Fuks Z, Kaplan HS, et al. Non-Hodgkin's lymphomas: results of radiotherapy. *Cancer* 32:683–691, 1973.

113. Hellman S, Chaffey JT, Rosenthal DS, et al. The place of radiation therapy in the treatment of non-Hodgkin's lymphoma. *Cancer* 39:843–851, 1977.

114. Burgers JMV, Taal BG, Van Heerde P, Somers R, Den Hartog Jager FCA, Hart AAM. Treatment results of primary stage I and II non-Hodgkin's lymphoma of the stomach. *Radiother Oncol* 11:319–326, 1988.

115. Hande KR, Fisher RI, DeVita VT, Chabner RA, Young RC. Diffuse histiocytic lymphoma involving the gastrointestinal tract. *Cancer* 41:1984–1989, 1978.

116. List AF, Greer JP, Cousar JC, et al. Non-Hodgkin's lymphoma of the gastrointestinal tract: an analysis of clinical and pathologic features affecting outcome. *J Clin Oncol* 6:1125–1133, 1988.

117. Toonkel LM, Fuller LM, Gamble JF, et al. Laparomy staged I and II non-Hodgkin's lymphomas: preliminary results of radiotherapy and adjunctive chemotherapy. *Cancer* 45:249–260, 1980.

118. Schein P, Chabner BA. Potential for prolonged disease-free survival following combination chemotherapy of non-Hodgkin's lymphoma. *Blood* 43:181–189, 1974.

119. DeVita VT, Cancellos GP, Chabner BA, et al. Advanced diffuse histiocytic lymphoma, a potentially curable disease: results with combination chemotherapy. *Lancet* 1:248–250, 1975.

120. Al-Katib A, Koziner B, Kurland E, et al. Treatment of diffuse poorly differentiated lymphocytic lymphoma: an analysis of prognostic factors. *Cancer* 53:2404–2412, 1984.

121. Nissen NI, Ersboll J, Hansen HS, et al. A randomized study of radiotherapy versus radiotherapy plus chemotherapy in stage I-II non-Hodgkin's lymphoma. *Cancer* 52:1–7, 1983.

122. Ossenkoppele GJ, Mol JJ, Snow GB, et al. Radiotherapy versus radiotherapy plus chemotherapy in stages I and II non-Hodgkin's lymphoma of the upper digestive and respiratory tract. *Cancer* 60:1505–1509, 1987.

123. DeVita VT. Human models of human disease: breast cancer and the lymphomas. *Int J Radiat Oncol Biol Phys* 5:1855–1867, 1979.

124. Randall J, Obeid M, Blackledge GRP. Hemorrhage and perforation of gastrointestinal neoplasms during chemotherapy. *Ann R Coll Surg Engl* 68:286–289, 1986.

125. Aozasa K, Ueda T, Kurata A, et al. Prognostic value of histologic and clinical factors in 56 patients with gastrointestinal lymphomas. *Cancer* 61:309–315, 1988.

126. Shimm DS, Dosoretz DE, Anderson T, Linggood RM, Harris NL, Wang CC. Primary gastric lymphoma: an analysis with emphasis on prognostic factors and radiation therapy. *Cancer* 52:2044–2048, 1983.

127. Skandalakis JE, Gray SW, Shepard D, et al. *Smooth muscle tumors of the alimentary tract*. Springfield, IL: Charles C Thomas, 1962.

128. Shiu MH, Farr GH, Papachristou DN, Hajdu SI. Myosarcomas of the stomach: natural history, prognostic factors and management. *Cancer* 49:177–187, 1982

129. Abramson DJ. Leiomyoblastomas of the stomach. *Surg Gynecol Obstet* 136:118–125, 1973.

130. Shiu MH, Brennan MF. Soft tissue sarcoma of the gastrointestinal tract. In: Shiu MH, Brennan MF, eds. *Surgical Management of Soft Tissue Sarcoma*. Philadelphia: Lea & Febiger, 1989: 172–180.

131. Lee YNM, Silverman H, Deck KB. Leiomyosarcomas of the gastrointestinal tract: should we consider metastasis to regional lymph nodes? *J Surg Oncol* 15:319, 1980.

132. Russel WO, Cohen J, Enzinger F, Hajdu SI. A clinical and pathological staging system for soft tissue sarcomas. *Cancer* 40:1562–1570, 1977.

133. Hajdu SI. *Pathology of soft tissue tumors*. Philadelphia: Lea & Febiger, 1979: 35–55, 311–320.

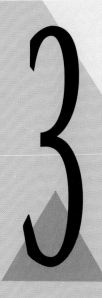

Colorectal Polyps

Michael O'Brien,
Sidney J. Winawer,
and Jerome D. Waye

Polyp is a general descriptive term applied to any protuberance above the surface of the bowel (Fig. 3.1). The great majority (66.5 percent) of such lesions encountered in the colon and rectum at endoscopy are adenomas, 11 percent are hyperplastic polyps, and the remainder (22 percent) are a miscellaneous group that includes mucosal polyps (normal mucosa), inflammatory polyps, juvenile polyps, hamartomas, and a variety of non-mucosal lesions (1).

ADENOMAS

Adenomas of the colon and rectum occur in more than 25 percent of the U.S. population over 50 years of age (2) (Figs. 3.2 and 3.3). They are unique among polyps of the large bowel in that they have the inherent capacity to evolve into invasive adenocarcinoma. Adenomas, then, are benign neoplasms with malignant potential.

Epidemiology

An impressively consistent statistic in relation to geographic variation of colorectal cancer incidence is the high degree of correlation with adenoma prevalence (3–11) (Fig. 3.4). Adenomas are common in populations with high colorectal cancer incidence and rare in those among whom colorectal cancer is seldom seen. Furthermore, when populations migrate from a low-risk to a high-risk environment, an increase in the frequency of adenomas parallels this new jeopardy (12). We now believe that almost all of the approximately 150,000 new cases of cancer of the colon and rectum that are diagnosed in the United States each year (13) arise in pre-existing adenomas.

Etiology
ENVIRONMENTAL FACTORS

The epidemiology of colorectal neoplasia suggests that this is largely an environmental disease, and the food we eat, rather than alcohol, tobacco, smokestack emission, or factory effluent, is most likely to account for the observed variations in its incidence. Fat, animal protein, and total caloric consumption as well as dietary fiber have all been linked to colon cancer mortality (14). Their proposed roles can be either protective, as in the case of dietary fiber, or conducive, which appears to be the effect of high fat, high total calories, and perhaps high meat consumption. While international comparisons of per capita fat intake and colon cancer mortality show a significant correlation (15,16), case control studies are inconclusive on the significance of dietary fat (17,18). Also, the putative relationship of meat consumption to colon carcinogenesis is challenged by time trend data that show that although beef consumption over the last 40 years has more than doubled in the U.S., the incidence of colon cancer over the same period has remained relatively stable (19). However, a recent study using dietary information obtained prospectively from a large cohort of U.S. women aged 34 to 59 provided evidence that a high intake of animal fat significantly increases the risk for colorectal cancer (14). It is difficult, especially in epidemiolog-

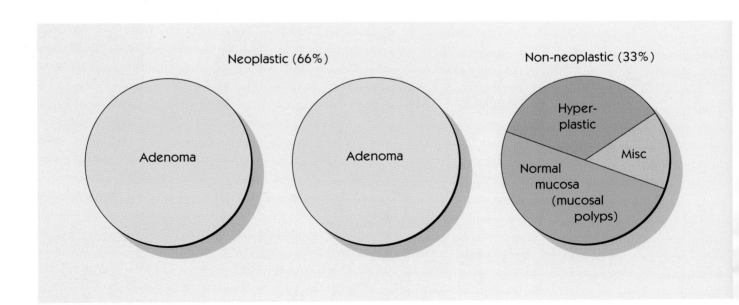

FIGURE 3.1 The types of polyps that are seen at colonoscopy. Data from the National Polyp Study (reference 1).

FIGURE 3.2 The relative frequency of small, intermediate, and large adenomas at colonoscopy. Data from the National Polyp Study (reference 1).

FIGURE 3.2 The relative frequency of small, intermediate, and large adenomas at colonoscopy. Data from the National Polyp Study (reference 1).

Frequency %

| 38% | 36% | 26% |

Small (≤0.5cm)   Medium (0.5–1.0cm)   Large (>1.0cm)

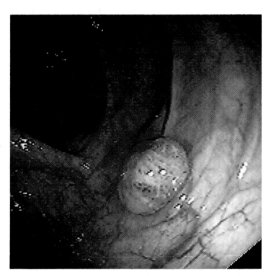
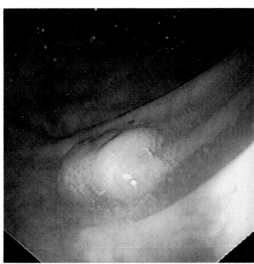

FIGURE 3.3 Typical colorectal adenomas as seen at endoscopy.

FIGURE 3.4:
COMPARISON OF COLORECTAL CANCER INCIDENCE AND ADENOMA PREVALENCE IN MALES AT MULTIPLE GEOGRAPHIC LOCATIONS

LOCATION	REF.	COLON CANCER INCIDENCE	PREVALENCE (%) ADENOMAS
Hawaii (Japanese)	(4)	Very high	64
Scotland (Aberdeen)	(3)	Very high	39
England (Liverpool)	(5)	High	37
U.S. (New Orleans)	(7)	High	36
Norway (Oslo)	(8)	High	34
Norway (Tromso)	(8)	Intermediate	40
Japan (Akita)	(7)	Intermediate	36
Spain (Barcelona)	(9)	Intermediate	29.3
Japan (Miyagi)	(7)	Low	14
Colombia (Cali)	(7)	Low	11
Finland (Kuopio)	(3)	Low	10

ic studies, to separate the effects of highly interrelated factors such as dietary fat, animal protein, and total calories (20). More definitive insights into these relationships may ultimately await controlled intervention studies. A working hypothesis that finds support in recent experimental studies (18,20–22) is that the findings in relation to meat and fat may in fact be reflections of an active association between colorectal neoplasia and total calories (5). (See Chapter 4.)

INHERITANCE AND COLORECTAL ADENOMAS

Familial adenomatous polyposis (FAP) (23) and the related Gardner's syndrome (24) are inherited disorders which have powerful associations with colorectal cancer that are attributable to the inheritance of a single gene (24). Dominant inheritance of a single gene probably also underlies hereditary nonpolyposis colon cancer (HNPCC) (25), a clinically distinct syndrome similarly marked by a high frequency of colon cancer. In both of these genetic entities, the pathogenesis of associated colon cancers is through the intermediary of colorectal adenomas. These familial disorders account for approximately 5 percent of cases of colorectal cancer seen each year (26) (Fig. 3.5).

A much larger role for inheritance, however, is suggested by reports that 16 percent to 26 percent of patients with colon cancer have at least one first-degree relative with the same disease (27–30). In other words, cancer of the large bowel occurs at least three times more often in the relatives of patients with this neoplasm than in the general population (31). Two recent studies of European tumor registries have shown that relatives of probands with colorectal adenomas *only*, who do not belong to either FAP or HNPCC categories, also show a markedly increased risk for colon cancer over that of the general population (32,33). (See Chapter 4.)

Adenoma Genesis (Fig. 3.6)

In the mucosa of the normal colon and rectum, DNA synthesis and cell division is largely confined to the lower part of the crypts of Lieberkuhn, predominantly the lower one-third (34). In the upper one-third and on the surface, the cells become fully mature and die or desquamate (35,36). With the development of an adenoma, the proliferative compartment moves to the upper part of the crypts

and the surface (34). The smallest adenoma identifiable to the microscopist is represented by immature proliferating (adenomatous) epithelium in the upper portion of a single crypt (37). From this single-crypt stage, the adenomatous epithelium spreads initially along the surface and into adjacent crypts replacing pre-existing normal epithelium, a phenomenon that has been referred to as a "snow-plow" effect (38). Concurrently, the adenomatous epithelium invaginates into the lamina propria by budlike tubular outgrowths mainly in the upper part of the mucosa, to produce the earliest polypoid elevation discernible to the endoscopist. With continued growth there is elongation and further branching of adenomatous glands and, as the lesion continues to expand toward the bowel lumen, peristalsis may cause the adenoma to acquire a pedicle or stalk of normal mucosa and submucosa.

CELL KINETICS

Several stages of abnormality of cell kinetics between normal and adenomatous have been described in the histologically normal mucosa (35). The most severe of these consists of an upward shift of the proliferative compartment and an increase in the relative numbers of proliferating cells (35) (see Fig. 3.1). Abnormalities of this type in histologically normal mucosa have been found in individuals with familial adenomatous polyposis (37–41). Such changes have also been described by some but not all investigators in patients with sporadic colon carcinoma (41) and adenomas (35). With the formation of an adenoma, there is a diffuse increase in proliferation with actively proliferating cells fairly uniformly distributed throughout the lesion so that the constituent cells show comparable degrees of proliferation whether located on the surface, in glands deep in the adenoma, or on the crests of villi (42).

CLONALITY

It is important to establish whether benign adenomas represent a continued hyperproliferative process or a mutational event. Fearon and associates employed recombinant DNA technology to convincingly show that colorectal adenomas are monoclonal (43). Their methodology involved the demonstration of a monoclonal pattern of X-chromosome inactivation. Using X-linked restriction fragment length polymorphisms, they found evi-

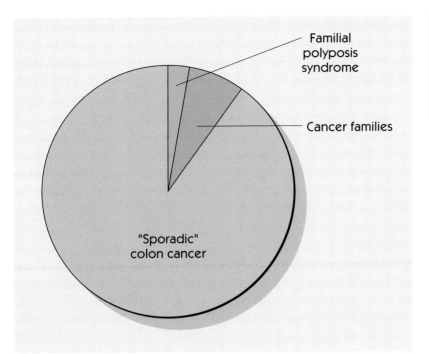

FIGURE 3.5 Relative contribution of defined inherited syndromes to new cases of colorectal cancer. (From Lynch H, Rozen P, Schelke GS. Hereditary colon cancer: polyposis and non-polyposis variants. *CA* 35:95–115, 1985.)

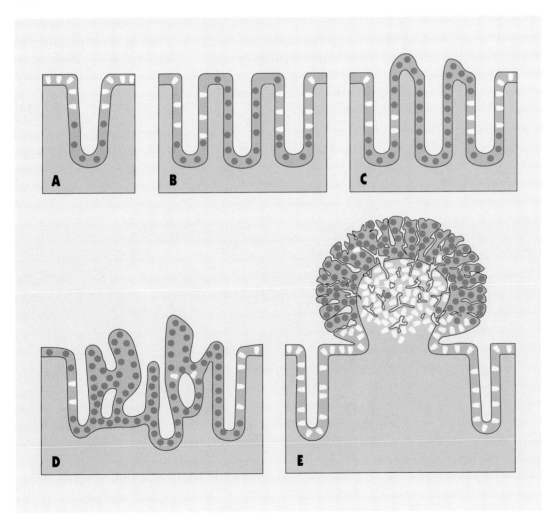

FIGURE 3.6 Histogenesis of adenomas. In the mucosa of the normal colon cell, division is largely confined to the lower part of the crypt. The smallest adenoma identifiable under the microscope is represented by immature proliferating (adenomatous) epithelium in the upper portion of a single crypt (**A**). The adenomatous epithelium buds and invaginates to form a tubular adenoma (**B–E**).

dence of monoclonality in 30 polyps, which included both sporadic adenomas and adenomas from FAPC patients.

Classification of Adenomas

GROWTH PATTERNS

Adenomas are classified as tubular, villous, or tubulovillous. A tubular adenoma is a polyp composed of straight or branched tubules lined by adenomatous (dysplastic) epithelium (Fig. 3.7). In endoscopy surveys, this category represents more than 80 percent of all adenomas encountered (1,44,45). Villous growth is defined as adjacent crypts or folia that are elongated to give an appearance of fingerlike extensions of adenomatous mucosa. When this histology is found in greater than 75 percent of the polyp, it is said to be villous (Fig. 3.8). An intermediate category, tubulovillous, is represented by a villous (Fig. 3.9) component of 25 percent to 75 percent of the polyp according to standard classification nomenclature (46). Villous and tubulovillous comprise 3 percent to 5 percent and 10 percent to 15 percent, respectively, of adenomas (1,45).

RELATIONSHIP OF TUBULAR TO VILLOUS GROWTH PATTERNS

Several clinicopathologic studies (45,47,48) including, most recently, an analysis of the pathol-ogy database of the National Polyp Study (U.S.) (1) have found a strong correlation between the extent of villous component and adenoma size. This favors the interpretation that as adenomas increase in size they progressively adopt a more villous growth pattern. Three-dimensional reconstructions of adenomas performed by Japanese investigators have shown that continued proliferation within the saccules of a tubular adenoma can produce elongation with compression of intervening stroma into thin septa to give a villous structure (49). Both very large tubular adenomas and very small villous adenomas may be encountered (but are rare), and risk for malignant transformation in adenomas can be independently related to both size and villous component. It remains to be shown, therefore, whether villous growth is merely a function of duration and/or rate of growth of adenomas or represents an intrinsic biologic characteristic of the component cells that may even have in some cases an acquired genetic basis, as part of a continuum of adenoma progression.

DYSPLASIA IN ADENOMAS

All adenomas by definition show at least mild dysplasia, and a proportion (6 percent) have more severe degrees of dysplasia or carcinoma in situ or are found to have a component of invasive ade-

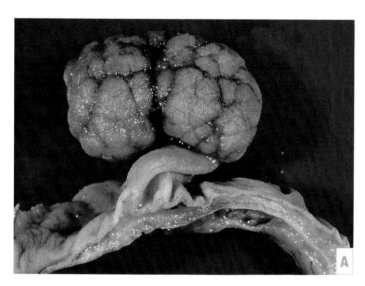

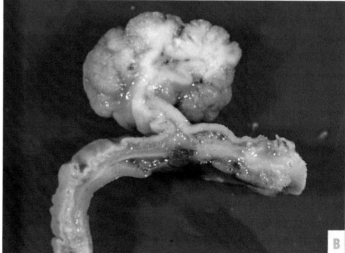

FIGURE 3.7 Tubular adenoma. (A) Illustrates the typical lobulated appearance of a tubular adenoma. The adenoma is attached to the bowel wall by a short pedicle. **(B)** Cross-section to show the adenoma anatomy.

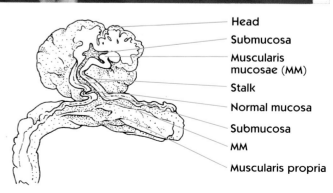

- Head
- Submucosa
- Muscularis mucosae (MM)
- Stalk
- Normal mucosa
- Submucosa
- MM
- Muscularis propria

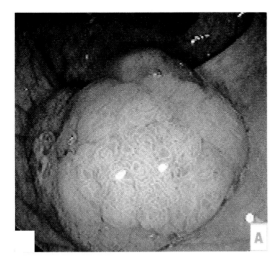

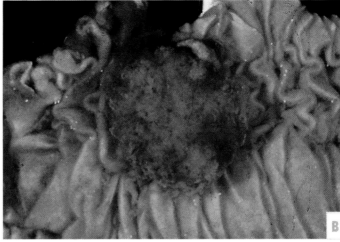

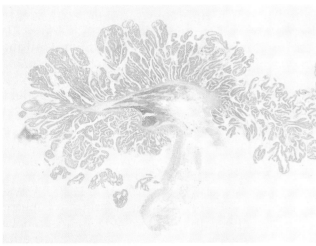

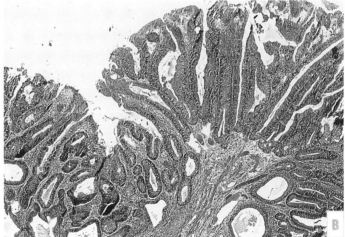

FIGURE 3.8 Villous adenoma. (A) Endoscopic appearance of a large villous adenoma. **(B)** This resection specimen highlights the villous character of the adenoma surface. **(C)** Shows the typical villous histology on H&E sections.

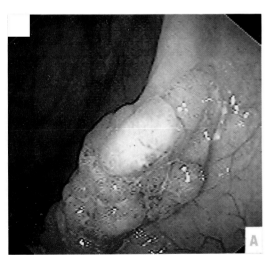

FIGURE 3.9 (A) Tubulovillous adenoma in the ascending colon. This polyp extends along the ridge of a haustral fold. **(B)** Tubulovillous adenoma, with line drawing of the adenoma.

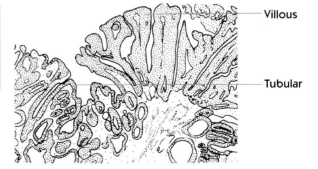

Villous

Tubular

nocarcinoma (2.5 percent) (44) (Fig. 3.10). Dysplasia is a morphologic term, descriptive in this context of cytologic atypia and architectural abnormality that resembles that of carcinoma. Classification of dysplasia (Fig. 3.11) is according to the degree of cytologic atypia and architectural abnormality of the glands. Severe dysplasia or carcinoma in situ represent the extreme end of this spectrum. Many authorities eschew the use of the term *carcinoma in situ* here because of the unwarranted implication of malignant biologic behavior and the attendant danger of overtreatment. The WHO classification (46) employs the term *severe dysplasia* to encompass this upper range of abnormality that is short of invasive carcinoma. An alternative and compatible term recognized by the current edition of the WHO classification (46) that we recommend is *high-grade dysplasia*. This term is also used in the classification of dysplasia in ulcerative colitis proposed by Riddel and associates (50), and it has been adopted by the National Polyp Study in recent publications (1). Low-grade dysplasia similarly corresponds to previously used mild and moderate categories. High-grade dysplasia represents the extreme end of the spectrum of abnormal histologic changes short of invasive carcinoma, and is encountered in 5 percent to 6 percent of endoscopically removed colorectal adenomas. This histologic abnormality is strongly associated with contiguous invasive carcinoma (51). The natural history of high-grade dysplasia

is not known from prospective observation in the colon, and it is possible that some lesions regress or do not progress to invasion. However there is considerable evidence that in most, if not all cases, it represents an intermediate stage in the evolution to invasive carcinoma and that it is a valid marker of malignant transformation (52).

LOW-GRADE DYSPLASIA Low-grade dysplasia incorporates the categories of mild and moderate dysplasia. In mild dysplasia, the crypts show branching or elongation, and some reduction of interglandular stroma may be apparent. Cell nuclei are oval, regularly overlapping, and basally located. Nuclear membranes are regular, the chromatin pattern is fine, and nucleoli are inconspicuous. In moderate dysplasia, glands show some loss of basal polarization of nuclei. Nuclear membranes are more irregular, and chromatin patterns are moderately uneven with more prominence of nucleoli.

HIGH-GRADE DYSPLASIA High-grade dysplasia incorporates the criteria of severe dysplasia and carcinoma in situ, which were separate in the initial working classification of the National Polyp Study. These combined categories (high-grade dysplasia) are also the equivalent of the WHO category of severe dysplasia..

High-grade dysplasia is present when there is complex irregularity of glands and papillary infolding, often with marked reduction of interglandular

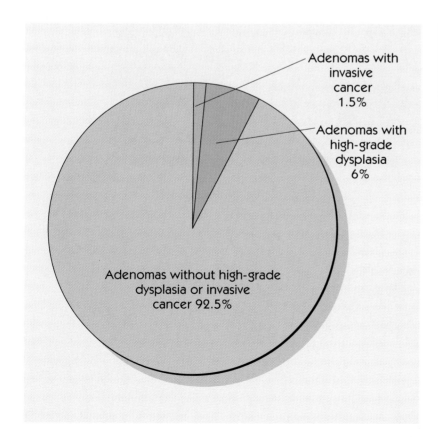

Adenomas with
invasive
cancer
1.5%

Adenomas with
high-grade
dysplasia
6%

Adenomas without high-grade
dysplasia or invasive
cancer 92.5%

FIGURE 3.10 Relative frequency of a finding of high-grade dysplasia and invasive carcinoma in a polyp resected at colonoscopy. Based on National Polyp Study Data (reference 1).

stroma; glands may show cribriform or back-to-back patterns. Cytologic abnormalities of high-grade dysplasia include marked irregularity of nuclear membranes; nuclear chromatin cleared, vesicular, irregularly clumped, or densely hyperchromatic; and large and irregular nucleoli.

MALIGNANT POLYPS (FIG. 3.12)

Adenomas with invasive carcinoma are known as malignant polyps. An adenoma is considered to have invasive carcinoma only when malignant cells have penetrated beyond the muscularis mucosae. The carcinoma has thus gained access

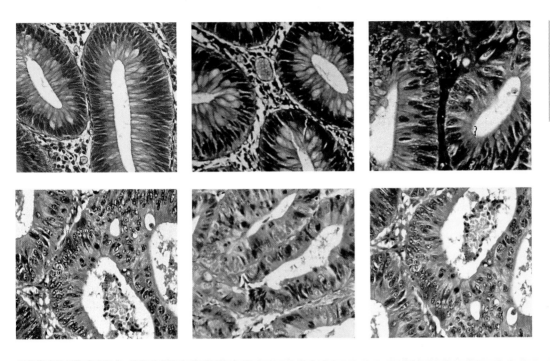

FIGURE 3.11 Classification of dysplasia. Top row indicates examples of low-grade dysplasia; high-grade examples are shown in bottom row.

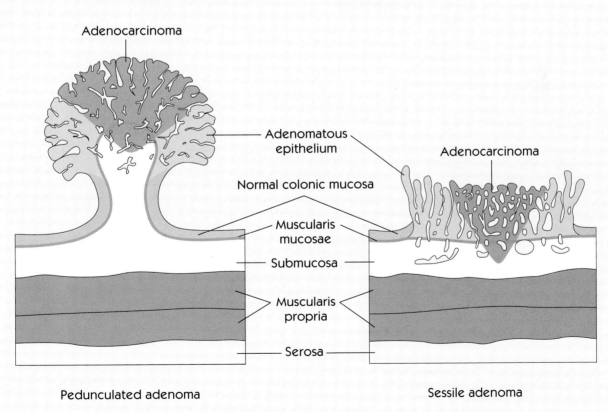

FIGURE 3.12 Structure of malignant polyps.

to the lymphatic-rich submucosa of the colon or rectum. In pedunculated adenomas, the submucosa of the bowel wall is in continuity with the core of the stalk and head of the polyp. In sessile adenomas, invasive carcinoma implies invasion directly into the submucosa of the underlying bowel wall. The term *intramucosal carcinoma* is sometimes used to describe a rare finding of invasion outside the basement membrane of glands, into the lamina propria of the mucosal component of the polyp, but without invasion beyond the muscularis mucosae. This finding has no proven clinical significance and has not been linked to a potential for distant spread. A separation of this entity from high-grade dysplasia in clinical classifications does not, therefore, appear warranted or desirable.

Distribution of Adenomas

Two-thirds (53) of colorectal adenomas, according to National Polyp Study data, occur in the left colon and rectum (Fig. 3.13). Endoscopy series may slightly underestimate the relative frequency of rectal adenomas since patients with large rectal lesions may be referred directly to a surgical specialist rather than to an endoscopist.

The distribution of adenomas in the general population is similiar to but does not correspond exactly to that of carcinoma. Colon carcinoma shows a marked left-sided predominance with 58 percent of all cancers located in the sigmoid colon and rectum (according to data from the NCI's Surveillance, Epidemiology, and End Results program, 1973–77) (54). Although adenomas also show a left-sided predominance (45,55) this is a less-marked predominance than in carcinomas. Multiple regression analysis of the National Polyp Study database has indicated that high-grade dysplasia in a left-sided adenoma occurs almost three times as often as in a right-sided adenoma. However, the same data also suggest that when controls are established for size and villous component, left-sided location does not independently increase the risk of malignant transformation (1). This may support the hypothesis of Hill and colleagues (56) that the main effect of distal location on colorectal adenomas is to enhance adenoma growth rather than to affect the progression directly to high-grade dysplasia and cancer.

Adenoma Progression to Carcinoma

The first use of the term *adenoma-carcinoma sequence* has been attributed to Jackman and Mayo in the title of a paper published in 1951 (57,58). The concept itself, that the large majority of colorectal cancers evolve from benign polyp precursors, is considerably older than this, and both the concept and its clinical implications have been put forward by a succession of investigators from St. Mark's Hospital, London, for more than 60 years (59–61). The evidence for the adenoma-carcinoma sequence has been frequently reviewed (62,63) and includes data from epidemiologic studies that have related adenoma prevalence to carcinoma incidence (12). The concept is also supported by the high concurrence rate of carcinoma and adenomas—approximately one-third of surgical resections for carcinoma will be found to harbor one or more adenomas (64,65) (Fig. 3.14). The frequent finding of contiguous benign adenoma in a carcinoma provides additional more direct evidence (63,66,67), although the frequency will depend on the stage of the carcinoma. When carcinoma is confined to the submucosa, residual adenoma will be found in 60 percent of cases (66,67). Convincing support for the adenoma-carcinoma sequence is also to be found in the natural history of inherited predispositions to colon cancer, both FAP and related syndromes and HNPCC. The gene for FAP and Gardner's syndrome (GS) has been defined (68,69,221,222), and it is likely that an acquired mutation of this gene may be involved in sporadic adenoma genesis. The precise identification of this gene or one at some alternative locus that is responsible for sporadic adenoma formation may provide a genetic label for adenomas, so that the frequency with which this label or marker is identified by a recombinant DNA probe in the genome of infiltrating carcinomas may be the ultimate measure of the significance of the adenoma-carcinoma sequence. The most recent evidence for the stepwise progression of colorectal cancer from adenoma to carcinoma is the discovery of specific *acquired* genetic abnormalities that are consistently associated with identifiable early, intermediate (large adenoma), and late stages of this progression.

DETERMINANTS OF MALIGNANT TRANSFORMATION

Given the high prevalence of adenomas in Western populations (see Fig. 3.4) it is evident that only a fraction of all adenomas will give rise to colon carcinoma. Eide (70) has estimated, based on Norwegian data, that the conversion rate for adenomas, defined as the average number of colorectal cancers each year as a percentage of the estimated number of adenoma-bearing individuals in the population, is 0.25 percent per year.

We have little or no knowledge of the biologic mechanisms that underlie whether a particular adenoma will evolve into carcinoma. However statistical analysis of the polyp and patient characteristics in large surgical series (51,71) and, more recently, colonoscopy studies (45) have identified clinical and anatomic factors that are associated with a greater likelihood of an individual adenoma harboring high-grade dysplasia or invasive cancer. Analysis of the National Polyp Study database of more than 5000 polyps from almost 2000 patients

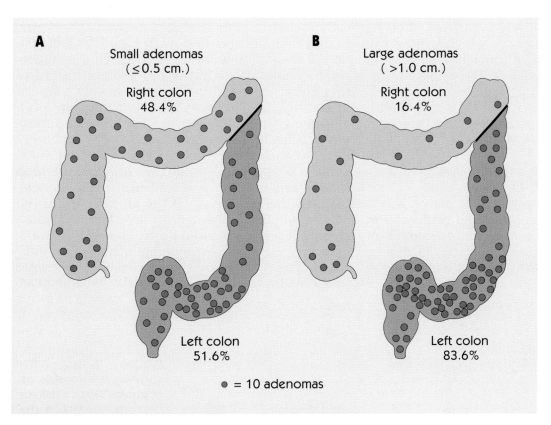

A
Small adenomas
(≤0.5 cm.)

Right colon
48.4%

Left colon
51.6%

B
Large adenomas
(>1.0 cm.)

Right colon
16.4%

Left colon
83.6%

● = 10 adenomas

FIGURE 3.13 (A) Anatomic distribution of adenomas. (B) Comparison of distribution of small and large adenomas. Data from the National Polyp Study (reference 1).

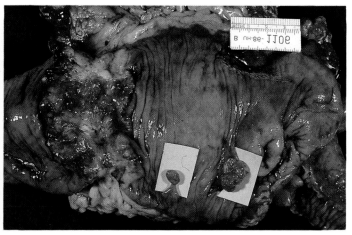

FIGURE 3.14 This resected colon harbors two pedunculated polyps in addition to an advanced carcinoma.

(1) has confirmed that polyp size is a major determinant of the likelihood that high-grade dysplasia will be found in a colorectal adenoma (1) (Fig. 3.15). The amount of villous growth in the adenoma is also an independent determinant of this risk, with an effect of comparable magnitude to that of size (1). Furthermore, the effects of size and villous component have been found to be multiplicative, that is, their combined effect is greater than the sum of their individual effects (1). Frequency of high-grade dysplasia in adenomas is unrelated to gender of the patient, according to the National Polyp Study data analysis, but logically appears to increase significantly with advancing age. When a patient has multiple adenomas, which will be the case in almost 50 percent of the adenoma-bearing population, the patient's risk of harboring an adenoma with high-grade dysplasia is proportionately increased, but this increased risk from multiplicity appears to be dependent on anatomic factors such as size and villous component only (Fig. 3.16).

THE MOLECULAR GENETICS OF THE ADENOMA-CARCINOMA SEQUENCE (FIG. 3.17)

The earliest step in the neoplastic process is a mutation that leads to a monoclonal proliferation of mucosal epithelial cells called an adenoma. In the case of familial polyposis this step is dependent on a prezygotic mutation involving a gene located on the long arm of chromosome 5

(68,69,221,222). Continued growth of the adenoma(s) is promoted by intraluminal factors, which exert their strongest effect in the distal colon. Large size and/or villous growth, increasing age of an adenoma, or multiplicity of adenomas increase the likelihood of further random mutations that will confer a selective growth advantage on a subclone of the adenoma constituent cells. In some cases a point mutation in a proto-oncogene may be the mechanism, for example, a mutation involving Ki-ras gene (72). Ras genes encode a plasma membrane-bound protein (p21) that tightly binds guanine nucleotides and exhibits weak GTPase (guanosine triphosphatase) activity, properties that execute its role in growth signal transduction across the cell membrane (73). Specific mutations produce alterations of the p21 protein that cause this growth control function to go awry. Recent studies (72,74,75) have reported ras-gene point mutations, predominantly in Ki-ras and at codon 12 of the gene, in over 40 percent of colon cancers. In many of the cancers revealing a ras mutation, the same mutation was found in adjacent residual benign adenoma. These findings would indicate that a Ki-ras gene mutation is an early event that precedes the development of invasive malignancy, making it a likely candidate to be a key mutation driving the adenoma-carcinoma sequence in many cases. The morphologic correlate of this stage of progression in the adenoma may be high-grade

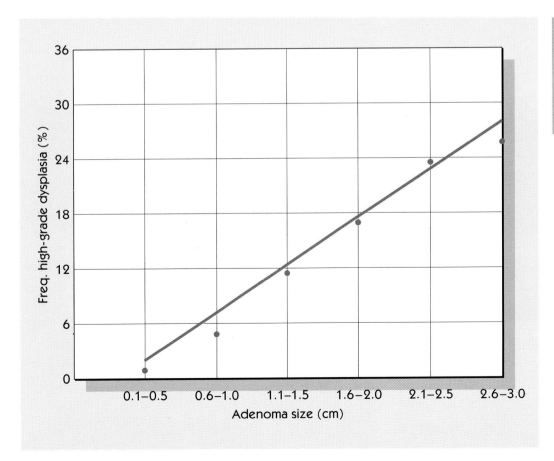

FIGURE 3.15 Graph showing relationship of adenoma size to risk for high-grade dysplasia in adenoma. Data fron National Polyp Study (reference 1).

dysplasia in a large adenoma (72). The development of invasive cancer is associated with further genetic alteration. Activation of additional oncogenes, by processes such as point mutations, gene amplification, or gene rearrangement, are among the possible mechanisms of progression. However, recent advances point to a major role for deletion of suppressor genes at this stage of colon carcinogenesis. Vogelstein and colleagues have found a high frequency of specific chromosomal deletions in colon cancer that cannot be explained by chance alone (72). One of these, a deletion of a segment of chromosome 17 (found in 77 percent of colon cancer patients but seldom in those with

adenomas) has been shown (72) to result in loss of a gene designated p53 that encodes a protein with known tumor-suppressing (or anti-oncogene) activity. Other deletions of genetic information encountered with high frequency in colon cancer, which may result in a similar loss of tumor-suppressor effects, include chromosome 5q21-q22 (in 35 percent of colon carcinomas) and chromosome 18q21-qter (in more than 80 percent of colon carcinomas) (76). The chromosome 18 candidate-gene has also recently been cloned (77) and is identified as DCC (deleted in colorectal carcinoma). It is thought to function in cell surface interactions (77). The current view is that loss of these suppressor genes

FIGURE 3.16:
RISK FACTORS FOR HIGH-GRADE DYSPLASIA IN COLORECTAL ADENOMAS

POLYP	PATIENT
Size	Age
Villous component (distal location)	Multiplicity

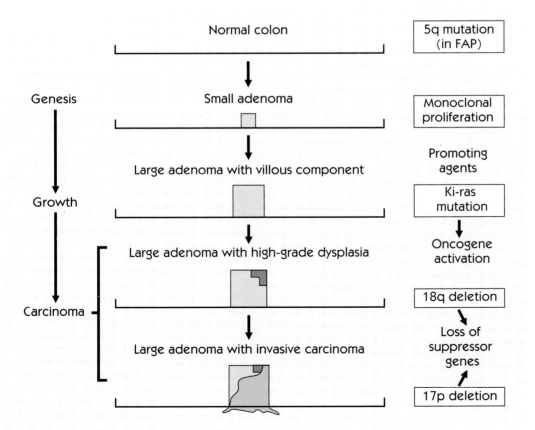

FIGURE 3.17
Molecular genetics of the adenoma-carcinoma sequence.

may be critical in the development of invasive carcinoma in an adenoma. There are numerous other genetic changes that occur during adenoma evolution and cancer progression. The minimum number of mutations that are necessary between normal mucosa and the development of invasive carcinoma is estimated to be eight to ten. In the majority of patients with colon cancers, very large numbers of genetic changes are seen. The specific genetic changes we have discussed here are considered likely to be pivotal because of the high frequency with which they are encountered in the various stages of the adenoma-carcinoma sequence.

Detection of Adenomas

DETECTION OF BLEEDING

Most colorectal polyps are not symptomatic, but some may reveal themselves by bleeding, presenting either as blood mixed in with the stool or as small flecks of blood in or on the surface of the stool. Visible blood is unlikely in proximal polyps, although occult bleeding occurs. Rectal bleeding is always abnormal, and its cause should be adequately investigated since it is difficult to predict the presence of neoplasia based on the history and sigmoidoscopic findings alone (78). In a patient who is at risk for colorectal cancer or polyps, total colonoscopy is now considered the best tool to be used as the primary investigation.

BARIUM ENEMA

The barium enema is widely available, inexpensive, and relatively risk-free. It has long been the only means of nonoperative large bowel investigation, but comparative studies have demonstrated its limitations in the diagnosis of polyps.

COLONOSCOPY

Adenomas may be missed on barium enema x-ray examination, but polyps and cancers may also be missed on colonoscopy. Approximately 10 percent to 15 percent of small polyps are missed during colonoscopy (79). The ability to reach the cecum is extremely operator-dependent and varies from 75 percent to 95 percent (80). Many adenomas will be undiagnosed in the absence of total colonoscopy.

Colonoscopic Polypectomy

ENDOSCOPIC ASSESSMENT

Pedunculated polyps may be attached to the colon with a pedicle that may be thin, thick, short, or long. Sessile polyps are attached directly to the wall and have been described in the following ways: marble type with a narrow base and round configuration; mountain type, with a broad attachment to the colon wall, typically multilobulated; clam shell, a polyp wrapped along a fold, extending both proximally and distally along the edge of a fold; a carpet type, a relatively flat polyp that may be particularly difficult to ensnare and whose margins may be indistinguishable from areas of normal mucosa (Fig. 3.18).

Three percent to 5 percent of polyps may show features of malignancy that include an irregular surface contour, ulceration, firm (or hard) consistency when the head is pushed with a snare or forceps, and broadening of the stalk (81,82) (Figs. 3.19–3.22).

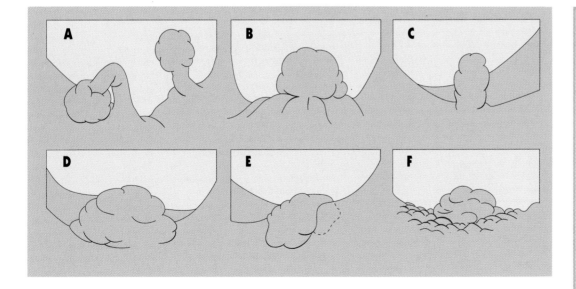

FIGURE 3.18 Schematic representation of polyp types as seen endoscopically. (A) Pedunculated polyps. The polyp at left has a long pedicle. **(B)** Sessile polyp with broad base and pseudopedicle. **(C)** Marble-type polyp with a small attachment to the wall. **(D)** Mountain-type polyp with a wide base. **(E)** Clamshell polyp wrapped around a fold. **(F)** Extended polyp consisting of a carpet-type flat polyp with a large sessile component.

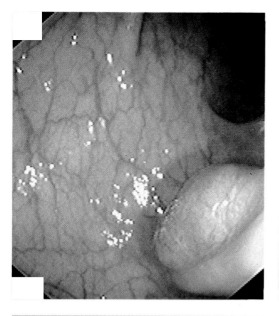

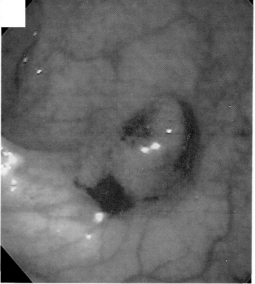

FIGURE 3.20 In the rectum this small irregularly shaped polyp with a central ulceration contained well-differentiated adenocarcinoma with invasion of the submucosa. The tumor was present at the cauterization line. A subsequent endoscopic ultrasound demonstrated that there was no evidence of residual tumor following polypectomy.

FIGURE 3.19 Malignant polyp with a benign appearance.

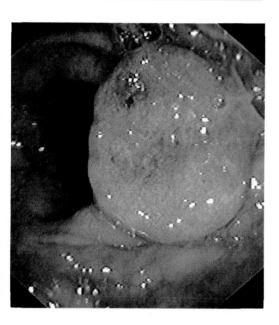

FIGURE 3.21 This flat ulcerated polyp was thought to contain invasive carcinoma and was sent for surgical rather than endoscopic resection. It was found to have infiltrating adenocarcinoma to the muscularis propria.

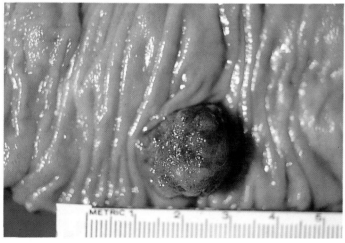

FIGURE 3.22 Surgical resection of a 2-cm malignant polyp extensively replaced by invasive adenocarcinoma. The surface erosion, the broadening of the base, and the firm-to-hard consistency as appreciated through the endoscope forceps by the endoscopist suggested a malignant polyp or a polypoid cancer unlikely to be adequately resected endoscopically.

TECHNIQUE

Once polyps are identified during colonoscopy, the polyp should be removed at the time of its discovery. Polyps may be endoscopically removed with hot biopsy forceps or through the wire snare and cautery method. Hot biopsy forceps are an insulated pincer with cup-shaped jaws through which electrical current can be passed to thermally cauterize the polyp base at the edge of the forceps (Fig. 3.23). Since current passes around the small polyp held within the forceps cups, the tissue is not damaged, and a biopsy can be done for histopathologic identification. Polyps less than 7 mm in size can be biopsied and simultaneously ablated using this technique. Cautery of the base seals the vessels to prevent bleeding. Larger polyps must be resected with the snare loop. If pedunculated, the loop can be placed around the stalk, and the pedicle separated by a combination of guillotine force (pulling on the wire), along with disruption of tissue by the thermal effect of heat generated by the electrosurgical unit. Sessile polyps with a small base can be transected in similar fashion, but those attached to the wall with a broad base (greater than 1.5 cm) are usually removed in a piecemeal fashion, with successive portions of the polyp being resected until all or most of the adenomatous tissue has been removed from the wall.

INDICATIONS FOR A SURGICAL APPROACH

Using a surgical rather than an endoscopic approach to remove colonic polyps depends on the size of the area over which the polyp is attached. Polyps with a base that extends over greater than one-third of the circumference of the bowel are usually not good candidates for colonoscopic resection nor are those whose linear extent involves two adjacent interhaustral septae. However, under certain circumstances, such as a rectal location, resection of polyps with a wide base can be attempted in a piecemeal fashion. In the proximal colon, where a piecemeal approach is safest for polyps over 1.5 cm in diameter, many flat polyps may be amenable to endoscopic resection

COMPLICATIONS OF COLONOSCOPY (FIG. 3.24)

In addition to the risks incurred during diagnostic colonoscopy, the complications of endoscopic polypectomy include hemorrhage, perforation, and postpolypectomy syndrome (83,84). Hemorrhage or perforation occurs in approximately 1.8 percent of patients, with hemorrhage being the most common complication, related to bleeding at the polypectomy site. Immediate postpolypectomy hemorrhage should be controlled at the time it is recognized, before blood fills the field and obscures vision. Immediate bleeding from a tran-

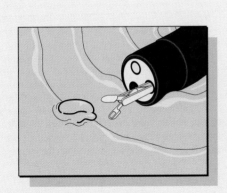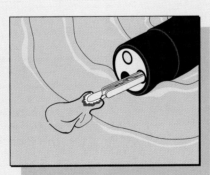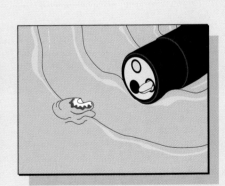

FIGURE 3.23 Schematic representation of hot biopsy forceps grasping a small polyp and pulling it away from the submucosa before thermal energy is applied. Forceps withdrawal provides a histologically intact fragment for microscopic evaluation.

sected pedicle may be controlled by regrasping the stalk with the snare and applying tourniquet-type pressure to promote hemostasis. If bleeding occurs after five minutes of stalk compression, pressure should be reinstituted for one or more further increments. Bleeding from a sessile base may also be treated with the snare if the area can be "bunched-up" to include sufficient tissue around the bleeding site. Failing snare hemostasis, the site may be coagulated using a monopolar (hot biopsy forceps) technique, a heater probe, laser, or injection of large volume epinephrine (dilution 1:10,000) around the polypectomy site.

Hemorrhage is a known and accepted complication of endoscopic polypectomy and can occur without any mishaps or untoward events. It may also be caused by closure of the snare resulting in polyp transection by a guillotine effect without electrocoagulation or from inadequate power to result in hemostasis.

Perforation occurs in 0.3 percent of polypectomies when the wall is cut through with the snare during cautery current or from thermal necrosis of the bowel wall. If free perforation occurs, and x-ray reveals a large amount of abdominal gas, the patient should have immediate laparotomy with closure of the perforation. If a small amount of air is detected on a postpolypectomy x-ray in an asymptomatic patient, and it does not accumulate, the patient may be given antibiotics and treated conservatively.

Postpolypectomy syndrome (84) is a combination of pain, tenderness, and leukocytosis with or without fever following endoscopic polypectomy. This syndrome is related to a thermal injury of the full thickness of the bowel wall, with serosal irritation giving rise to symptoms and signs of an acute inflammatory process, with varying degrees of localized pain, tenderness, rebound, with occasional fever and leukocytosis. The thermal damage must be differentiated from a colonoscopic perforation (which it clinically resembles) by obtaining an abdominal x-ray to rule out the possibility of free air. These patients should be observed carefully. Those with severe symptoms should be hospitalized, given nothing by mouth, and started on antibiotics in case a through-and-through perforation occurs. Symptom onset is within four to 12 hours following polypectomy, and usually rapidly subsides after 48 hours. Surgery is not necessary in postpolypectomy syndrome patients, but careful observation is necessary since perforation through the site of tissue damage may ensue.

FIGURE 3.24:
COMPLICATIONS OF COLONOSCOPIC POLYPECTOMY

REFERENCE	NUMBER OF POLYPECTOMIES	HEMORRHAGE N(%)	PERFORATION N(%)	MORTALITY N(%)
Rogers et al. (1975)	6214	115 (1.9)	18 (0.29)	0
Smith (1979)	7393	71 (1.0)	39 (0.5)	1 (0.01)
Frühmorgen and Demling (1979)	7365	165 (2.2)	25 (0.3)	8 (0.1)
Shinya (1982)	5500	24 (0.4)	2 (0.04)	0
Nivatvongs and Fang (1982)	1200	7 (0.5)	0	0
Macrae et al. (1983)	1795	48 (2.6)	2 (0.1)	0
Gilbert et al. (1984)	1901	42 (2.2)	2 (0.1)	0
Total	31368	472 (1.5)	88 (0.3)	9 (0.03)

From Cohen LB, Waye JD. Treatment of colonic polyps—practical considerations. *Clin Gastroenterol* 15(2):359–376, 1986.

Initial Management of Patients with Polyps (Fig. 3.25)

The management of patients with colorectal polyps can be divided into initial management and follow-up (85,86). After detection, the index polyp should be removed completely to eliminate all neoplastic tissue, and the entire specimen should be submitted for microscopic examination. Polypectomy of larger polyps can be accomplished with the cautery snare, while small sessile polyps should be biopsied and ablated with hot biopsy forceps. Pedunculated polyps and sessile polyps with a small attachment to the colon wall can be removed completely with one application of the cautery snare.

If a sessile polyp with a wide-based attachment is not completely removed at the initial polypectomy, additional endoscopy may be required to remove the rest of the tumor. Endoscopic excision of a polyp may not be possible when it is located in an inaccessible site or if the polyp is larger than 2 cm in diameter and sessile, especially with a broad area of implantation onto the colonic wall. If complete endoscopic resection cannot be per-formed, surgical resection may be required. This, however, is necessary in only a very few cases. Since the frequency of additional (synchronous) adenomas in patients with a demonstrated adenoma at the time of diagnosis is approximately 40 percent to 50 percent (1), the initial management of a patient with an identified adenoma should include total colonoscopy with removal of all polyps. This policy may be modified, however, in the presence of significant medical problems.

EXAMINATION OF RESECTED POLYP (FIG. 3.26)

After endoscopic resection, every effort must be made to retrieve the entire specimen for examination and classification. It is important to record clinical and anatomic features, such as the number of polyps and their size, gross morphology (pedunculated or sessile), and anatomic sites. An attempt should be made to identify the base of the polyp. Contraction of the muscularis mucosae may cause a specimen to curl into a ball, making subsequent identification of the resection site extremely difficult. To avoid this, sessile polyps

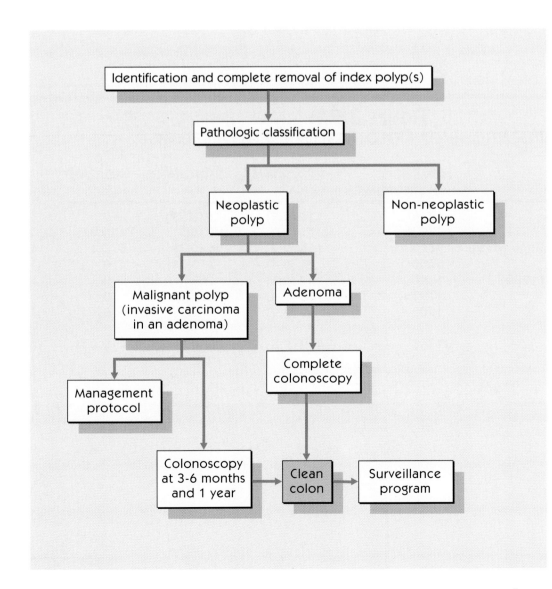

FIGURE 3.25 Initial management algorithm.

may be placed flat on a piece of cardboard, thick paper, an absorbable gelatin sponge (Gelfoam), or a frosted glass slide before insertion into fixative. The base of polyps that are pedunculated or have a small site of attachment to the colon may be identified with India ink or with a pin inserted at the line of resection.

Histologic sections are made from stepwise sagittal blocks of the entire polyp, taking care to represent the stalk and polyp resection margin. Adenomas should be classified by histologic type (tubular, villous, or tubulovillous). High-grade dysplasia should be recorded when present. The terms *carcinoma in situ, intramucosal carcinoma,* or *focal carcinoma* should not be used in the report, as discussed earlier. When invasive adenocarcinoma is encountered in the polyp, that is, carcinoma invasive through muscularis mucosa, the report should include the grade of differentiation of the carcinoma, lymphatic or vascular space permeation, volume of polyp replaced by carcinoma, depth of invasion, and status of resection margin.

Pseudoinvasion with adenoma misplaced into the stalk or submucosa should be distinguished from true invasive carcinoma. Reporting should include whether the excision appears complete. Frequently this determination cannot be accurately made without discussion and correlation of endoscopic and pathologic findings.

Follow-up Management

Patients who have had an adenoma removed have an increased risk of developing subsequent adenomas (metachronous). Prior to fiberoptic colonoscopy, the reported rate of recurrence ranged from 20 percent to 50 percent. Although the patients in the original studies did not have an examination of the entire colonic mucosa to exclude synchronous lesions, investigations performed with colonoscopy have confirmed the previous observations. The National Polyp Study has generated data on identified adenomas found after complete clearing of all synchronous adenomas in a cohort that had not

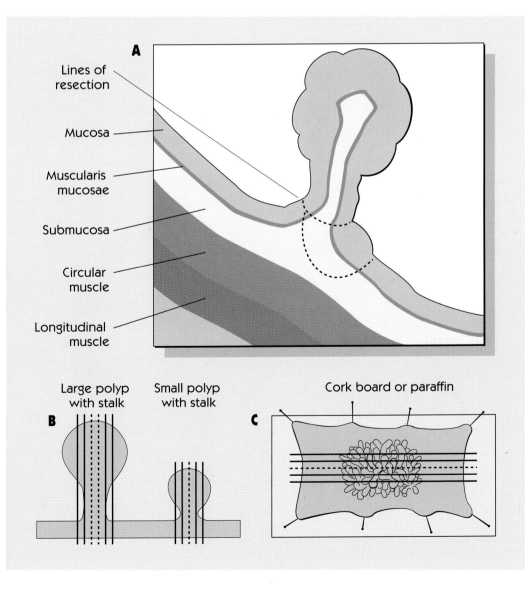

FIGURE 3.26 Pathologic evaluation of polypectomy specimen. (A) This diagrammatic representation of a polyp shows important architectural landmarks and questions that should be addressed so that an informed decision regarding adequacy of resection and prognosis can be made. **(B)** The key to proper handling of a polypectomy specimen with a stalk is a precise cut along the long axis of the stalk. In a small polyp this should bisect the stalk. In the larger polyp the key is a 2-mm section from the center of the stalk with multiple parallel cuts at 2-mm intervals. **(C)** A sessile adenoma should, ideally, be fixed in a pinned-out position before section. Multiple longitudinal cuts including resection margin should then be taken at 2-mm intervals.

had any prior intervention. In this population, it was noted that adenomas were detected at a rate of 29 percent to 35 percent, depending on the interval from their initial colonoscopy. Adenomas at follow-up tended to be small (Fig. 3.27), mostly tubular, without high-grade dysplasia, and uniformly distributed throughout the colon compared with the distal distribution of larger adenomas with more varied histology seen at initial diagnosis (44) (Fig. 3.28). About 50 percent of the adenomas found at follow-up are new; the rest are polyps missed at the initial examination.

Long-Term Follow-up

Colonoscopy is the preferred method of follow-up examination after removal of an initial adenoma. An annual fecal occult blood test has been used in the follow-up period but is of questionable value.

The objective of a surveillance program is to prevent the development of colorectal cancer. The recurrence rate of adenomas in patients after initial polypectomy is high enough to justify periodic follow-up. Ideally, all synchronous adenomas are removed at the time of the initial polypectomy. The frequency of missed synchronous lesions, however, has been estimated to be 10 percent to 15 percent. A proper surveillance schema should, therefore, offer the opportunity of finding these missed lesions and new metachronous adenomas but must be designed to protect the patient from the risk and cost of unnecessary examinations and

an overwhelming of medical resources. Several studies have been investigating follow-up strategies in these patients.

The endoscopist must be confident that a "clean colon," free of adenomas, has been established before instituting long-term follow-up. Frequently, repeated examinations may be indicated after incomplete or piecemeal removal of some large or sessile lesions, for patients with numerous polyps, or after a technically unsatisfactory examination. Following apparently complete removal of a pedunculated malignant polyp, judged on combined endoscopic and histologic grounds, most endoscopists perform repeat examination at three months and one year before reverting to routine follow-up.

Current information suggests that after establishing a clean colon, there can usually be an interval of three years before repeat examination. Some centers present predictive evidence of increased risk in patients with multiple adenomas and recommend a follow-up examination every year in those with two or more adenomas but every three years in those with a single adenoma.

Management of Malignant Polyps
ENDOSCOPIC EVALUATION

Although polyps with features listed in Figure 3.29 are not invariably malignant and many malignant polyps are indistinguishable endoscopically from adenomas, the endoscopist should pay special

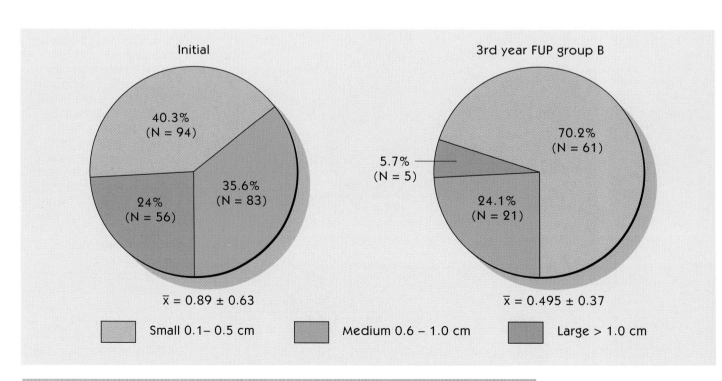

$\bar{x} = 0.89 \pm 0.63$ $\qquad$ $\bar{x} = 0.495 \pm 0.37$

Small 0.1– 0.5 cm $\qquad$ Medium 0.6 – 1.0 cm $\qquad$ Large > 1.0 cm

FIGURE 3.27 Comparison of adenoma size at initial examination and on follow-up after a three-year interval. Data from the National Polyp Study (reference 1).

attention to any lesion with malignant characteristics since they may be managed somewhat differently than the routine adenoma. If cancer is suspected by any of the above criteria, the snare should be placed more toward the wall when resecting a predunculated polyp than toward the head as is the usual practice. Special care must be directed toward recovering all of the fragments for histopathologic evaluation, and to localize the polyp's precise position in the colon should subsequent surgery be needed.

Precise localization of the polypectomy site may be desirable even if surgery is not to be performed, and the patient is to be followed endoscopically. Reliance on the centimeter distance of colonoscopy insertion is unreliable as are intraluminal landmarks. The best method for localizing the polypectomy site is by India ink injection (20), whereby a dilute suspension of sterile black carbon particles is injected at the site. The area is stained forever and can be readily detected by the surgeon and by the endoscopist on repeat examination.

PEDUNCULATED MALIGNANT POLYPS

The pedunculated malignant polyp has by long convention been placed in a different category than the sessile malignant polyp by many clinicians. When polyps are pedunculated, the submucosa of the polyp is separated from the submucosa of the colon wall by a thin tubular segment of submucosa, whereas in sessile polyps the submucosa of the polyp is directly contiguous with the submucosa of the colon wall (see Fig. 3.12). The literature on malignant polyps is inconsistent, with several authors utilizing their own

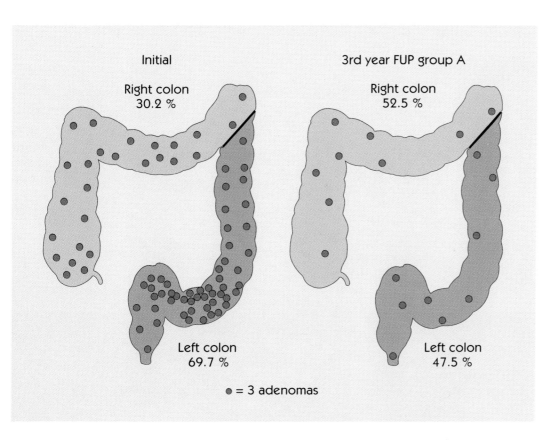

Initial

Right colon
30.2 %

Left colon
69.7 %

3rd year FUP group A

Right colon
52.5 %

Left colon
47.5 %

● = 3 adenomas

FIGURE 3.28 Comparison of distribution of adenomas on initial examination and on follow-up with examinations at one year and three years. Data from the National Polyp Study (reference 1).

FIGURE 3.29: ENDOSCOPIC FEATURES OF MALIGNANT POLYPS

Irregular surface contour
Ulceration or erosion
Firm or hard consistency
Stalk broadening
Friability

classification system for depth of invasion, rendering it difficult to compare extent of tumor invasion and its significance from one paper to another. Some reports mix the results from surgically resected specimens with those removed colonoscopically, which tends to unfavorably skew the outcomes by including cases that would not have been considered for endoscopic resection.

Guidelines for endoscopic polypectomy are fairly well accepted when discussing pedunculated polyps. When certain favorable clinical and histologic criteria are met following removal of pedun-

FIGURE 3.30:
HISTOLOGIC RISK FACTORS IN MALIGNANT POLYPS

	FAVORABLE (LOW RISK)	UNFAVORABLE (HIGH RISK)
Degree of differentiation	Well or moderate	Poor
Vascular or lymphatic invasion in polyp	Absent	Present
Resection margin	Clear or 2-mm margin	Involved

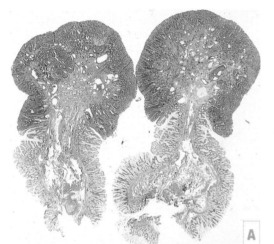
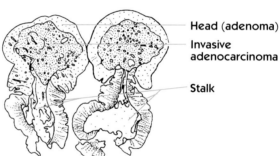

Head (adenoma)
Invasive adenocarcinoma
Stalk

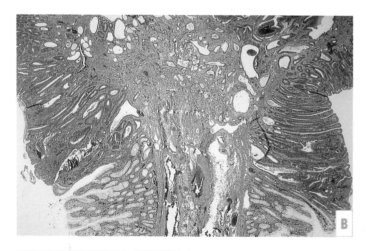
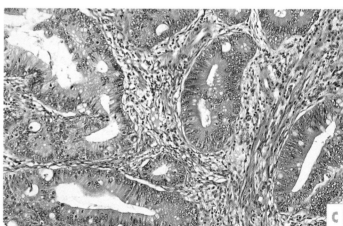

FIGURE 3.31 Pedunculated malignant polyp with favorable histologic features. (A) A section of a bisected malignant polyp with a long pedicle. The line drawing outlines a wedge of invasive adenocarcinoma extending to the submucosa at the junction of the head and stalk (the polyp neck). **(B)** This detail shows the lower limit of the invasive adenocarcinoma and no evidence of vascular space invasion. **(C)** The histology is well to moderately differentiated.

culated malignant polyps, it is the general consensus of the literature on this subject that surgery should not be performed since the risk of having residual cancer at the site or nodal metastasis is extremely low and less than the mortality from surgical resection (see Fig. 3.3). These favorable criteria are that the tumor be well or moderately differentiated, the resection margin be clear of malignant cells, and the cancer not invade lymphatic channels or vascular spaces within the polyp (Figs. 3.30 and 3.31).

Poorly differentiated carcinoma is rare in malignant polyps, but is seen in 15 percent of surgical resection specimens for colorectal carcinoma (87). Poor differentiation appears to be a feature that can be correlated with tumor mass and with vascular space invasion. Its presence in malignant polyps is an ominous prognostic sign and mandates surgical resection if the patient's clinical condition does not preclude it.

Invasion of lymphatics or veins within the submucosa of the polyp head or stalk is also a relatively rare phenomenon and is thought to be a poor prognostic sign, although there have not been enough cases reported to constitute a series that would bear a statistical analysis of its impact, independent of other negative factors. A recent report (88) indicates that this type of vessel invasion is found more frequently if a combination of H&E and elastin stains is used (Fig. 3.32).

The acceptable distance from invasive carcinoma to the endoscopic diathermy burn is variable among many reports in the literature. Some authors (89) mention that the margin must be "healthy," while others insist upon a minimum of a 1-mm margin (90), a 2-mm margin (91,92), or a 3-mm margin (82). Lipper (93) states that the presence of malignant cells at the resection margin is the only criterion that reliably predicts a poor outcome. Morson (87) has found good long-term results in cases

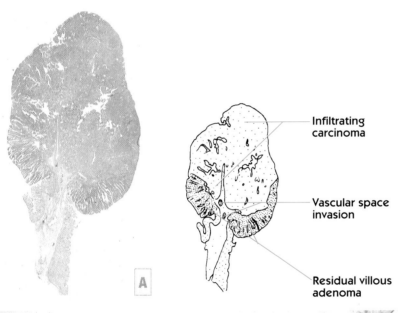

Infiltrating carcinoma

Vascular space invasion

Residual villous adenoma

A

FIGURE 3.32 Pedunculated polyp with unfavorable histologic features. (A) A pedunculated adenoma whose head is extensively replaced by infiltrating poorly differentiated adenocarcinoma. In the submucosa at the neck of the polyp permeation of a lymphatic space by tumor is seen. Line drawing shows the main features of the polyp. **(B)** Detail of polyp showing residual villous adenoma and poorly differentiated adenocarcinoma. **(C)** Detail showing lymphatic space invasion.

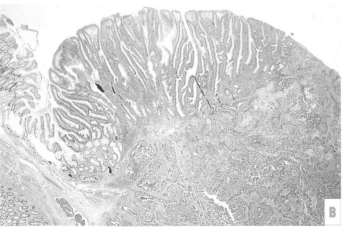

B

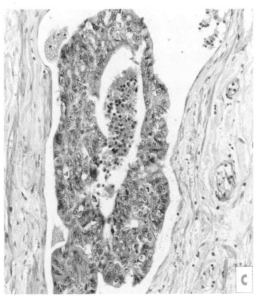

C

with a tumor at the resection margin that were deemed to be safe because the endoscopist considered that all abnormal tissue had been removed during colonoscopy. Morson felt that in such cases the diathermy burn caused sufficient cell necrosis to eradicate all residual malignant cells at the margin of the tumor.

SESSILE MALIGNANT POLYPS

Sessile malignant polyps are often considered separately by both clinicians and pathologists. The concern is that malignant cells that cross the muscularis mucosa of a sessile polyp are actually invading into the portion of the submucosa that is directly contiguous with the rest of the bowel wall submucosa and are not protected by a "buffer zone" of submucosa as in pedunculated polyps.

Many authors feel, however, that there is no sound basis for this assertion and that malignant polyps which are sessile should not be considered any differently from those that are pedunculated (87,89,93,94). A review of the literature in 1988 (91) drew the conclusion that sessile and pedunculated malignant polyps did not differ in their risk for residual or metastatic disease if favorable criteria were applicable. However, Wilcox (95), in a paper on decision analysis and the therapeutic options in malignant polyps, concluded that all sessile malignant polyps should have an operative resection if the patient is a good-risk candidate. Christie (81) agreed, in spite of the low frequency of residual or nodal cancer in the patients he himself reported with sessile malignant polyps. Other authors have also expressed the view that sessile malignant polyps should be treated by further surgical resection (82,95–98). Cooper (99) reported that sessile malignant polyps had a high frequency of residual or nodal cancer, but all eight of the cases in his series found to have residual disease also had positive resection margins. Langer (94) contended that only sessile malignant polyps resected in a piecemeal fashion should be subjected to surgery because of the possibility of error in orienting tissue received by the pathologist.

There is a consensus that if no unfavorable criteria are present in pedunculated malignant polyps, there is a low or nonexistent risk of residual tumor or lymph node metastases (81,90,100,101) and therefore surgery is not indicated. Many also contend that this equally applies even if the polyp is sessile (87,94,102), but it is reasonable to consider a resection in these patients if their surgical risk is low. Some authors have attempted to add other risk factors to the above-mentioned criteria such as deep stalk invasion (102) or extensive tumor invasion of over one-third of the polyp's submucosa (90).

Endoscopic Follow-up

If the decision for endoscopic follow-up of a malignant polyp has been made, a full repeat colonoscopy need not be undertaken soon after the index colonoscopy if the initial examination was completed to the cecum (unless the malignant polyp was located in the right colon). Endoscopy for evaluation of the polypectomy site may be performed in four to 12 weeks to assess completeness of resection and again in three to six months. If no recurrent tumor is present, annual examinations should then be performed for two years, after which routine polyp follow-up is recommended. If recurrent tumor is seen at the polypectomy site, surgical bowel resection should be carried out.

India ink may be injected into the mucosa as a permanent marker to guide the surgeon in locating the area to be resected or to aid in relocating a polypectomy site during future examinations. Circumferential injections are of greater help in subsequent surgical localization than single mucosal injections because the endoscopist cannot predict which surface of the bowel will be directed upward toward the surgeon's view.

HYPERPLASTIC POLYPS

Hyperplastic polyps are small sessile mucosal elevations of the colon and rectum with a distinctive histologic appearance. They seem to be caused by focal defects in the process of crypt cell maturation and luminal dehiscence.

Epidemiology

There is considerable variation in the prevalence of hyperplastic polyps in various populations and geographic locations. Hawaiian-Japanese appear to have the highest reported prevalence of hyperplastic polyps—73 percent of males and 51 percent of females (5) compared with 15 percent for white males and 14 percent for black males in a New Orleans study (8).

Figure 3.33 summarizes the published data on adenoma and hyperplastic polyp prevalence and colon cancer incidence in multiple geographic locations. The occurrence of hyperplastic polyps in the various populations studied shows a significant association with the prevalence of adenomas, despite some exceptions (8,10). Statistical analysis also confirms adenoma prevalence as a significant predictor of colon cancer incidence. Hyperplastic polyp prevalence, however, also appears to be significantly related to colon cancer incidence based on analysis of these data, but further study shows that this association is *not independent but contingent* on the significant association that exists between the prevalence of hyperplastic polyps and that of adenomas. Thus, the epidemiologic data provide some support for an association between the occurrence of hyperplastic polyps and adenomas but suggests that the factor(s) underlying this association are independent of those linked to adenoma progression and cancer evolution.

Pathogenesis

In the normal colorectal mucosa, as we have described above, as stem cell progeny from the crypt base mature, they migrate to the surface where they are ultimately extruded. Hayashi and colleagues (103) on the basis of ultrastructural and in vitro cell kinetic studies proposed that a hyperplastic polyp results from a disturbance of this cycle so that detachment of mature cells is delayed or impeded, and the retained epithelium becomes hypermature. As evidence for this, the surface epithelium of the hyperplastic polyp is characterized by increased height, increased numbers of tall microvilli, a thickened fibroblastic sheath, and other ultrastructural features that suggest hypermaturity (103,104). In the basal portion of the glands of the hyperplastic polyp, cells of intermediate differentiation predominate (104). When mitoses are found they are usually confined to the middle or basal zones of the glands (105). Cell kinetic studies confirm that, in common with normal glands, cell proliferation is largely confined to the basal zone, but upward migration of cells is, in fact, considerably slower than normal, and the number of cells labelled is less than normal (103). This is in sharp contrast to adenomas where cell replication occurs equally in deep and superficial portions of tubules or glands (34,42).

Patient Characteristics

Hyperplastic polyps appear earlier in the colon and rectum than do adenomas. Arthur (106) found one or more hyperplastic polyps in the rectum of six of 25 individuals aged 10 to 40 years at autopsy but found no adenomas. An examination of other autopsy studies show hyperplastic polyps appearing with comparable frequency in the fifth, sixth, and seventh decades. There is either no correla-

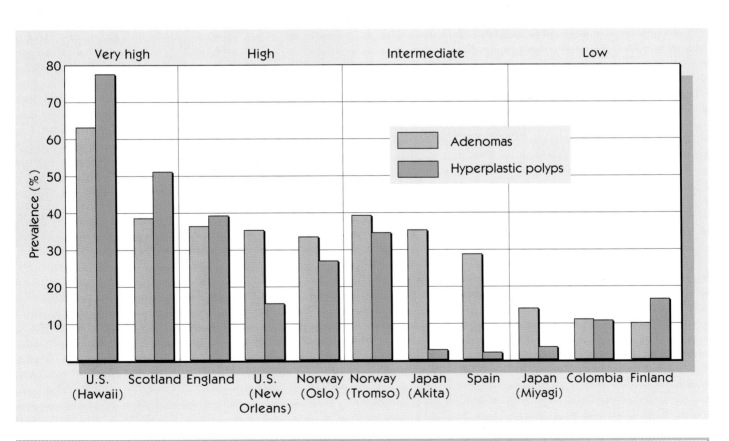

FIGURE 3.33 Prevelance of hyperplastic polyps compared to that of adenomas in populations with reported very high, high, intermediate, and low incidence of colon carcinoma, at multiple geographic locations. (Adapted from references 4,6,8–10.)

tion or a weak association (4) with increasing age, and in several studies the prevalence in the very elderly was found to be less than in the middle-aged (6–9). The prevalence of adenomas, however, increases significantly with advancing age (7–9). A majority of autopsy studies reviewed found that hyperplastic polyps tend to be more prevalent in males than females (4,7–9), although some studies show no significant gender difference (4).

Endoscopic Appearance

The hyperplastic polyp is typically a broad-based, flat, pale nodule (Fig. 3.34) often with a papillary surface that blends with the normal mucosa at the periphery. This contrasts with adenomas that range up to 5 mm in size, and typically have a globular shape, reddish color, and in some instances a short pedicle (Fig. 3.35). It is difficult to distinguish accurately between hyperplastic polyps and adenomas when polyps are 5 mm or less at endoscopy, according to experienced endoscopists (108) and recent studies that have specifically addressed the issue (109–111).

Microscopic Appearance

Hyperplastic polyps are typically composed of elongated funnel-shaped nonbranching crypts. The cells in the basal portion of the crypts are cuboidal, of intermediate type, lacking in mucin; mitoses are common. Argentaffin cells and, rarely, Paneth cells may be found. The upper portion of the crypts show micropapillary infolding of tall columnar cells and goblet cells, the former usually predominant. Invagination of crypts deep to muscularis mucosae may also be seen giving an inverted appearance, as described by Sobin (67).

Differential Diagnosis

The hyperplastic polyp submitted to the pathologist for diagnosis is typically a 3-mm or smaller tissue fragment that has been obtained by hot biopsy forceps with its attendant pressure or heat artifact. The differential diagnosis is usually between adenoma, hyperplastic polyp, and polyps consisting only of normal mucosa (mucosal tags). The small biopsy is frequently poorly oriented. In terms of classification (Fig. 3.36), the most crucial area to be represented is the surface, where if

FIGURE 3.34: CLASSIFICATION OF SMALL (≤ 5 MM) COLORECTAL POLYPS

	RELATIVE FREQUENCY (%)
Adenomas	50
Hyperplastic polyps	20
Other	
Mucosal tags (normal tissue)	25
Indeterminate	1–3
Inflammatory	1–2
Miscellaneous	1–2

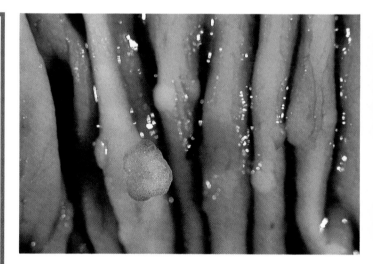

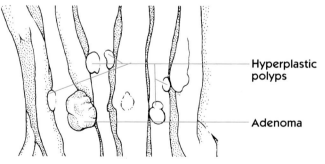

Hyperplastic polyps

Adenoma

FIGURE 3.35 Several hyperplastic polyps are seen, which tend to be located near the apex of the mucosal folds as is typical. The slightly larger adenoma reveals its nature by its red hue and slightly bosselated, irregular surface. (From reference 107.)

immature epithelium can be identified the lesion can be accurately diagnosed as an adenoma. The surface portion of the mucosa is equally crucial to diagnosis in hyperplastic polyps where the serrated (in vertical section) or stellate (in horizontal section) outline of the upper portion of the gland is characteristic. Frequently the diagnostic features are present in a focal area of the biopsy (Fig. 3.37), even confined to a portion of a single gland. Examination of ribbon serial sections will, therefore, enhance accuracy of the classification and tend to diminish the "normal mucosa" category as will orientation of the specimen by the endoscopy assistant prior to formalin immersion.

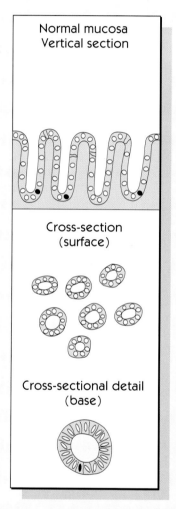
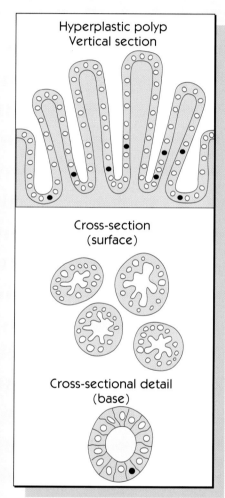
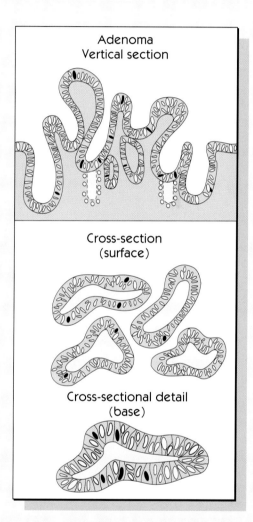

FIGURE 3.36 Schematic of small polyps. (Adapted from original drawing by J. Kasznica, MD, Mallory Institute of Pathology, Boston.)

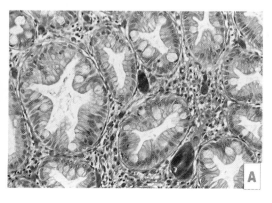
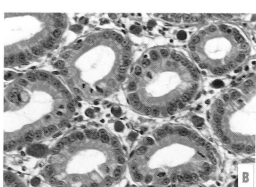

FIGURE 3.37 Hyperplastic polyps. (A) Polyps in tangential section of surface. **(B)** Cross-section through base of hyperplastic polyps.

MIXED HYPERPLASTIC POLYPS AND ADENOMAS

Adenomatous change may sometimes be encountered in an otherwise typical hyperplastic polyp (112–115) and, conversely, areas resembling a hyperplastic polyp may be seen in adenomas. In view of the high prevalence of both lesions in the rectum and sigmoid, occasional juxtapositioning of both entities might be expected, and a hyperplastic gland may be no more resistant to adenomatous transformation than a normal gland. Longacre and Fenoglio (116) have recently drawn attention to a variant of adenoma that resembles the architecture of a hyperplastic polyp for which they suggested the term *serrated adenoma*. A study from St. Mark's Hospital (112) examined the claim that foci with histologic features of hyperplastic polyps were encountered frequently in small villous adenomas implying a possible precursor role in the genesis of such adenomas (116). This experienced group noted the occurrence of this phenomenon in less than 1 percent of 500 adenomas, a figure comparable to the experience of Cooper and co-workers (114), although an Italian study reported such a finding in 10 percent of adenomas that they studied (117). The distinctive morphologic features of hyperplastic polyps (which may be attributable not to hyperplasia but to hypermaturation) might be expected to be found in other pathologic contexts and are, in fact, occasionally found within inflammatory and juvenile polyps and in relation to ischemic mucosal injury (112). Morphologic studies, therefore, provide essentially no support for the hypothesis that hyperplastic polyps may have some precursor role in adenoma development.

Distribution in the Colon and Rectum

The distribution of hyperplastic polyps less than 5 mm in size is concentrated in the lower sigmoid and rectum (Fig. 3.38). For small adenomas of the same size there tends to be uniform distribution from cecum to rectum. Tedesco and associates (118) noted that 77 percent of hyperplastic polyps occurred distal to the splenic flexure, and 52.9 percent were located in the rectosigmoid. Church and colleagues (119) found that 55 percent of hyperplastic polyps removed during total colonoscopy were located in the sigmoid and rectum. In the National Polyp Study, where complete examination of the colon and removal of all polyps encountered for histologic examination are requirements, 78 percent of all hyperplastic polyps were found in the rectum and sigmoid compared with 50 percent of all adenomas (120). Autopsy studies (8,9) have also confirmed the relative predominance of hyperplastic polyps located in the lower sigmoid and rectum. Williams and co-workers (6) found hyperplastic polyps in the rectum in 86 percent of the autopsies they performed. In an autopsy study by Eide and co-workers (9) the tendency to form hyperplastic polyps, expressed as frequency per cm length of bowel segment, was 4.3 in the rectum compared with an overall mean value for the large bowel of 1.8. In this regard, the predominance of hyperplastic polyp localization in the distal segments has been compared with the distribution of colorectal cancer (121). However, the distribution is not entirely analogous, in that cancers are relatively more frequent in the upper rectum and sigmoid whereas peak clustering of hyperplastic polyps is seen in the middle and lower rectum.

Clinical Significance of Hyperplastic Polyps

Recently, several studies (119,122,123) have questioned the existence of a clinically significant association between hyperplastic polyps and adenomas. Achkar and colleagues (123) reported that adenomas or hyperplastic polyps found during flexible sigmoidoscopy were equally reliable as harbingers of proximal adenomas, when total colonoscopy was undertaken. Furthermore, this association was significantly greater than in a control group that consisted of patients with a mucosal tag found on initial flexible sigmoidoscopy. In a retrospective study, Ansher and colleagues (122) found that the percentage of patients harboring an adenoma in the absence of a hyperplastic polyp was 15 percent compared with 49 percent when a hyperplastic polyp was also present. In addition, they found that the likelihood of an isolated right-sided adenoma was significantly increased when a left-sided hyperplastic polyp was present. Church and co-workers reported similiar associations (119), while Provenzale and co-workers did not (124).

As has been pointed out by Waye (108) and by Winawer (125), the main difficulty in interpreting the significance of these studies is the absence of a control group of patients with normal findings in the sigmoid and rectum and lack of standardized pathology. The National Polyp Study data analysis permitted the comparison of a large cohort of 3406 patients with no lesion on the left (distal to splenic flexure) to a group of 1507 with adenomas on the left and 184 with hyperplastic polyps only on the left. Adenomas on the left were shown to be a predictor of adenomas on the right, particularly so when multiple adenomas were present. However, the frequency of right-sided adenomas was similiar when hyperplastic polyps only or no lesions were found on the left. The study, therefore, strongly suggests that a hyperplastic polyp in the rectum and sigmoid is not an indication per se to perform a total colonoscopy (120).

Relative Frequency of Polyp Categories

The relative frequency of hyperplastic polyps among small lesions (5 mm or less) seems to be considerably less than earlier estimates. The perception that more than 90 percent of small polyps are hyperplastic polyps appears to be attributable mainly to Lane and colleagues (105) who reported in 1971 on 2000 polyps recovered from resection specimens and sigmoidoscopic excisions. One-third were less than 3 mm in size and more than 90 percent of these were hyperplastic polyps. This appeared to corroborate the figures from an earlier autopsy study by Arthur (106) of micronodules in 51 rectums from individuals over age 40 in which the frequency of hyperplastic polyps was four times that of adenomas (75 percent vs. 18 percent) and 90 percent of the lesions harvested were hyperplastic polyps. Although these studies dealt with the distal large bowel or rectum, where hyperplastic polyps are most frequent (see Fig. 3.38), they appear to greatly overestimate the relative frequency of hyperplastic polyps encountered in current clinical practice, possibly because of the extremely small size of the polyps sampled. Endoscopic studies show that, among small polyps from the large bowel overall, adenomas are found at least as frequently as hyperplastic polyps (118,126) and three recent series (119,127,128) found the ratio of adenomas to hyperplastic polyps among small polyps was approximately 3:1. In the rectum or rectosigmoid, this ratio changes so that the hyperplastic polyps may outnumber adenomas; however, even at this location a ratio of 1:2 is not exceeded in these series (see Fig. 3.3). Ryan and co-workers (129) found that in the distal 10 cm small polyps were least likely to be adenomas. In the National Polyp Study analysis, hyperplastic polyps represented 11.5 percent of all polyps harvested and 16.4 percent of small polyps (see Fig. 3.3). The proportion of hyperplastic polyps among small polyps of the rectum was 37.4 percent. At present, the most reasonable approach to patients with small colonic polyps is complete colonoscopy, and then placement under follow-up surveillance those individuals in whom the polyps are adenomatous. Individuals with only hyperplastic polyps do not require colonoscopy or follow-up surveillance.

OTHER POLYPS
Mucosal Polyps

On histopathologic examination of biopsies taken from small mucosal excrescences, approximately 20 percent will be composed of normal mucosa. These polyps are not in the category of neoplastic growths nor are they hyperplastic polyps. These small mucosal tags have no clinical significance; if they could be recognized as such removal is not necessary. However, there are no distinguishing endoscopic characteristics that differentiate these

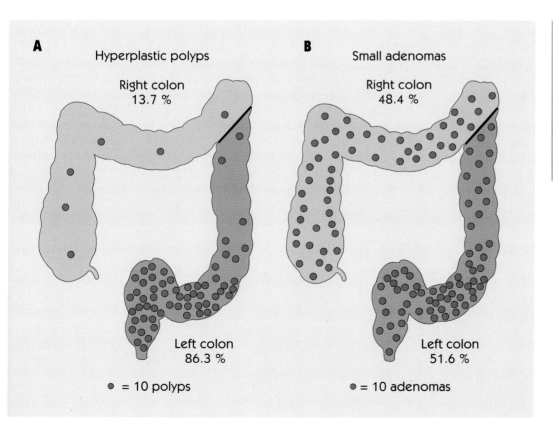

A Hyperplastic polyps

Right colon
13.7 %

Left colon
86.3 %

● = 10 polyps

B Small adenomas

Right colon
48.4 %

Left colon
51.6 %

● = 10 adenomas

FIGURE 3.38 Comparison of distribution of hyperplastic polyps and small adenomas. (A) Hyperplastic polyp distribution. (B) Small adenoma distribution. Data from National Polyp Study (reference 1).

from adenomas or hyperplastic polyps, all of which may appear to be relatively pale or the same color as the surrounding mucosa.

Juvenile Polyps

Juvenile polyps, so called because they are most frequently found in children, are variously considered to be hamartomatous (130) or inflammatory (131) in nature. They are also referred to as *retention polyps*, a name that relates to the theory that the cystic dilation of mucus-filled glands typical of these lesions is due to inflammatory occlusion of the crypt necks. While the majority of patients with juvenile polyps are under 20 years of age and have solitary lesions located in the distal rectum, these polyps are also encountered in adults (132). The prevalence of juvenile polyps in individuals under 20 years based on an autopsy series by Helwig is approximately 1 percent (133). Numerous polyps of this type widely distributed in the colon and rectum suggest the familial juvenile polyposis syndrome (134).

ENDOSCOPIC AND GROSS APPEARANCE
Juvenile polyps are usually spheroid in shape, 1 to 3 cm in diameter, and pedunculated (Fig. 3.39A). They have a bright red granular surface that may bleed on contact. When the resected specimen is sectioned, it reveals multiple mucus-filled cysts in a congested stroma (Fig. 3.39B).

MICROSCOPIC FEATURES
The surface of a juvenile polyp is a monolayer of columnar cells interrupted by frequent, often extensive erosions and associated inflammation. The stroma is voluminous relative to the normal mucosa of adenomas and separates tubules that range in caliber from that of normal crypts to the macroscopically visible dilated cysts. All are lined by columnar or cuboidal epithelium with numerous goblet cells. Reparative changes may be prominent focally and mimic adenomatous change. The stroma and frequently the tubules also contain numerous neutrophils and eosinophils (Fig. 3.39C).

DIAGNOSIS AND MANAGEMENT
The most common presentation is the passage of bright red blood in the stool of a child or adolescent (131,132). In as many as 10 percent of cases the polyp is spontaneously shed from its stalk and is retrieved from the stool (131). This propensity to autoamputation is attributed to the lack of anchoring extensions of muscularis mucosa into the polyp head, which characterizes adenomas, for example. Anal prolapse of the polyp during defecation may also be the initial presentation. Additional polyps are found at re-examination in three percent to eighteen percent of cases (132,135).

Inflammatory Polyps

Inflammatory polyps are attributable to mucosal ulceration and repair. There are three categories that can be defined. The first type, which is accurately described as a pseudopolyp, is produced by confluent ulceration isolating ragged islands of residual inflamed mucosa (Fig. 3.40). A second type, which also occurs in the context of acute colitis, is due to undermining ulceration giving rise to polypoid inflamed mucosal tags. The third type, referred to by Kelly and co-workers (137) as mature inflammatory polyps, is derived from repair and regeneration of these mucosal tags.

Inflammatory polyps occur most frequently in the context of idiopathic chronic inflammatory bowel disease, most frequently in ulcerative colitis but also in Crohn's disease. In clinical series such polyps are seen in 12.5 percent to 19 percent of patients with ulcerative colitis (138–140) but in surgical resection specimens inflammatory polyps are found in over 50 percent of patients (137,141). Inflammatory polyps are described in association with several other inflammatory disorders including bacillary dysentery and amoebic colitis; they are frequent in schistosomiasis; they have been reported in ischemic colitis, with stercoral ulcers and in the vicinity of ureterosigmoidostomies (142). Inflammatory polyps may be single or multiple, occasionally myriad in number and may be segmental or diffuse in distribution.

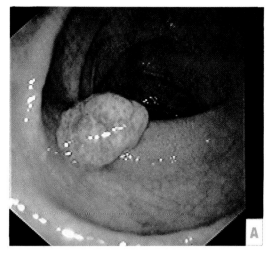

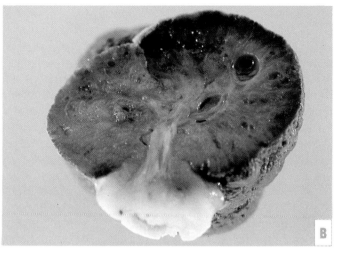

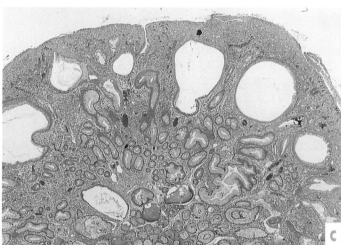

FIGURE 3.39 Juvenile polyp. (A)
Endoscopy: small juvenile polyp with
typical mottled appearance (due to cystic glands). **(B)** Cross-section to show
cystic glands. (From reference 107.) **(C)**
Surface and glands are lined by columnar, nondysplastic mucosa. There is
abundant stroma between the glands.

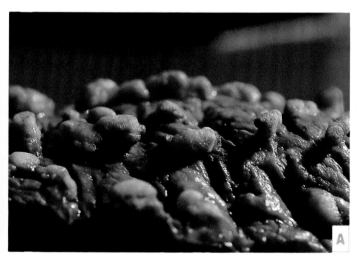

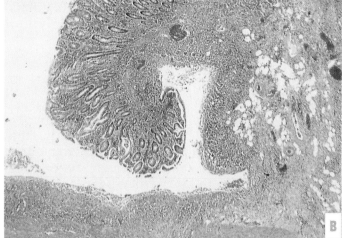

FIGURE 3.40 Inflammatory pseudopolyp. (A) Pseudopolyps produced by confluent ulceration isolating ragged islands of residual inflamed mucosa. **(B)** Microscopic view showing ulceration undermining pseudopolypoid inflamed mucosa.

ENDOSCOPIC AND GROSS APPEARANCE

Inflammatory polyps typically are of uniform width from base to head and have an appendage-like appearance on endoscopy (Fig. 3.41). In some, bulbous enlargement of the head may be seen, which may show ulceration. Bifid forms are also quite common as are tubular bridges between adjacent polyps and mucosa. Arborescent forms may also be seen.

MICROSCOPIC FEATURES

The appearance of inflamed mucosal tags is clearly indistinguishable from inflamed pseudopolyps in acute colitis. Mature inflammatory polyps are covered by mucosa that encloses a core of muscularis mucosa and submucosa. The mucosal component may be entirely normal or show regenerative changes or mixed inflammatory or regenerative changes. Pure granulation tissue polyps and polyps devoid of a submucosal core may also be seen (137).

DIAGNOSIS AND MANAGEMENT

The nature of inflammatory polyps can be readily ascertained by colonoscopy. Myriad polyps can produce a mass effect. When polyps are numerous, removal of all polyps is neither practical nor necessary. A sample of polyps should be removed to confirm their nature histologically. There is general agreement (137) that dysplastic and malignant change is no more likely to supervene in inflammatory polyps than in the adjacent nonpolypoid mucosa.

GIANT INFLAMMATORY POLYPS

When inflammatory polyps exceed 1.5 cm in length they are said to be giant inflammatory polyps (143). These may be multiple and involve the entire length of colon, but frequently they involve a short segment of colon 15 cm or less (144). They have the same histologic appearance as smaller mature inflammatory polyps and also often show tissue ulceration and granulation at the tip. They are encountered most frequently in the transverse colon and, as with their smaller counterparts, are least common in the rectum.

Giant inflammatory polyps are usually multiple, segmental, and circumferential. They may suggest a neoplasm on barium enema, and rarely cause incomplete obstruction, retrograde obstruction of barium flow, or intussusception. They may also be associated with abdominal pain and blood loss. Surgical resection may be indicated if morbidity warrants it. Williams and co-workers have reported endoscopic treatment of giant polyps in schistosomiasis as a strategy for management of patients with significant associated morbidity (145).

INFLAMMATORY CLOACOGENIC POLYP

A distinctive appearing polyp, which is inflammatory in nature and occurs in the distal rectum, has been labelled by Lobert and Appleman as inflammatory cloacogenic polyp (146). The surface epithelium consists of variable proportions of squamous, columnar epithelium and variable proportions of squamous or transitional epithelium. Crypts are hyperplastic, and the lesion may be mistaken for a tubular or tubulovillous adenoma. The stroma has a distinctive fibromuscular character. This type of polyp has been reported in association with solitary rectal ulcer syndrome and Crohn's disease as well as in other clinical settings (147). Patients with this lesion should, in view of the former association, be evaluated for the presence of occult or overt mucosal prolapse. A similar pathogenesis due to mucosal prolapse may underlie a rare polyplike entity described as polypoid prolapsing colonic mucosal folds, which is occasionally seen in diverticular disease (148,149). A condition characterized by numerous polyps with features similar to the above and restricted to the rectosigmoid has recently been described by Burke and colleagues as eroded polypoid hyperplasia of the rectosigmoid (150).

Peutz–Jeghers Polyps

A polyp that is characterized by normal mucosal elements draped on a treelike scaffolding of muscularis mucosa is a Peutz–Jeghers polyp (151) (Fig. 3.42). Such polyps are characteristic of the familial polyposis syndrome. They are hamartomatous overgrowths of normal components, appropriate to their specific location in the gastrointestinal tract. They are usually most numerous in the small intestine but are also found in the stomach and colon and usually total less than 100. The mucosa of the colonic polyp is represented by normal mucus goblet and absorptive cells with argentaffin cells and, less commonly, Paneth cells in mildly irregular crypts.

Lymphoid Polyps

A localized hyperplasia of mucosal and submucosal lymphoid tissue may present as a single or, less commonly, multiple polyps and is most frequently encountered in the lower rectum (152). Physiologic reactive changes distinguish this entity from lymphomatous involvement.

Small lymphoid nodules are a common normal finding in the colon and rectum with high-resolution barium contrast studies (153) and in normal colorectal tissue examined histologically. A marked increase in size and number of lymphoid aggregates can produce striking nodularity (154) or an appearance of diffuse polyposis.

Submucosal Lesions
Carcinoid Tumors
Carcinoid tumors involving the mucosa and submucosa may present as a small polypoid nodule. These lesions are essentially limited to the sigmoid and rectum. They are composed of columnar or cuboidal cells arranged in trabeculae or lobules

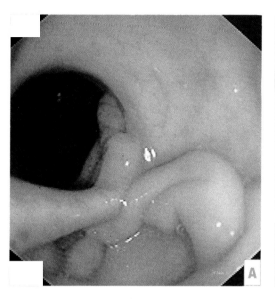

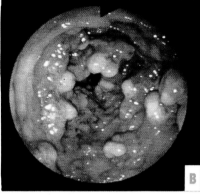
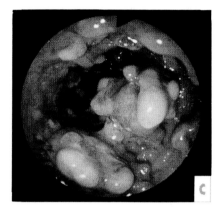

FIGURE 3.41 Inflammatory polyp. (A) Long filamentous inflammatory polyps in a patient with ulcerative colitis. **(B,C)** Exuberant pseudopolyps with white areas of slough on their surface. (From reference 136.)

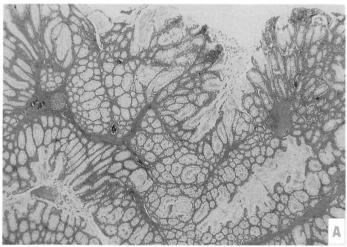
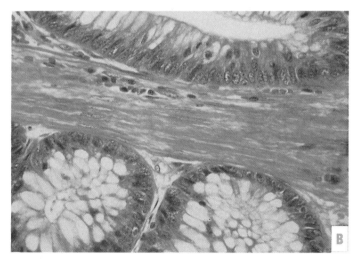

FIGURE 3.42 (A) The arborescent pattern of this 2-cm Peutz-Jeghers polyp is quite evident in this specimen (x4). **(B)** At high power, normal-appearing colonic epithelium and normal smooth muscle are juxtaposed (x100). (From reference 107.)

with a fibromuscular stroma (Fig. 3.43). They show neuroendocrine properties on histochemical and immunochemical staining.

There have been several recent studies that have addressed the management of carcinoid tumors (155–158), and there appears to be unanimity that carcinoid tumors of the sigmoid and rectum, when less than 2 cm in diameter and confined to mucosa and submucosa, are biologically benign and are appropriately treated by endoscopic resection alone. Malignant carcinoid tumors of the colon and rectum, on the other hand, are invariably advanced at time of diagnosis and show mitotic activity and deep mural invasion (155,158).

LIPOMAS (FIG. 3.44)
The majority of lipomas in the intestinal tract occur in the colon, mostly around the ileocecal valve. These submucosal tumors are composed of adipose tissue supported by a fibrous stroma. Although usually single, multiple lipomatosis of the large bowel has been reported. The size ranges from 0.5 cm to 15.0 cm. Most lipomas are asymptomatic but large lesions may give rise to abdominal pain related to peristaltic propulsion causing traction.

Lipomas may be diagnosed radiographically by their smooth, changeable configuration as well as their radiolucency on barium enema examinations. On endoscopic examination they are covered by normal surface mucosa with an interlacing blood vessel pattern, are somewhat yellowish in color, and indent easily (pillow-sign) when palpated with a biopsy forceps. When the surface is denuded by progressively deeper biopsies, fat may be seen bulging through the mucosal rent. Although endoscopic removal is not suggested, this approach may be acceptable when the lipoma is pedunculated and symptomatic.

OTHER MESENCHYMAL LESIONS
A leiomyoma is sometimes discovered as an incidental yellowish white polyp that usually measures less than 1.5 cm in diameter and is benign. Other mesenchymal lesions include neural tumors, polypoid ganglioneuroma, and submucosal neurofibroma or schwannoma. Multiple gastrointestinal neurofibromas may be encountered in von Recklinghausen's disease, but in most reported cases the location of these tumors has been extraluminal (serosal) (159). Multiple ganglioneuromas as a manifestation of an inherited disorder may be seen in von Recklinghausen's disease, in association with multiple endocrine neoplasia, type 2, or as an isolated abnormality (160).

POLYPOSIS SYNDROMES
Familial Adenomatous Polyposis (FAP)
Familial adenomatous polyposis (FAP) is an inherited condition characterized primarily by the presence of hundreds to thousands of polyps (adenomas) throughout the colon and rectum (162) (Fig. 3.45). According to Bussey (163), the first documented description of FAP was that of Corvisart in 1847 (164); Cripps described the condition in siblings in 1882 (165), and Handfort, in 1890, appears to have been the first to note the high incidence of associated carcinoma of the colon and rectum (166). In 1930, Dukes (167) published a comprehensive review of familial polyposis, and later he and Lockhart-Mummery clearly established that the disease had an autosomal dominant pattern of inheritance with a high degree of penetrance (168). In the 1950s Eldon J. Gardner described a syndrome similiar to FAP but with the additional component of distinctive extracolonic lesions, most notably osteomas of the skull, dentigerous cysts, retinal pigmentation spots (CHRPE), multiple epidermal cysts, and desmoid tumors (162,169–171). A further twist to the clinical story was provided by Turcot and colleagues (172) who reported in 1959 the occurrence of central nervous system tumors in two siblings with FAP; several further reports of this association, termed *Turcot syndrome*, have since appeared (173–175). There is debate as to whether Turcot syndrome is a separate entity or a variant of FAP (26). The distribution of the disease in several families also has suggested that it may be an autosomal recessive disorder (26). Other extra-gastrointestinal malignancies have also been reported in FAP and GS, including primary tumors of the thyroid (176), biliary tract (177), and liver (178).

Pathology of Colorectal Adenomas in FAP
Patients with FAP have myriad polyps in the range of over 100 to over 5000; 90 percent are less than 0.5 cm in diameter and only 1 percent are more than 1.0 cm in diameter (163). The adenomas are evenly distributed throughout the colon but larger adenomas tend to have a more distal location (163). The histologic subtypes of FAP adenomas are similiar to that of sporadic adenomas of the same size range—they are predominantly tubular with tubulovillous and, rarely, pure villous represented in the larger polyps (163). The frequency of a finding of a carcinoma in an individual adenoma is

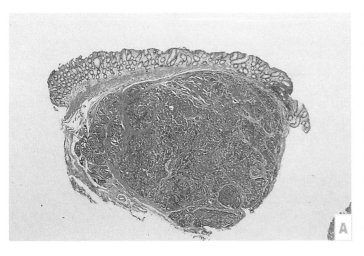

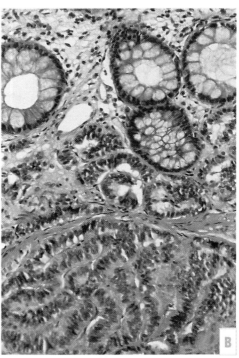

FIGURE 3.43 (A) This rounded mass of a 0.7-cm rectal carcinoid was almost entirely confined by the submucosa (x4). **(B)** The carcinoid, which appears to "bud off" the base of the crypts, assumes a typical ribbonlike appearance in the submucosa (x66). (From reference 107.)

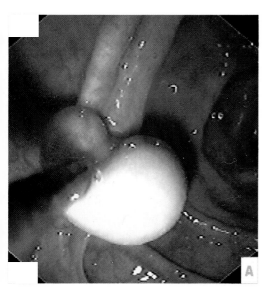

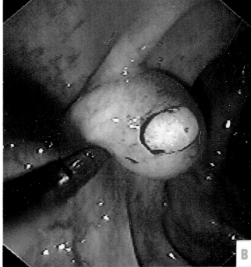

FIGURE 3.44 (A) A biopsy forceps indenting a submucosal lipoma (pillow sign). **(B)** Fat bulging from the surface of a lipoma after denuding the mucosal layer by taking multiple spot biopsies.

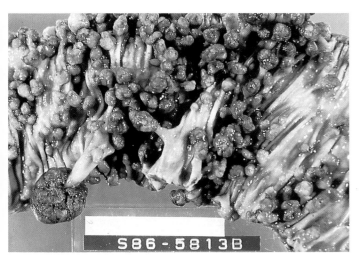

FIGURE 3.45 The varying appearance of tubular adenomas at different stages of development is evident in this colon from a patient with FAP. (From reference 107.)

related to adenoma size and is very similiar to the frequency in comparable sporadic adenomas. One hundred or more polyps is widely accepted as an essential criterion for the diagnosis of FAP (179). Nonetheless, FAP families have been described in which some members have fewer than 100 polyps (26,180).

ADENOMA CARCINOMA SEQUENCE IN FAP

The incidence of colorectal carcinoma in untreated FAP patients approaches 100 percent (60). The mean age at diagnosis of propositus FAP patients in the St. Mark's Hospital series is 26 to 28 years for patients without associated carcinoma and 39.2 years when cancer is also present (181). For screened relatives with FAP, the respective figures are 23.7 years and 33.0 years (181). These data suggest an approximate ten-year interval between the formation of adenomas and the development of advanced cancers. This interval length is comparable to that proposed for adenoma to invasive carcinoma evolution in the general population (45). The distribution of the cancers both in high-incidence countries such as Britain and low-incidence countries such as Japan is also similiar to that of sporadic cancers (182). The extremely high incidence of colorectal cancer in FAP appears to be a function, therefore, of the numbers of adenomas present and is modulated by environmental phenomena similiar to those operating in sporadic adenomas. Fifty percent of FAP patients have more than one cancer at the time of diagnosis (163) compared with 3.2 percent in the general population of patients with colorectal cancer (66).

UPPER GASTROINTESTINAL TRACT POLYPS IN FAP

The mucosal growth disorder that underlies FAP and Gardner's syndrome is also manifested throughout the small intestine and particularly in the second part of the duodenum where multiple small adenomas, albeit in smaller numbers than in the colon, are found in a majority of patients (182–188). Gastric polyps are also frequently found. These may be adenomas but are much more likely to be minute hamartomas called fundic gland hyperplasia, or both types of polyps may be seen (184–189). There may be a slightly increased risk for gastric carcinoma in Japanese with FAP, but this is not the case for affected individuals in Western countries (160). There is, however, in all populations, a well-documented increase in duodenal and periampullary carcinoma in patients with FAP (162) (Fig. 3.46). The overall risk is in the region of 5 percent for FAP and may be no higher in Gardner's syndrome (162,190). Malignant transformation of small bowel adenomas distal to the duodenum is very uncommon.

Gardner's Syndrome

The gastrointestinal manifestations in FAP and Gardner's syndrome are essentially identical (162,190). Indeed, the reported finding of subclinical evidence of some of the extracolonic stigmata of Gardner's syndrome in many FAP patients and the identification of kindreds with both syndromes have led to the emergence of the view that the familial adenomatous polyposis coli syndromes may represent essentially one disease. The explanation of perceived differences is likely to be offered ultimately by molecular genetic studies, which can determine whether variable expression of the extragastrointestinal manifestations reflects the pleiotropic effect of a single gene (169).

Molecular Genetics of FAP

Herrera and colleagues reported in 1986 (191) a cytogenetic finding of an interstitial deletion in the long arm of chromosome 5 (5q) in the karyotype of a patient with Gardner's syndrome. Prompted by this finding, two groups, one in London and the other in Utah, independently used similiar recombinant DNA methodologies to determine whether the gene could be linked to segments on the long arm of chromosome 5 for which DNA probes were available (68,69). They examined DNA preparations for restriction fragment length polymorphisms (RFLP) generated by the restriction enzyme Taq 1. They had available for study DNA harvested from multiple members of a total of 18 FAP or Gardner's syndrome kindreds. They discovered that one particular probe (C11P11) identified an RFLP that showed profound segregation with the disease. They had proof, therefore, of linkage of this RFLP to the FAP-GS gene. In addition they demonstrated its location in a specific chromosomal region, 5q22 (68). With this development, precise identification of the gene and the nature of its product appeared to be only a matter of time. Identification and characterization of the FAP gene was reported in 1991 (221,222).

Screening and Surveillance

Screening for colonic polyposis should be performed in all individuals at risk for this condition. It should begin between the ages of ten and 12 years, be performed yearly until age 40, and continue every three years thereafter (26). Flexible proctosigmoidoscopy is the preferred screening procedure. Surveillance for gastric, duodenal, and periampullary polyps should begin when the diagnosis of colonic polyposis is made and should continue every one to three years thereafter. Side-viewing endoscopy is the screening modality of choice (26).

NONADENOMATOUS POLYPOSIS (FAMILIAL) SYNDROMES

Peutz–Jeghers Syndrome

The first report of the association of familial gastrointestinal polyps and pigmentations of the skin and mucous membranes was by Peutz in 1921 (192). The syndrome and its clinical significance was detailed by Jeghers in 1949 (193).

DIAGNOSIS AND MANAGEMENT

Abnormal pigmentation of Peutz–Jeghers syndrome, which develops in infancy and early childhood and tends to fade at puberty, consists of round to oval macules 1 to 12· mm in diameter on the lips (96 percent) (Fig. 3.47), buccal mucosa (83 percent) (where it is most persistent), and less commonly on digits, eyelids, nose, gingiva, and hard palate. Pigmented macules may be found also on the anal mucosa and genital area. The syndrome has a mendelian dominant pattern of inheritance. Within affected families, patients are found with pigmentation and no polyps and, conversely, with polyps without pigmentation (194).

The most frequent clinical presentation of this syndrome is abdominal colic due to intussusception of a small intestinal polyp, and many patients undergo several abdominal explorations over a lifetime. The risk of gastrointestinal cancer is small, estimated by Reid to be in the range of 2 percent to 3 percent (195). Bilateral microscopic sex cord tumors with annular tubules (SCAT) (196,197) are frequently found in females with this disorder. Most examples of gastrointestinal cancer have been

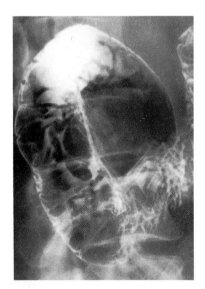
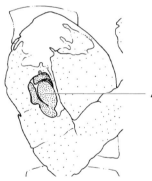

Adenoma

FIGURE 3.46 A villous adenoma surrounding the ampulla shown by hypotonic duodenography in a patient with FAP. (From reference 161.)

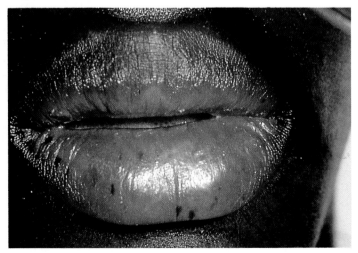

FIGURE 3.47 The characteristic flat pigmented lesions of Peutz–Jeghers syndrome are due to an increase in melanin and melanocytes. Here they are present on the lips and the mucosa of the tongue. (From reference 107.)

found in the duodenum and gastric antrum (195, 198), but there have also been reports of colon cancer in a young age group (199). It has been suggested (200,201) that such cancers arise from coincidental adenoma. However, the rare finding of dysplastic change and in situ and early cancers in Peutz–Jeghers polyps suggests that this is a possible mechanism of gastrointestinal cancer evolution in the syndrome (198,200,202). In either event, this outcome is so infrequent that prophylactic surgery is not a consideration in the management of Peutz–Jeghers syndrome.

Juvenile Polyposis

Juvenile polyposis coli is a disorder characterized by the presence of multiple (more than ten) (160) juvenile polyps in the colon and rectum (Fig. 3.48). It may be associated in some patients with similar polyps in the stomach and small intestine. Approximately 25 percent of cases are familial with an automosomal dominant pattern of inheritance (179). The disease was first separated from FAP by McColl and colleagues (134). It presents with clinical symptoms, such as bleeding, anemia, and growth retardation, usually in childhood and at an earlier age than FAP. Its distinction from FAP is important because in FAP there is an extremely high risk of colon cancer, whereas in juvenile polyposis the risk for colon cancer is very much less but still may not be inconsequential (179). Approximately 9 percent of patients with this syndrome according to a review of published cases by Järvinen and Franssilla (203) have developed colon cancer, in many cases before age 40. These authors also noted a history of gastrointestinal cancer in almost two-thirds of affected families.

PATHOLOGY

The typical polyp of juvenile polyposis is identical to the sporadic juvenile polyp; however, a lobulated appearance is more often seen, and the stromal component may be less voluminous. Several reports (204–206) have drawn attention to the development in this syndrome of focal adenomatous change within some juvenile polyps, which may become extensive or predominant *within* an individual polyp. High-grade dysplasia has been reported in some of these polyps, and this is a presumed pathway for colorectal cancer development. It has not been possible to estimate the overall frequency of this phenomenon.

DIAGNOSIS AND MANAGEMENT

Most publications have eschewed prophylactic colectomy on the basis of the small risk of malignant transformation. A conservative approach is certainly indicated for patients with small numbers of polyps that can be managed by colonoscopic polypectomy. In patients with large numbers of polyps, colectomy may sometimes be indicated to control blood loss or anemia. In patients with numerous polyps, Järvinen and Franssila (203) have suggested that the risk of colorectal cancer at an early age justifies prophylactic colectomy with ileorectal anastomosis. Prophylactic surgery may certainly be a consideration in those patients with numerous polyps where polypectomies or biopsies have shown adenomatous change or where there is a strong family history of colorectal cancer. Although prophylactic colectomy remains a moot point in the management of these patients in general, it is generally accepted that the level of risk for colon cancer in juvenile polyposis warrants lifetime colonoscopic surveillance.

RECOMMENDATIONS FOR SURVEILLANCE IN JUVENILE POLYPOSIS AND PEUTZ–JEGHERS SYNDROME

Rectal bleeding or gastrointestinal symptoms require thorough evaluation in those at risk for familial juvenile polyposis or Peutz–Jeghers syndrome. Presymptomatic screening in at-risk individuals should begin in the second decade of life, if symptoms have not occurred by then, and include annual fecal occult blood testing and every-three-year flexible proctosigmoidoscopy. Every-three-to-five-year endoscopic investigation of the upper and lower gastrointestinal tract is indicated once the diagnosis is made, to survey and remove large, dysplastic, or bleeding polyps. Small bowel x-ray should be done at a similar interval. Periodic physical examination, including breast palpation, should be done in Peutz–Jeghers patients in view of the reported increased frequency of extraintestinal malignancies.

Cowden's Disease

This is a rare dominantly inherited disorder described by Lloyd and Dennis in 1963 (207). It is characterized by multiple facial trichilemmomas, acral keratoses, and oral mucosal polyps and reported to be associated with benign and malignant breast and thyroid neoplasms (208,209).

Multiple small polyps (2 to 5 mm) located in the rectosigmoid are a common feature (208,210). These, like the mucocutaneous lesions, have been described as hamartomas (208). They consists of a near-normal epithelium, which may show mild reparative type changes, a fibrotic stroma, and disorganized proliferation of smooth muscle in the base of the polyp. These lesions are distinct from the Peutz–Jegher's polyp and have no propensity for malignant change. Hamartomatous polyps are also described in the esophagus and proximal gastrointestinal tract (210).

Hereditary Nonpolyposis Colon Cancer Syndrome

Hereditary nonpolyposis colon cancer syndrome (HNPCC) was first defined in the 1960s by Henry Lynch (211) in a kindred that had been studied for its cancer propensity by Aldred Warthin at the beginning of the century (212). It is characterized by the development of colon cancer at a young age; the tumors are frequently multiple and favor a proximal location (Fig. 3.49). The syndrome may be associated with the occurrence of other adenocarcinomas, particularly cancers of the endometrium, ovary, and stomach (213); the two categories are often distinguished as Lynch syndrome I and II, respectively. The pattern of inheritance suggests autosomal dominant transmission with a high degree of penetrance (169,209, 214–216). In a large series of HNPCC patients, the mean age at which colon carcinoma was diagnosed was 41 years. Almost 25 percent of patients had multiple colon cancers and 60 percent of the colonic tumors were located in the right colon (compared with 34 percent in a control series) (214). HNPCC also tends to be more poorly differentiated and appears to be more likely to show mucin production (215). HNPCC may account for as many as 4 percent to 6 percent of colon cancers (217).

Adenomas in HNPCC

Although this syndrome is referred to as nonpolyposis (214) to distinguish it from familial polyposis syndromes, polyps (adenomas) are, in fact, found in association with colon cancer in HNPCC patients with a frequency comparable to that seen with sporadic carcinomas (215,217). Recent studies support the view that the pathway to cancer is through an adenoma intermediary. The adenomas from HNPCC patients are found to be larger and show a higher frequency of villous histology and high-grade dysplasia than sporadic adenomas (215), and a recent pathologic study of 50 cases of carcinoma in patients with HNPCC found residual adenoma in 12 percent. It has been suggested that "flat adenomas" (218) may occur with some frequency in the HNPCC syndrome (219).

The basic biologic defect in HNPCC has not been identified. An abnormal increase in cell turnover in crypts of the colorectal mucosa has been found by some (41) but not by all investigators (220). One study of children from affected kindreds found a spectrum of in vitro, cell-mediated, immunologic defects that suggested diminished capacity to recognize or kill incipient cancer cells (113). In view of the findings in relation to associated adenomas, a compelling hypothesis is that the basic genetic defect is one which promotes the growth of sporadically occurring adenomas.

Diagnosis

Because of the lack of a distinctive phenotype, it may be difficult to be certain if an adenoma or cancer in an individual is random, or if the lesion is occurring as part of HNPCC syndrome. A precise family history is, therefore, critical. It will often demonstrate whether the colon cancer is isolated, part of an HNPCC family, or part of a partially penetrant familial cluster of cases. To make matters more difficult, there is some evidence of even greater heterogeneity among familial cases of colon cancer than these three categories. There may be a spectrum of inherited susceptibilities ranging from those with a very

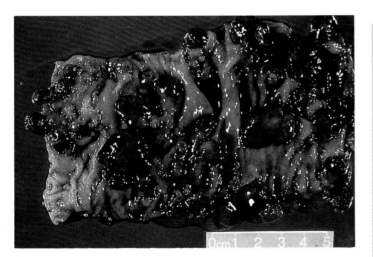

FIGURE 3.48 This segment of rectosigmoid contains numerous typical juvenile polyps; the total number present in the colon was 63. (From reference 107.)

Figure 3.49:
Hereditary Nonpolyposis Colorectal Carcinoma (HNPCC)

MAIN CLINICAL FEATURES
Early presentation (mean 41 years)
Proximal location (54% right colon)
Multiplicity frequent (24%)
Mucinous differentiation common (35–39%)

From references 215 and 217.

low to those with a very high expression of polyps and cancer. Several investigators have noted, for example, that multiple adenomas are associated with a higher familial risk. This situation may represent an intermediate syndrome yet to be well characterized. In view of such findings, it is important to define the individual familial risk within each pedigree or kindred (Fig. 3.50). Screening can then be tailored to the phenotypic characteristics occurring in the specific family situation, even if the genetic risk category cannot be well defined. Lynch syndrome II may be even more difficult to distinguish from random cancer cases because of its additional association with otherwise common extraintestinal malignancies.

Surveillance

Individuals at risk for HNPCC should have an annual fecal occult blood test and full colonoscopy every two years beginning at age 25, or beginning at an age five years younger than the age of the earliest colon cancer diagnosis in the family. Colonoscopy should be performed annually after age 35 (26).

FIGURE 3.50:
SCREENING OF RELATIVES OF THOSE WITH COLORECTAL CANCER

One first-degree relative affected with colon cancer	**Standard screening should begin by 35 to 40 years of age (annual digital rectal exam and fecal occult blood test, and, every three to five years, colonoscopy)**
Two first-degree relatives affected with colon cancer	**Annual fecal occult blood test and colonoscopy every three to five years beginning by age 35 to 40 years, or at an age five years younger than the age of the earliest colon cancer in relatives, whichever comes first**
Three or more first-degree relatives affected with the colon cancer but not polyposis coli	**HNPCC should be the presumed diagnosis until screening, as outlined for HNPCC, proves otherwise**
First-degree relative of an individual with colon cancer diagnosed at an age younger than 30 years	**Inherited syndromes (one of the polyposes or HNPCC) should be suspected**

References

1. O'Brien MJ, Winawer SJ, Zauber AG, et al., and The National Polyp Study Workgroup. The National Polyp Study: patient and polyp characteristics associated with high-grade dysplasia in colorectal adenomas. *Gastroenterology* 98: 371–379, 1990.

2. Rex DK, Lehman GA, Hawes RH, Ulbright TM, Smith JJ. Screening colonoscopy in asymptomatic average-risk persons with negative fecal occult blood tests. *Gastroenterology* 100: 64–67, 1991.

3. Stemmerman GN. Geographic epidemiology of colorectal cancer: the role of dietary fat in colorectal cancer. In: Seitz HK, Simanowski UA, Wright NA, eds. *Colorectal Cancer: Pathogenesis to Prevention*. New York: Springer-Verlag, 1989: 3–23.

4. Clark JC, Collan Y, Eide TJ, et al. Prevalence of polyps in an autopsy series from areas with varying incidence of large bowel cancer. *Int J Cancer* 36:179–186, 1985.

5. Stemmermann GN, Yataui R. Diverticulosis and polyps of the large intestine. *Cancer* 31:1260–1270, 1973.

6. Williams AR, Balasooriya BAW, Day DW. Polyps and cancer of the large bowel: a necropsy study in Liverpool. *Gut* 23: 835–842, 1982.

7. Morten H, Vatn MH, Stalsberg H. The prevalence of polyps of the large intestine in Oslo: an autopsy study. *Cancer* 49:819–825, 1982.

8. Correa P, Sting JP, Reiff A, Johnson WD. The epidemiology of colorectal polyps. Prevalence in New Orleans and international comparisons. *Cancer* 39:2258–2264, 1977.

9. Eide TJ, Stalsberg H. Polyps of the large intestine in northern Norway. *Cancer* 42:2839–2848, 1978.

10. Bombi JA. Polyps of the colon in Barcelona, Spain. An autopsy study. *Cancer* 61:1472–1476, 1988.

11. Haghighi P, Nasr K, Mohallatee EA, et al. Colorectal polyps and carcinoma in southern Iran. *Cancer* 39(1)274–278, 1977.

12. Correa P. Epidemiology of polyps and cancer. In: Morson BC, ed. *The Pathogenesis of Colorectal Cancer*. Philadelphia: W.B. Saunders, 1978:126–152.

13. Silverberg E, Lubera JA. Cancer statistics, 1988. *CA* 38:3–22, 1988.

14. Willett WC, Stampfer MJ, Colditz GA, Rosner BA, Splizer FE. Relation of meat, fat and fiber intake to the risk of colon cancer in a prospective study among women. *N Engl J Med* 323:1664–1672, 1990.

15. Armstrong B, Doll R. Environmental factors and cancer incidence and mortality in different countries with special reference to dietary practices. *Int J Cancer* 15:617–631, 1975.

16. Howel MA. Diet as an etiological factor in the development of cancers of the colon and rectum. *J Chronic Dis* 28:67–80, 1975.

17. Stemmermann G, Nomura AMY, Heilbrun LK, Mower H, Hayashi T. Colorectal cancer in Hawaiian Japanese men: a progress report. *Natl Cancer Inst Monogr* 69:125–131, 1985.

18. Kolonel LN. Fat and colon cancer: how firm is the epidemiologic evidence? *Am J Clin Nutr* 45:336–341, 1987.

19. Graham S, Dayal H, Swanson M, Mittleman A, Wilkinson G. Diet in the epidemiology of cancer of the colon and rectum. *J Natl Cancer Inst* 61(3):709–714, 1978.

20. Nauss KM, Locniskar M, Newberne PM. Effect of alteration in the quality and quantity of dietary fat on 1,2-dimethylhydrazine-induced colon tumorigenesis in rats. *Cancer Res* 43:4083–4090, 1983.

21. Nauss KM, Jacobs LR, Newberne PM. Dietary fat and fiber: relationship to caloric intake, body growth and colon tumorigenesis. *Am J Clin Nutr* 45:243–251, 1987.

22. Kritchevsky D, Weber MM, Buck CL, Klurfeld DM. Calories, fat and cancer. *Lipids* 21(4):272–274, 1986.

23. Bussey HJR. *Familial polyposis coli*. Baltimore: The Johns Hopkins University Press, 1975.

24. Gardner EJ. A genetic and clinical study of intestinal polyposis, a predisposing factor for carcinoma of the colon and rectum. *Am J Hum Genet* 3:167–176, 1951.

25. Lynch HT, Lynch PM, Albano WA, Lynch JF. The cancer family syndrome: a status report. *Dis Colon Rectum* 24:311–322, 1981.

26. Burt RW, Bishop DT, Lynch HT, Rozen P, Winawer SJ. Risk and surveillance of individual with heritable factors for colorectal cancer. *WHO Bulletin*, in press.

27. Woolf CM. A genetic study of carcinoma of the large intestine. *Am J Hum Genet* 10:42–52, 1958.

28. Macklin MT. Inheritance of cancer of the stomach and large intestine in man. *J Natl Cancer Inst* 24:551–571, 1960.

29. Lovett E. Family studies in cancer of colon and rectum. *Br J Surg* 63:13–28, 1976.

30. Duncan JI, Kyle J. Family incidence of carcinoma of the colon and rectum in North-East Scotland. *Gut* 23:169–171, 1982.

31. Anderson DE. Risk in families of patients with colon cancer. In: Winawer S, et al., eds. *Colorectal Cancer: Prevention, Epidemiology and Screening*, New York: Raven Press, 1980, 109–115.

32. Maire P, Morichau-Beauchant M, Drucker J, Barboteau, MA, Barbier J, Matuchansky C. Prevalence familiale due cancer du colon et du rectum: Resultats d'une enquete "castemoins" de 3 ans. *Gastroenterol Clin Biol* 8:22–27, 1984.

33. Ponz de Leon M, Ascari A, Antonioli A, et al. Frequency of colorectal cancer among the first-degree relatives of patients with cancer or polyps of the large bowel. *Gut* 26:A1153, 1985.

34. Maskens AP. Histogenesis of adenomatous polyps in the human large intestine. *Gastroenterology* 77:1245–1251, 1979.

35. Deschner EE, Lewis CM, Lipkin M. In-vitro study of human rectal epithelial cells. I. Atypical zone of H3-thymidine incorporation in mucosa of multiple polyposis. *J Clin Invest* 42:1922–1928, 1963.

36. Maskens AP, Deschner EE. H3-thymidine incorporation into epithelial cells of normal appearing colorectal mucosa of cancer patients. *J Natl Cancer Inst* 58:1221–1224, 1977.

37. Deschner AP. Mechanisms of adenoma formation in the colon. In: Levin B, Riddel RH, eds. *Frontiers in Gastrointestinal Cancer*. New York: Elsevier, 1984:249–259.

38. Lane N, Lev R. Observations on the origin of adenomatous epithelium of the colon. *Cancer* 16:751–764, 1963.

39. Usugane M, Fujita M, Lipkin M, Palmer R, Friedman E, Augenlicht L. Cell proliferation in explant cultures of human colon. *Digestion* 24:224–233, 1982.

40. Lipkin M, Blattner WE, Gardner EJ, et al. Classification and risk assessment of individuals with familial polyposis, Gardner's syndrome, and familial non-polyposis colon cancer from H3-thymidine labelling patterns in colonic epithelial cells. *Cancer Res* 44:4201–4207, 1984.

41. Lipkin M, Blattner WE, Fraumeni JF Jr, Lynch HT, Deschner EE, Winawer S. Tritiated thymidine labelling distribution as a marker for hereditary predisposition to colon cancer. *Cancer Res* 43:1899–1904, 1983.

42. Johnston PJ, O'Brien MJ, Dervan PA, Carney DN. Immunohistochemical analysis of cell kinetic parameters in colonic adenocarcinomas, adenomas and normal mucosa. *Hum Pathol* 20(7):696–700, 1989.

43. Fearon ER, Hamilton SR, Vogelstein B. Clonal analysis of human colorectal tumours. *Science* 238:193–196, 1987.

44. Winawer SJ, Zauber A, Diaz B, et al. The National Polyp Study: overview of program and preliminary report of patient and polyp characteristics. In: Steele GJ, Burt R, Winawer SJ, Karr J, eds. *Basic and Clinical Perspectives of Colorectal Polyps and Cancer*. New York: Alan R. Liss, 1988.

45. Konishi F, Morson BC. Pathology of colorectal adenomas: a colonoscopic survey. *J Clin Pathol* 35:830–841, 1982.

46. Jass JR, Sobin LH. *World Health Organization international classification of tumors, histological typing of intestinal tumors*. New York: Springer-Verlag, 1989.

47. Fung CHK, Goldman H. The incidence and significance of villous change in adenomatous polyps. *Am J Clin Pathol* 53: 21–25, 1970.

48. Hermanek P, Frühmorgen P, Guggenmoos-Holzmann I, Altendorf A, Matek W. The malignant potential of colorectal polyps—a new statistical approach. *Endoscopy* 15:16–20, 1983.

49. Takahashi T, Iwama N. Three dimensional microstructure of gastrointestinal tumours: gland pattern and its diagnostic significance. *Pathol Annu* 1:419–440, 1985.

50. Riddel RH, Goldman H, Ransohoff DF, et al. Dysplasia in inflammatory bowel disease: standardized classification with provisional clinical applications. *Hum Pathol* 14:931–968, 1983.

51. Muto T, Bussey HJR, Morson BC. The evolution of cancer of the colon and rectum. *Cancer* 36:2251–2270, 1975.

52. Berge T, Ekelund G, Meffner C, Phil B, Wenckert A. Carcinoma of the colon and rectum in a defined population. *Acta Chir Scand* 438 (Suppl): 1–86, 1973.

53. O'Brien MJ, Gottlieb LS, Sternberg SS, Winawer SJ, Zauber A, Diaz B, and the NPS workgroup. National Polyp Study, relevance of anatomic location to the evolution of colorectal adenomas. *Lab Invest* 58 (Abstract):68A, 1988.

54. National Cancer Institute. *Surveillance, epidemiology, and end results, incidence and mortality data 1973–1977.* NIH Publication No. 81-2330: 66–67, 1981.

55. Matek W, Hermanek P, Demling L. Is the adenoma-carcinoma sequence contradicted by the differing location of colorectal adenomas and carcinomas? *Endoscopy* 18:17–19, 1986.

56. Hill MJ, Morson BC, Bussey HJR. Aetiology of adenoma-carcinoma sequence in large bowel. *Lancet* i:245–247, 1978.

57. Jackman RJ, Mayo CW. The adenoma-carcinoma sequence in cancer of the colon. *Surg Gynecol Obstet* 93:327–330, 1951.

58. Stryker SJ, Wolff BE, Culp CE, Libbe SD, Ipstrup DM, MacCarty RL. Natural history of untreated colonic polyps. *Gastroenterology* 93:1009–1013, 1987.

59. Lockhart-Mummery JP, Dukes C. The precancerous changes in the rectum and colon. *Surg Gynecol Obstet* 46:591–596, 1928.

60. Morson BC. The polyp-cancer sequence in the large bowel. *Proc R Soc Med* 67:451–457, 1974.

61. Dukes CE. Simple tumours of the large intestine and their relation to cancer. *Br J Surg* 13:720–733, 1926.

62. Lane N. The precursor tissue of ordinary large bowel carcer. *Cancer Res* 36:2669–2671, 1976.

63. Morson BC. The evolution of colorectal carcinoma. *Clin Radiol* 35:425–431, 1984.

64. Day DW, Morson BC. The adenoma-carcinoma sequence, In: Morson BC, ed. *The Pathogenesis of Colorectal Cancer.* Philadelphia: W.B. Saunders, 1978:58–71.

65. Eide TJ. Remnants of adenomas in colorectal carcinomas. *Cancer* 51:1866–1872, 1983.

66. Heald RJ, Bussey HJR. Clinical experience at St Mark's Hospital with multiple synchronous cancers of the colon and rectum. *Dis Colon Rectum* 18:6–10, 1975.

67. Sobin LH. Inverted hyperplastic polyps of the colon. *Am J Surg Pathol* 9:265–272, 1985.

68. Bodmer WF, Bailey CJ, Bodmer J, et al. Localization of the gene for familial adenomatous polyposis on chromosome 5. *Nature* 328:614–619, 1987.

69. Leppert M, Dobbs M, Scambler P, et al. The gene for familial polyposis coli maps to the long arm of chromosome 5. *Science* 238:1411–1413, 1987.

70. Eide TJ. Risk of colorectal cancer in adenoma-bearing individuals within a defined population. *Int J Cancer* 38:173–176, 1986.

71. Grinnell RS, Lane N. Benign and malignant adenomatous polyps and papillary adenomas of the colon and rectum. An analysis of 1856 tumours in 1335 patients. *Int Abst Surg* 106:519–538, 1958.

72. Vogelstein B, Fearon ER, Hamilton SR, et al. Genetic alterations during colorectal tumor development. *N Engl J Med* 319:525–532, 1988.

73. Lowy DR, Willamsen BM. The ras gene family. *Cancer Surv* 5:275–289, 1986.

74. Bos JL, Fearon ER, Hamilton SR, et al. Prevalence of ras gene mutations in human colorectal cancers. *Nature* 327:293–297, 1987.

75. Forrester K, Almoguira C, Han K, Grizzle WE, Perucho M. Detection of high incidence of K-ras oncogenes during human colon tumorigenesis. *Nature* 327:298–303, 1987.

76. Stanbridge EJ. Identifying tumor suppressor genes in human colorectal cancer. *Science* 274:12–13, 1990.

77. Fearon ER, Cho KR, Nigro JM, et al. Identification of a chromosome 18 gene that is altered in colorectal cancers. *Science* 247:49–55, 1990.

78. Mant A, Bokey EL, Chapuis PH, et al. Rectal bleeding. Do other symptoms aid in diagnosis? *Dis Colon Rectum* 32(3): 191–196, 1989.

79. Waye JD, Braunfeld S. Surveillance intervals after colonoscopic polypectomy. *Endoscopy* 14:79–81, 1982.

80. Bat L, Williams CB. Usefulness of pediatric colonoscopes in adult colonoscopy. *Gastrointest Endosc* 35:329–332, 1989.

81. Christie JP. Polypectomy or colectomy? Management of 106 consecutively encountered colorectal polyps. *Am Surg* 54: 93–99, 1988.

82. Williams CB, Whiteway JE, Jass JR. Practical aspects of endoscopic management of malignant polyps. *Endoscopy* 19: 31–37, 1987.

83. Cohen LB, Waye JD. Treatment of colonic polyps–practical considerations. *Clin Gastroenterol* 15(2):359–376, 1986.

84. Waye JD. The post polypectomy coagulation syndrome. *Gastrointest Endosc* 27:1984, 1981.

85. Lambert R, Sobin LH, Waye JD, Stadler GA. The management of patients with colorectal adenomas. In: Holleb A, ed. *Third International Symposium on Colorectal Cancer.* New York: American Cancer Society, 1984:43–52.

86. Winawer SJ, Williams C, Frühmorgen P, Grigioni W, Kronborg O, Morson BC. Colorectal adenoma patients. Risk of cancer and results of follow-up. *ROMA 88 Working Team Report* - No. 11 (Summary). Rome, Italy, Sept. 4–11.

87. Morson BC, Whiteway JE, Jones EA, Macrae FA, Williams CB. Histopathology and prognosis of malignant colorectal polyps treated by endoscopic polypectomy. *Gut* 25:437–444, 1984.

88. Muller S, Chesner IM, Egan MJ, et al. Significance of venous and lymphatic invasion in malignant polyps of the colon and rectum. *Gut* 30:1385–1391, 1989.

89. Rossini FP, Ferrari A, Coverlizza S, et al. Large bowel adenomas containing carcinoma—a diagnostic and therapeutic approach. *Int J Color Dis* 3:47–52, 1988.

90. Sugihara K, Muto T, Morioka Y. Management of patients with invasive carcinoma removed by colonoscopic polypectomy. *Dis Colon Rectum* 32:829–834, 1989.

91. Ehrinpreis MN, Kinzie JL, Jaszewski R, Peleman RL. Management of the malignant polyp. *Gastroenterol Clin North Am* 17:837–850, 1988.

92. Cranley JP, Petras RE, Carey WD, Paradis K, Sivak MV. When is endoscopic polypectomy adequate therapy for colonic polyps containing invasive carcinoma? *Gastroenterology* 91:419–427, 1986.

93. Lipper S, Kahn LB, Ackerman LV. The significance of microscopic invasive cancer in endoscopically removed polyps of the large bowel. A clinicopathologic study of 51 cases. *Cancer* 52:1691–1699, 1983.

94. Langer JC, Cohen A, Taylor BR, Stafford S, Jeejeebhoy KN, Cullen JB. Management of patients with polyps containing malignancy removed by colonoscopic polypectomy. *Dis Colon Rectum* 27:6–9, 1984.

95. Wilcox GM, Beck JR. Early invasive cancer in adenomatous colonic polyps ("malignant polyps"). Evaluation of the therapeutic options by decision analysis. *Gastroenterology* 92:1159–1168, 1987.

96. Riddell RH. Hands off "cancerous" large bowel polyps. *Gastroenterology* 89:432–435, 1985.

97. Fried GM, Hreno A, Duguid WP, Hampson LG. Rational management of malignant colon polyps based on long-term follow-up. *Surgery* 96:815–821, 1984.

98. Haggitt RC, Glotzbach RE, Soffer EE, Wruble LD. Prognostic factors in colorectal carcinomas arising in adenomas: implications for lesions removed by endoscopic polypectomy. *Gastroenterology* 89:328–336, 1985.

99. Cooper HS. Surgical pathology of endoscopically removed malignant polyps of the colon and rectum. *Am J Surg Pathol* 7:613–623, 1983.

100. Eckardt VF, Fuchs M, Kanzler G, Remmele W, Stienen U. Follow-up of patients with colonic polyps containing severe atypia and invasive carcinoma. *Cancer* 61:2552–2557, 1988.

101. Richards WO, Webb WA, Morris SJ, et al. Patient management after endoscopic removal of the cancerous colon adenoma. *Ann Surg* 205:665–672, 1987.

102. Greenburg AG, Saik RP, Coyle JJ, Peskin GW. Mortality and gastrointestinal surgery in the aged. *Arch Surg* 116:788–791, 1981.

103. Hayashi T, Yatani R, Apostol J, Stemmerman GN. Pathogenesis of hyperplastic polyps of the colon: a hypothesis based on ultrastructure and in vitro cell kinetics. *Gastroenterology* 66:347–356, 1974.

104. Kay GI, Fenoglio CM, Pascal RR, Lane N. Comparative electron microscopic features of normal, hyperplastic and adenomatous human colonic epithelium. *Gastroenterology* 64: 926–945, 1973.

105. Lane N, Kaplan H, Pascal RR. Minute adenomatous and hyperplastic polyps of the colon: divergent patterns of epithelial growth with specific associated mesenchymal changes. *Gastroenterology* 60:537–551, 1971.

106. Arthur JF. Structure and significance of metaplastic nodules in the rectal mucosa. *J Clin Pathol* 21:735–743, 1968.

107. Mitros FA. *Atlas of gastrointestinal pathology.* New York: Gower Medical Publishing, 1988.

108. Waye JD. Hyperplastic colon polyps—are they markers? *Ann Intern Med* 109:851–852, 1988.

109. Chapuis PH, Goulston KJ. Clinical accuracy in the diagnosis of small polyps using the flexible fiberoptic sigmoidoscope. *Dis Colon Rectum* 25:669–672, 1982.

110. Neale AV, Demers RY, Budev H, Scott RO. Physician accuracy in diagnosing colorectal polyps. *Dis Colon Rectum* 30:247–250, 1987.

111. Norfleet RG, Ryan ME, Wyman JP. Adenomatous and hyperplastic polyps cannot be reliably distinguished by their appearance through the fiberoptic sigmoidoscope. *Dig Dis Sci* 33(9):1175–1177, 1988.

112. Williams GT, Arthur JF, Bussey HJR, Morson BC. Metaplastic polyps and polyposis of the colorectum. *Histopathology* 4:155–170, 1980.

113. Urbanski SJ, Kossakowska AE, Marcon N, Bruce WR. Mixed hyperplastic adenomatous polyps—an underdiagnosed entity. Report of a case of adenocarcinoma arising within a mixed hyperplastic adenomatous polyp. *Am J Surg Pathol* 8:551–556, 1984.

114. Cooper HS, Patchefsky AS, Marks G. Adenomatous and carcinomatous changes within hyperplastic colonic epithelium. *Dis Colon Rectum* 22:152–156, 1979.

115. Franzin G, Novelli P. Adenocarcinoma occurring in a hyperplastic (metaplastic) polyp of the colon. *Endoscopy* 14:28–30, 1982.

116. Longacre Teri A, Fenoglio-Preiser CM. Mixed hyperplasia adenomatous polyps/serrated adenomas. *Am J Surg Pathol* 14:524–537, 1990.

117. Franzin G, Zamboni G, Scarpa A, Dina R, Iannucci A, Novelli P. Hyperplastic (metaplastic) polyps of the colon. A histologic and histochemical study. *Am J Surg Pathol* 8: 687–698, 1984.

118. Tedesco FJ, Hendrix JC, Pickens CA, Brady PG, Mills LR. Diminutive polyps: histopathology, spatial distribution, and clinical significance. *Gastrointest Endosc* 28:1–5, 1982.

119. Church JM, Fazio VW, Jones IT. Small colorectal polyps.

Are they worth treating? *Dis Colon Rectum* 31:50–53, 1988.

120. Zauber A, Winawer SJ, Diaz B, O'Brien M, et al. The National Polyp Study (NPS): the association of colonic hyperplastic polyps and adenomas. *Am J Gastroenterol* 83 (Abstract): 1060, 1988.

121. Jass JR. Relation between metaplastic polyp and carcinoma of the colorectum. *Lancet* 1:28–30, 1983.

122. Ansher AF, Lewis JH, Fleischer DE, et al. Hyperplastic colonic polyps as a marker for adenomatous colonic polyps. *Am J Gastroenterol* 84:113–117, 1989.

123. Achkar E, Carey W. Small polyps found during fiberoptic sigmoidoscopy in asymptomatic patients. *Ann Intern Med* 109:880–883, 1988.

124. Provenzale D, Garrett JW, Condon SW, Sandler RS. Risk for colon adenomas in patients with rectosigmoid hyperplastic polyps. *Ann Intern Med* 113:760–763, 1990.

125. Winawer SJ. Views on the biology and clinical significance of hyperplastic polyps. *Am J Gastroenterol* 85(4):367–370, 1990.

126. Granqvist S, Gabrielsson N, Sundelin P. Diminutive colonic polyps: clinical significance and management. *Endoscopy* 11:36–42, 1979.

127. Waye JD, Lewis BS, Frankel A, Geller SA. Small colon polyps. *Am J Gastroenterol* 83:120–122, 1988.

128. Feczko PJ, Bernstein MA, Halpert RD, Ackerman LV. Small colonic polyps: a reappraisal of their significance. *Radiology* 152:301–303, 1984.

129. Ryan ME, Norfleet RG, Kirchner JP, et al. The significance of diminutive colonic polyps found at flexible sigmoidoscopy. *Gastrointest Endosc* 35(2):85–89, 1989.

130. Morson BC. Some peculiarities in the histology of intestinal polyps. *Dis Colon Rectum* 5:337–344, 1961.

131. Roth SI, Helwing EB. Juvenile polyps of the colon and rectum. *Cancer* 16:468–479, 1963.

132. Mazier WP, Bowman HE, Sun KH, Muldoon JP. Juvenile polyps of the colon and rectum. *Dis Colon Rectum* 17:523–527, 1974.

133. Helwig EB. Adenomas of large intestine in children. *Am J Dis Child* 72:289–295, 1946.

134. McColl I, Bussey HJR, Veale AMD, Morson BC. Juvenile polyposis coli. *Proc R Soc Med* 57:896–897, 1964.

135. Horrilleno EG, Eckert C, Ackerman LV. Polyps of the rectum and colon in children. *Cancer* 10:1210–1220, 1957.

136. Silverstein FE, Tytgat GNJ. *Atlas of gastrointestinal endoscopy.* New York: Gower Medical Publishing, 1987.

137. Kelly JK, Gabos S. The pathogenesis of inflammatory polyps. *Dis Colon Rectum* 30:251–254, 1987.

138. De Dombal FT, Watts JMcK, Watkinson G, Goligher JC. Local complications of ulcerative colitis: stricture, pseudopolyposis and carcinoma of the colon and rectum. *Br Med J* 1:1442–1477, 1966.

139. Jalan KN, Sircus W, Walker RJ, McManus JPA, Prescott RJ, Card WI. Pseudopolyposis in ulcerative colitis. *Lancet* 2:555–559, 1969.

140. Teague RH, Read AE. Polyposis in ulcerative colitis. *Gut* 16:792–795, 1975.

141. Goldgraber M. Pseudopolyps in ulcerative colitis. *Dis Colon Rectum* 8:335–363, 1965.

142. Levine DS, Surawiz CM, Spencer GD, Rohrmann CA, Silverstein FE. Inflammatory polyposis two years after ischemic colon injury. *Dig Dis Sci* 10:1159–1167, 1986.

143. Hinrichs HR, Goldman H. Localised giant pseudopolyps of the colon. *JAMA* 205:108–109, 1968.

144. Kelly JK, Langevin JM, Price LM, Hershfield NB, Share S, Blustein P. Giant and symptomatic inflammatory polyps of the colon in idiopathic inflammatory bowel disease. *Am J Surg Pathol* 10:420–425, 1986.

145. Hussein AM, Medany S, Abou-el-Madg AM, Sherif SM, Williams CB. Multiple endoscopic polypectomies for schitosomal polyposis of the colon. *Lancet* 1:673–674, 1983.

146. Lobert PF, Appleman HD. Inflammatory cloacogenic polyp: a clinical inflammatory lesion of the anal transition zone. *Am J Surg Pathol* 5:761, 1981.

147. Saul SH. Inflammatory cloacogenic polyp: relationship to solitary rectal ulcer syndrome/mucosal prolapse and other bowel disorders. *Hum Pathol* 18:1120–1125, 1987.

148. Kelly JK. Polypoid prolapsing colonic mucosal folds in diverticular disease. *AJCP* 94:500A, 1990.

149. Franzin G, Fratton A, Manfrini C. Polypoid lesions associated with diverticular disease of the sigmoid colon. *Gastrointest Endosc* 31:196–199, 1985.

150. Burke P, Sobin LH. Eroded polypoid hyperplasia of the rectosigmoid. *Am J Gastroenterol* 85:975–980, 1990.

151. Morson BC. Histopathology of the small intestine. *Proc R Soc Med* 52:6–10, 1959.

152. Price AB. Benign lymphoid polyps and inflammatory polyps. In: Morson BC, ed. *The Pathogenesis of Colorectal Cancer*. Baltimore: W.B. Saunders, 1978: 33–42.

153. Watanabe H, Margulis AR, Harter L. The occurrence of lymphoid cell nodules in the colon of adults. *J Clin Gastroenterol* 5:535–539, 1983.

154. Ranchod M, Kevin KJ, Dorfman RF. Lymphoid hyperplasia of the gastrointestinal tract: a study of 26 cases and review of the literature. *Am J Surg Pathol* 12:383–398, 1978.

155. Sauven P, Ridge JA, Quan SH, Sigurdson ER. Anorectal carcinoid tumors. Is aggressive surgery warranted? *Ann Surg* 211:67–71, 1990.

156. Federspiel BH, Burke AP, Sobin LH, Shekitka KM. Rectal and colonic carcinoids. A clinicopathologic study of 84 cases. *Cancer* 65:135–140, 1990.

157. Ishikawa H, Imanishi K, Otani JT, Okuda S, Tatsuta M, Ishiguro S. Effectiveness of endoscopic treatment of carcinoid tumors of the rectum. *Endoscopy* 21:133–135, 1989.

158. Burke M, Shepherd N, Mann CV. Carcinoid tumors of the rectum and anus. *Br J Surg* 74:358–361, 1987.

159. Hochberg FH, DaSilva AB, Galdabini J, Richardson EP. Gastrointestinal involvement in von Recklinghausen's neurofibromatosis. *Neurology* 24:1144–1151, 1974.

160. Haggitt RC, Reid BJ. Hereditary gastrointestinal polyposis syndromes. *Am J Surg Pathol* 10:871–887, 1986.

161. Misiewicz JJ, et al. *Atlas of clinical gastroenterology*. New York: Gower Medical Publishing, 1985.

162. Lewis RA, Crowder WF, Eierman LA, Naussbaum RL, Ferrell RE. The Gardner syndrome: significance of ocular features. *Ophthalmology* 91:916–925, 1984.

163. Bussey HJR, Morson BC. Familial polyposis coli. In: Lipkin M, Good RA, eds. *Gastrointestinal Tract Cancer*. New York: Plenum, 1978:275–294.

164. Corvisart L. Hypertrophie partielle de la muqueuse intestinale. *Bull Soc Anat* 22:400, 1847.

165. Cripps WH. Two cases of disseminated polyps of the rectum. *Trans Pathol Soc London* 33:165–168, 1882.

166. Handford H. Disseminated polypi of the large intestine becoming malignant. *Trans Pathol Soc London* 41:133, 1890.

167. Dukes C. The heredity factor in polyposis intestine or multiple adenomata. *Cancer Rev Brist* 5:241–256, 1930.

168. Lockhart-Mummery HE, Dukes CE. Familial adenomatosis of the colon and rectum. *Lancet* 2:586–589, 1939.

169. Goldman H, Ming S, Hickok DF. Nature and significance of hyperplastic polyps of the human colon. *Arch Pathol* 89:349–354, 1970.

170. Gardner EJ, Plenk HP. Hereditary pattern for multiple osteomas in a family group. *Am J Hum Genet* 4:31–36, 1952.

171. Gardner EJ, Richards RC. Multiple cutaneous and subcutaneous lesions occurring simultaneously with hereditary polyposis and osteomatosis. *Am J Hum Genet* 5:137–147, 1953.

172. Turcot J, Despres J-P, St. Pierre F. Malignant tumors of the central nervous system associated with familial polyposis of the colon: report of two cases. *Dis Colon Rectum* 2:465–468, 1959.

173. Banughman F, List CF, Williams JR, Muldoon JP, Segarra JM, Volkel JS. The glioma-polyposis syndrome. *N Engl J Med* 281:1345–1346, 1969.

174. Sayed AK, Jafri SZH, Shenoy SS. Intestinal polyposis and brain tumor in a family. *Dis Colon Rectum* 22:486–491, 1979.

175. Lewis JH, Ginsberg AI, Toomey KE. Turcot's syndrome, evidence for autosomal dominant inheritance. *Cancer* 51:524–528, 1983.

176. Thompson JS, Harned RK, Anderson JC, et al. Papillary carcinoma of the thyroid and familial polyposis coli. *Dis Colon Rectum* 26:583–585, 1983.

177. Järvinen H, Nyberg M, Peltokallio P. Upper gastrointestinal tract polyps in familial adenomatosis coli. *Dis Colon Rectum* 26:525–528, 1983.

178. Kingston JE, Herbert A, Draper GJ, et al. Association between hepatoblastoma and polyposis coli. *Arch Dis Child* 58:959–962, 1983.

179. Bussey HJR, Veale AMO, Morson BC. Genetics of gastrointestinal polyposis. *Gastroenterology* 74:1325–1330, 1978.

180. Lynch HT, Lynch PM, Follett KL, Harris RE. Familial polyposis coli: heterogeneous polyp expression in 2 kindreds. *J Med Genet* 16:1–7, 1979.

181. Bussey HJR. Polyposis syndromes. In: Morson BC, ed. *Pathogenesis of Colorectal Cancer*. Philadelphia: W.B. Saunders, 1978: 81–94.

182. Utsunomiya J, Iwama T. Adenomatosis coli in Japan. In: Winawer SJ, Schottenfeld D, Sherlock P, eds. *Colorectal Cancer: Prevention, Epidemiology and Screening*. New York: Raven Press, 1980.

183. Yao T, Iida M, Ohsato K, Watanabe H, Omae T. Duodenal lesions in familial polyposis of the colon. *Gastroenterology* 73: 1086–1092, 1977.

184. Burt RW, Berenson MM, Lee GR, Tolman KG, Freston JW, Gardner EJ. Upper gastrointestinal polyps in Gardner's syndrome. *Gastroenterology* 36:295–301, 1984.

185. Bulow S, Lauritsen KB, Johansen A, Svendsen LB, Sondergaard JO. Gastroduodenal polyps in familial polyposis coli. *Gastroenterology* 4:61–64, 1985.

186. Ranzi T, Castagnone D, Velio P, Bianchi P, Polli EE. Gastric and duodenal polyps in familial polyposis coli. *Gut* 22: 363–367, 1981.

187. Järvinen H, Nyberg M, Peltokallio P. Upper gastrointestinal tract polyps in familial adenomatosis coli. *Gut* 24:333–339, 1983.

188. Watanabe H, Enjoji M, Yao T, Ohsato K. Gastric lesions in familial adenomatosis coli: their incidence and histologic analysis. *Hum Pathol* 9:269–283, 1978.

189. Iida M, Tsuneyoshi Y, Itoh H, et al. Natural history of fundic gland polyposis in patients with familial adenomatosis coli/Gardner's syndrome. *Gastroenterology* 89:1021–1025, 1985.

190. Watne AL, Lai V-Y, Carrier J, Coppula W. The diagnosis and surgical treatment of patients with Gardner's syndrome. *Surgery* 82:327–333, 1977.

191. Herrera L, Kakati S, Gibas L, Pietrzak E, Sandberg A. Brief clinical report: Gardner syndrome in a man with an interstitial deletion of 5q. *Am J Med Genet* 25:473–476, 1986.

192. Peutz JLA. Over een zeer merkwaardige, gecombineerde familiaire polyposis van de slymoliezen van den tractus intestinalis met die van de neuskeelholte en gepaard met ligenaardige pigmentaties van huid-en slymoliezen. *Ned Nschn Geneesk* 10:134–146, 1921.

193. Jeghers H, McKusick VA, Katz KH. Generalized intestinal polyposis and melanin spots of the oral mucosa, lips and digits: a syndrome of diagnostic significance. *N Engl J Med* 241:993–1005, 1949.

194. Watne AL. Patterns of inheritance of colonic polyps. *Semin Surg Oncol* 3:71–76, 1987.

195. Reid JD. Intestinal Carcinoma in the Peutz-Jeghers syndrome. *JAMA* 7:833–834, 1974.

196. Scully RE. Sex cord tumor with annular tubules: a distinctive ovarian tumor of the Peutz-Jeghers syndrome. *Cancer* 25:1107, 1970.

197. Young RH, Welch WR, Dickersin GR, Scully SE. Ovarian sex cord tumor with annular tubules. Review of 74 cases including 27 with Peutz-Jeghers syndrome and 4 with adenoma malignum of the cervix. *Cancer* 50:1384, 1982.

198. Burdick D, Prior JT. Peutz–Jeghers syndrome: a clinicopathologic study of a large family with a 27-year follow-up. *Cancer* 50:2139–2146, 1982.

199. Hood AB, Krush MS. Clinical and dermatologic aspects of the hereditary intestinal polyposes. *Dis Colon Rectum* 8: 546–548, 1983.

200. Cochet B, Carrel J, Desbaillets L, Widgren S. Peutz-Jeghers syndrome associated with gastrointestinal carcinoma. Report of two cases in a family. *Gut* 20:169–175, 1979.

201. Wennstrom J, Pierce ER, McKusick VA. Hereditary benign and malignant lesions of the large bowel. *Cancer* 34:850–857, 1974.

202. Perzin KH, Bridge MF. Adenomatous and carcinomatous changes in hamartomatous polyps of the small intestine. Peutz-Jeghers syndrome: report of a case and review of the literature. *Cancer* 49:971–983, 1982.

203. Järvinen H, Franssila KO. Familial juvenile polyposis coli; increased risk of colorectal cancer. *Gut* 25:792–800, 1984.

204. Goodman ZD, Yardley JH, Milligan FD. Pathogenesis of colonic polyps in multiple juvenile polyposis. Report of a case associated with gastric polyps and carcinoma of the rectum. *Cancer* 43:1906–1913, 1979.

205. Ramaswamy G, Elhosseiny AA, Tchertkoff V. Juvenile polyposis of the colon with atypical adenomatous changes and carcinoma in-situ. *Dis Colon Rectum* 27:393–398, 1984.

206. Grotsky HW, Rickert RR, Smith WD, Newsome JF. Familial juvenile polyposis coli. A clinical and pathologic study of a large kindred. *Gastroenterology* 82:494–501, 1982.

207. Lloyd KN, Dennis M. Cowden's disease. A possible new symptom complex with multiple system involvement. *Ann Intern Med* 58:136–142, 1963.

208. Carlson GJ, Nivatvongs S, Snover DC. Colorectal polyps in Cowden's disease (multiple hamartoma syndrome). *Am J Surg Pathol* 8:763–770, 1984.

209. Brownstein MH, Wolf M, Bikowski JB. Cowden's disease: a cutaneous marker for breast cancer. *Cancer* 41:2393–2398, 1971.

210. Gorensek M, Matko I, Skralovnik A, Rode M, Satler J, Jutersek A. Disseminated hereditary gastrointestinal polyposis with orocutaneous hamartomatous. *Endoscopy* 16:59–63, 1984.

211. Lynch HT, Shaw MW, Magnuson CW et al. Hereditary factors in colon cancer. Study of two large Midwestern kindreds. *Arch Intern Med* 117:206–212, 1966.

212. Warthin AS. Heredity with reference to carcinoma: as shown by the study of the cases examined in the pathological laboratory of the University of Michigan, 1895–1913. *Arch Intern Med* 12:546–555, 1913.

213. Lynch HT, Rozen P, Schuelke GS. Hereditary colon cancer: polyposis and nonpolyposis variants. *CA* 35:95–115, 1985.

214. Mecklin JP, Järvinen HJ. Clinical features of colorectal carcinoma in cancer family syndrome. *Dis Colon Rectum* 29: 160–164, 1986.

215. Mecklin JP, Sipponen P, Järvinen HJ. Histopathology of colorectal carcinomas and adenomas in cancer family syndrome. *Dis Colon Rectum* 29:849–853, 1986.

216. Mecklin JP, Järvinen HJ, Peltolkallio P. Cancer family syndrome, genetic analysis of 22 Finnish kindreds. *Gastroenterology* 90:328–333, 1986.

217. Mecklin JP. Frequency of hereditary colorectal carcinoma. *Gastroenterology* 93:1021–1025, 1987.

218. Adachi M, Muto T, Morioka Y, Ikenaga T, Hara M. Flat adenoma and flat mucosal carcinoma (116 type)—a new precursor of colorectal carcinoma? *Dis Colon Rectum* 31:236–243, 1988.

219. Lynch HT, Smyrk T, Lanspa SJ, et al. Flat adenomas in a colon cancer-prone kindred. *J Natl Cancer Inst* 80:278–282, 1988.

220. Markowitz JF, Aiges HW, Cunningham-Rundles S, et al. Cancer family syndrome: marker studies. *Gastroenterology* 91: 581–589, 1986.

221. Groden J, Theiveris A, Samowitz W, et al. Identification and characterization of the familial adenomatous polyposis coli gene. *Cell* 66:589–600, 1991.

222. Kinzler KW, Nilbert MC, Su L, et al. Identification of FAP locus genes from chromosome 5q21. *Science* 253:661-664, 1991.

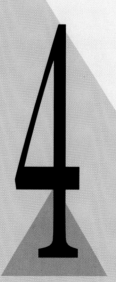

Colorectal Cancer

Sidney J. Winawer,
Warren E. Enker,
and Bernard Levin

Malignant tumors of the colon and rectum may be classified as either primary or metastatic. Primary malignant tumors are those arising within the colon and rectum. The most common malignant tumors of the colon and rectum are primary malignancies, and within this group adenocarcinoma is the most frequent. Epidermoid carcinomas of the anus and other primary adenocarcinomas of the rectum arising at the squamocolumnar junction are much less frequent (1).

Other types of tumors that rarely originate in to the large bowel include leiomyosarcomas, lymphomas, and malignant carcinoid tumors. In addition, lymphoma, leiomyosarcoma, malignant melanoma, and cancer of the breast, ovary, prostate, or lung, as well as other gastrointestinal tumors, can metastasize to the large bowel. This chapter will focus on primary colorectal cancer, especially adenocarcinoma.

Colorectal cancer is a neoplasm of worldwide importance, ranking among the three leading cancers with an incidence of approximately one million cases and a mortality of 500,000 annually worldwide (Fig. 4.1) (2). This cancer is particularly prevalent in Western countries (3). While the high incidence of colorectal cancer has always been a basis for intensive research, conceptual and technologic advances in recent years have added new dimensions to our understanding of this cancer. We now have a clearer insight, for example, into the premalignant adenoma stage, the role of genetic and environmental factors, mechanisms of growth regulation in the colonic mucosa, and high-risk groups. More effective endoscopic and surgical tools have also been developed, and we are beginning to realize benefits from these and other new modalities of treatment.

EPIDEMIOLOGY
Overall Incidence

The incidence of colorectal cancer varies widely around the world (Figs. 4.2–4.4). High rates are typical of more developed countries in North America, Western Europe, and New Zealand, while lower rates are found in Eastern Europe, most South American countries, Asia, and Africa. Incidence rates for colon cancer range from 1.3 cases per 100,000 in Nigeria to 30 per 100,000 in the United States. For cancer of the rectum, rates range from 1.2 per 100,000 in Nigeria to 18.2 per 100,000 in the United States. The rates of these two cancers generally parallel each other and hence they are often combined as colorectal cancer. In addition, many tumors are difficult to localize clinically to either the rectum or the colon.

Incidence rates have been correlated with other factors within countries. High rates have been linked with higher income and higher education levels. The higher rates previously reported in urban residents as compared to rural residents have disappeared, however, perhaps because more detailed approximations of dietary patterns have been obtained for both groups. Also, regional variations within countries usually cannot be explained purely by differences in socioeconomic levels or dietary patterns. Mortality rates parallel incidence rates worldwide (4). The five-year survival rate for colorectal cancer is now approximately 50 percent,

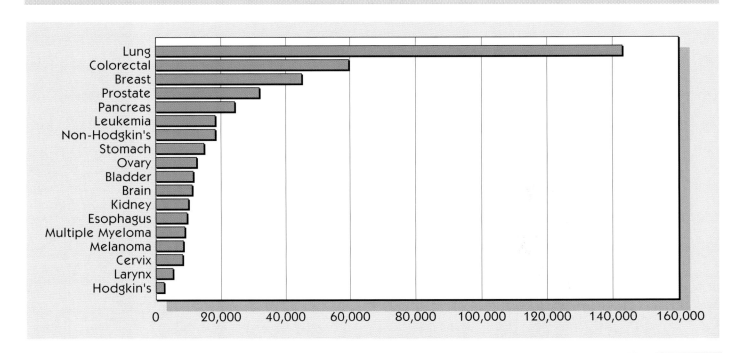

FIGURE 4.1 United States cancer mortality by anatomic site. Lung, colon-rectum, and breast are the leading three sites. Skin cancer is not included. (From reference 91.)

but a lower survival (34 percent) is seen for rectal cancer in blacks in the United States (3,4).

Age and Sex

The age-specific incidence rate of colorectal cancer begins to rise at age 40 and rises more steeply at age 50. Cancer in younger age groups usually occurs in conjunction with personal or familial risk factors. Colon cancer affects men and women at similar rates, while rectal cancer is more common in men (see Fig. 4.2) (4).

Time Trends

The incidence of colorectal cancer has been increasing worldwide during the past several decades. This increase has been seen not only in high-incidence Western countries such as the United States but also in countries such as Japan where the rate had been lower in the past. This may be due in part to Westernization of diet. On the other hand, the mortality rate has leveled off and has even shown a decline in some areas, including high-incidence countries such as the United States and Germany. The growing gap between rising incidence and declining mortality may be due to several factors, such as continued presence of environmental and dietary carcinogens, as well as the increased longevity of populations, is offset by earlier and more accurate diagnosis and improved surgical techniques (Fig. 4.5).

Trends in Anatomic Location

In countries with a high incidence of colorectal cancer, an anatomic clustering of colorectal cancer occurs in the sigmoid area, with a second cluster-

---

FIGURE 4.2:
AGE-STANDARDIZED INCIDENCE OF COLORECTAL CANCER IN REGIONS WITH THE HIGHEST AND LOWEST RATES

COLON

MALES		FEMALES	
Connecticut, USA	32.3	San Francisco, USA	
New York, USA	31.4	(Japanese)	27.4
Los Angeles, USA		New Zealand (non-Maori)	26.9
(Chinese)	31.3	Connecticut, USA	26.4
(Japanese)	30.8	New York, USA	26.3
Cali, Colombia	4.5	Singapore (Malays)	3.3
Bombay, India	3.5	Poona, India	2.8
Poona, India	3.1	Israel (non-Jews)	1.8
Dakar, Senegal	0.6	Dakar, Senegal	0.7

RECTUM

MALES		FEMALES	
Northwest Canada	22.6	Israel (U.S. or European	
Los Angeles, USA		Jewish immigrants)	13.4
(Japanese)	21.7	Neuchatel, Switzerland	13.4
Hawaii, USA		Israel (all Jews)	11.9
(Japanese)	21.4	Netherlands Antilles	7.6
Bas-Rhin, France	21.0	Cali, Colombia	2.3
Cali, Colombia	3.4	Israel (non-Jews)	1.5
Israel (non-Jews)	3.1	Dakar, Senegal	1.0
Dakar, Senegal	1.5		

Incidence per 100,000 population. Data from Waterhouse JAH, Muir CS, Shanmugaratam K, Powel J. *Cancer incidence in five continents*, Vol. 4. IARC Publication No. 42. Lyon, France: Lyon International Agency for Research on Cancer, 1982.

ing in the cecum and ascending colon. In recent years there has been a proximal shift of colorectal cancer, with a reduction in the sigmoid colon and an increase in the ascending colon and cecum. At present, the proportion of cancers in the rectosigmoid is 55 percent (Fig. 4.6) (4).

Etiology
Dietary Factors

Epidemiologic, case-control, and laboratory animal studies performed over the past few decades have established a strong connection between nutrition

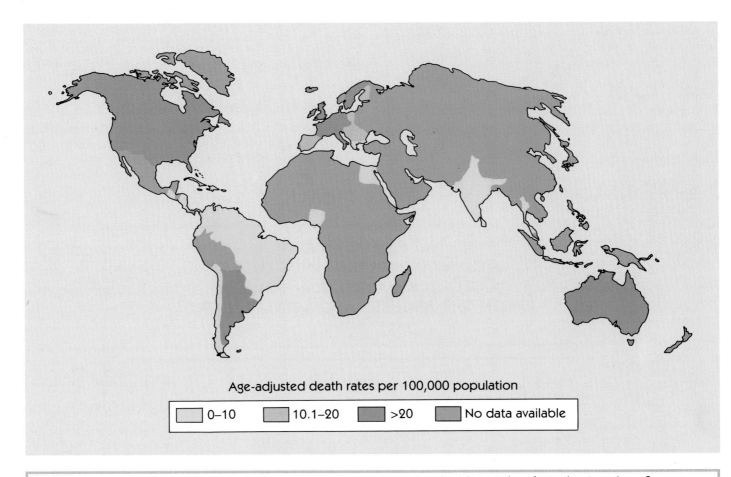

Age-adjusted death rates per 100,000 population

| | 0–10 | | 10.1–20 | | >20 | | No data available |

FIGURE 4.3 Geographic distribution of colorectal cancer. Age-adjusted death rates per 100,000 population. (Based on incidence data from the American Cancer Society's *Cancer facts and figures,* 1990.)

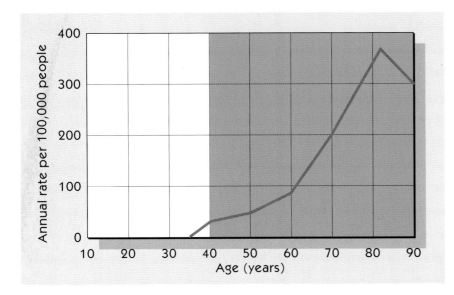

FIGURE 4.4 U. S. incidence of colorectal cancer. The risk begins to rise at age 40 and more sharply beginning at age 50. More than 80 million people are at risk. (Developed by the Memorial Sloan–Kettering Cancer Center and Health Learning Systems.)

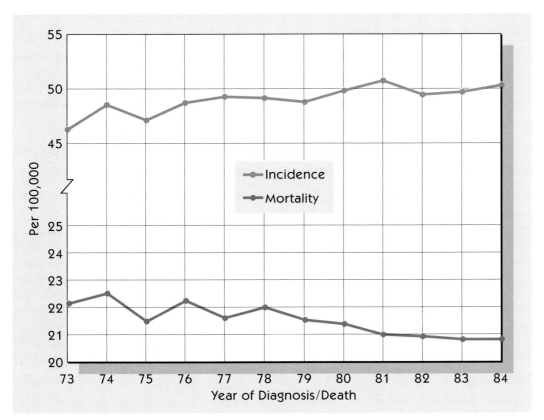

FIGURE 4.5 Time-trend of the incidence and mortality from colorectal cancer in the United States from 1950–1985. The trend toward a decreasing mortality in the presence of a continued rise in incidence is unique and may be a result of earlier detection, more accurate diagnosis, and more effective treatment. (From reference 3.)

FIGURE 4.5 Time-trend of the incidence and mortality from colorectal cancer in the United States from 1950–1985. The trend toward a decreasing mortality in the presence of a continued rise in incidence is unique and may be a result of earlier detection, more accurate diagnosis, and more effective treatment. (From reference 3.)

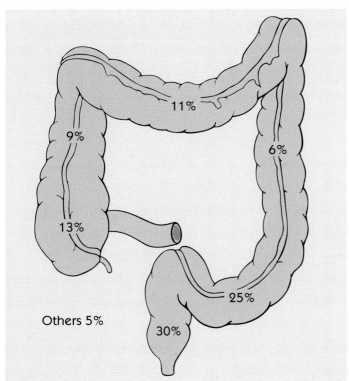

FIGURE 4.6 Frequency of adenocarcinoma in different anatomic segments of the colon and rectum. (From reference 5.)

and colorectal cancer (6–22). Various dietary constituents have been implicated in colorectal cancer, including fat, excess calories, lack of fiber, alcohol, and inadequate intake of vitamins such as retinoids, ascorbic acid, α-tocopherol, minerals (e.g., calcium), and trace elements (e.g., selenium). The worldwide variation in colorectal cancer incidence and mortality shows direct relationship with total dietary fat consumption. Populations with high dietary fat consumption have higher death rates (Fig. 4.7). People who move from a low-risk country (e.g., Japan) to a high-risk country (e.g., the U.S.) demonstrate an increase in risk to match that seen in the population of the new country (Fig. 4.8) (8,11–13,23–25). Most studies have not correlated colorectal cancer risk with any one specific type of fat, but rather with the total amount of fat consumed. Several mechanisms have been proposed to explain the cancer-promoting action of dietary fat, including 1) an increase in bil-

iary sterol excretion, which could have a deleterious effect on colonic epithelium (Fig. 4.9); 2) an increase in lipid peroxidation radicals generated from fat metabolism; 3) increased incorporation of fatty acids in cell membranes; 4) increased synthesis of prostaglandins, which can lead to increased cell proliferation; 5) alteration in gut bacteria; and 6) an increase in available calories.

The hypothesis that dietary factors may protect against colorectal cancer was first proposed by Burkitt (26), who observed that African blacks consuming a high-fiber diet had a lower death rate from large bowel cancer than African whites, whose fiber intake was low. Epidemiologic studies do not consistently support this finding, probably because dietary fiber is not a simple chemical entity but rather a diverse group of compounds that originate in plants and are resistant to human digestive enzymes (Fig. 4.10) (27–33). The mechanisms by which fiber may protect against colorectal cancer

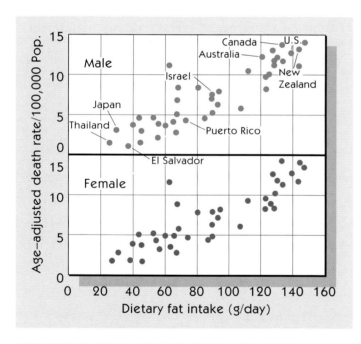

FIGURE 4.7 Positive correlations between the amount of fat available for consumption in grams per capita per day and age-adjusted mortality from cancers of the colon. (From Carroll KK, Khor HT. Dietary fat in relation to tumorigenesis. *Prog Biochem Pharmacol* 10:308, 1975.)

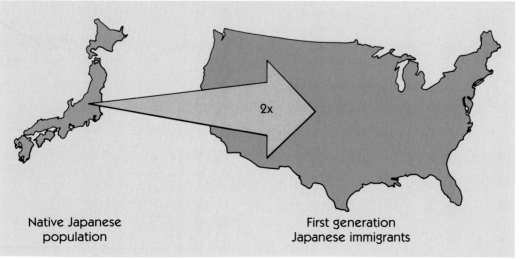

FIGURE 4.8 The increased incidence in first generation Japanese who have emigrated to the United States strongly suggests environmental factors in etiology. (Developed by the Memorial Sloan–Kettering Cancer Center and Health Learning Systems.)

have not been elucidated, but the following have been proposed: 1) reduced transit time of food, decreasing the exposure to carcinogens; 2) binding and dilution of carcinogens in the gut lumen; 3) an alteration in gut flora; 4) decrease in fecal pH, causing deionization of potentially harmful free fatty acids and bile acids. Of considerable current interest in chemoprevention studies are naturally occurring anticarcinogens such as those found in cruciferous vegetables (broccoli, cauliflower, etc.) and in other fruits and vegetables.

Animal studies and epidemiologic studies suggest that excessive body weight and calorie intake may also increase the risk of colorectal cancer (34). Certain vitamins, minerals, and trace elements have been proposed as having an effect on carcinogenesis. Calcium, for example, is thought to neutralize the damaging effects of bile acids and free fatty acids, which are considered to be strong cancer promoters in the colon. One of the first steps in carcinogenesis is a hyperproliferation of the lining epithelium of the bowel mucosa (Fig. 4.11), which appears to be stimulated by excess fat and can be reduced to a lower rate by supplemental dietary calcium (35). Vitamin A and related compounds have also been found to have a potential antineoplastic effect on the colon. Vitamin C has been shown to inhibit fecal mutagen formation, hence protecting the colonic mucosa. Both vitamin E and selenium are antioxidants and can also protect against carcinogenesis by neutralizing the damaging effect of free radicals, particularly those originating from fat metabolism. The average per capita selenium intake in 27 countries was found to be inversely correlated with the combined mortality from all cancers, including colorectal cancer (36).

Genetic Factors

Inherited susceptibility factors may be important in most cases of colon cancer (Figs. 4.12–4.15) (37). There are well-established inheritable syndromes of colorectal cancer which can be separated into two major categories: the polyposis syndromes and the hereditary nonpolyposis colorectal cancer syndromes. Both are inherited as autosomal-dominant syndromes. The polyposis syndromes include: familial adenomatous polyposis (FAP) and Gardner's syndrome (GS) (38,39); Peutz–Jeghers disease; and familial juvenile polyposis (37). (See Chapter 3.)

These well-defined inheritable syndromes account for about 6 percent (1 percent FAP and GS; 5 percent hereditary nonpolyposis colorectal cancer, or HNPCC) of new cases of colorectal cancer annually. In the past, the remaining 94 percent were considered to be "sporadic," without any inherited susceptibility. However, three large studies demonstrated that colorectal cancer occurred

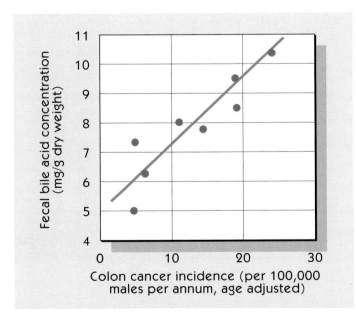

FIGURE 4.9 Correlation between fecal bile acid concentration and colon cancer incidence as found in three different studies. (From Hill MJ, Taylor AJ, Thompson MH, et al. Fecal steroids and urinary volatile phenols in 4 Scandinavian populations. *Nutr Cancer* 4:67–73, 1982.)

FIGURE 4.10: PHYSIOLOGIC PROPERTIES OF FIBER

CELLULOSE
1–4 β-D-glucose polymers
40% digestible by bacterial flora

HEMICELLULOSE
Various hexoses and pentoses
50% digestible
Bind cations and bile salts

PECTINS
Various hexoses and pentoses
95% digestible
Bind cations

LIGNIN
Nondigestible

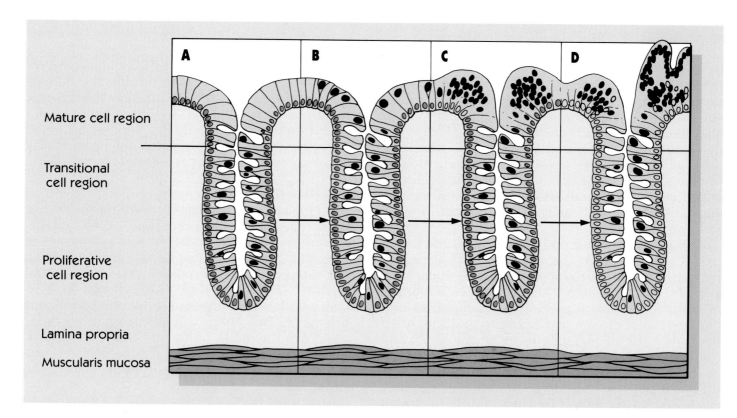

Mature cell region

Transitional cell region

Proliferative cell region

Lamina propria

Muscularis mucosa

FIGURE 4.11 Biopsies of the normal appearing flat mucosa can be obtained and radioautographs made by incubating the tissue with tritiated thymidine which is taken up by cells (*black dots*) that are in the DNA synthesis phase of the cell cycle and therefore capable of proliferating. This series of diagrams demonstrates: **(A)** normal crypts with proliferation confined to the lower two-thirds; **(B)** expansion of the proliferation zone to the surface as the field defect which precedes neoplastic change of the mucosa; **(C)** accumulation of cells at the surface as neoplasia begins; **(D)** beginning of a polyp. (From Lipkin M. Phase 1 and phase 2 proliferative lesions of chronic epithelial cells in diseases leading to colonic cancer. *Cancer* 34:878, 1974.)

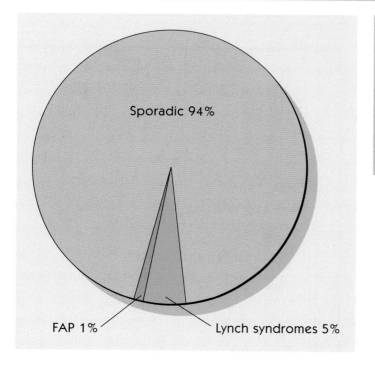

Sporadic 94%

FAP 1%   Lynch syndromes 5%

FIGURE 4.12 Pie diagram depicting the proportion of annual cases of colorectal cancer resulting from well-defined inherited syndromes such as familial adenomatous polyposis (FAP) and Lynch syndromes I and II and as "sporadic" cases, i.e., with no apparent familial factors. It is now believed that sporadic cases have an inherited basis, also providing susceptibility to environmental carcinogenesis. (Adapted from American Cancer Society, Inc. *Third international symposium on colorectal cancer—1983.* New York: ACS, 1984.)

in first-degree relatives (parents, children, siblings) of individuals with colorectal cancer approximately 3.5 times more frequently than expected by chance. Recent studies confirmed these observations and have also demonstrated an increased risk for adenomas in first-degree relatives of individuals with colorectal cancer and an increased risk in first-degree relatives with adenomas (37,41–43).

A recent genealogic data-base study gave a result

FIGURE 4.13:
RISK FACTORS FOR COLORECTAL CANCER

AVERAGE RISK

AGE
50 years and older; asymptomatic
  general population

HIGH RISK

PAST HISTORY
Sporadic colorectal adenomas
Colorectal cancer
Inflammatory bowel disease
Breast, ovarian, or endometrial cancer
Radiation therapy

HIGH RISK

FAMILY HISTORY
Familial adenomatous polyposis
Gardner's syndrome
Turcot's syndrome
Oldfield's syndrome
Juvenile polyposis
Hereditary nonpolyposis colorectal
  cancer syndromes (HNPCC)
"Flat" adenoma syndrome
"Sporadic" colorectal cancer
"Sporadic" colorectal adenoma

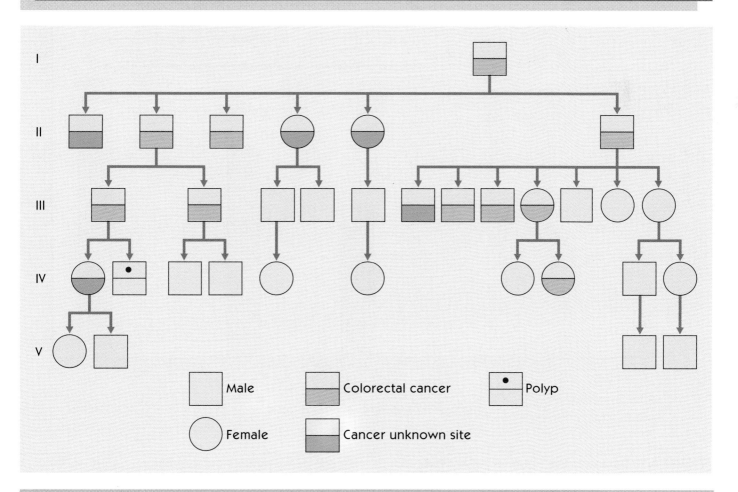

FIGURE 4.14 Pedigree of family with high prevalence of colorectal cancer.

similar to the various genetic epidemiologic studies cited above. Familial clustering of colorectal cancer and colorectal adenomatous polyps was observed in a large kindred, having multiple cases of colorectal cancer, but no apparent pattern of inheritance was found. Pedigree analysis showed that the familial excess of adenomas and cancer was a dominant inherited susceptibility. Additional studies in the same cohort have suggested that most adenomatous polyps arise from a common, partially pene-

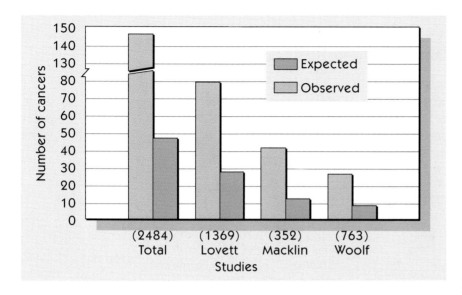

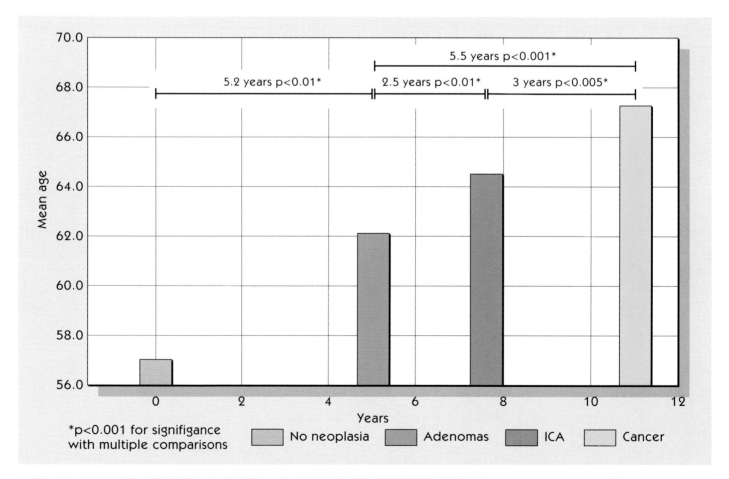

FIGURE 4.15 Familial aggregates in "sporadic" colorectal cancer. Three studies comparing observed and expected number of colorectal cancers in relatives of patients with colorectal cancer are summarized. (From Kussin SZ, Lipkin M, Winawer SJ. Inherited colon cancer: clinical implications. *Am J Gastroenterol* 72:448–457, 1979.)

FIGURE 4.16 Data from the National Polyp Study showing the mean age of patients with no neoplasia, adenomas, adenomas with invasive cancer (ICA) and gross cancer, demonstrating the long natural history of colon cancer as it evolves through the adenoma stage from a normal colon.

trant susceptibility gene (44,45). These studies support the concept that most of the "sporadic" colorectal cancers have inherited etiologic factors.

There has been considerable interest in the genetic variations found in adenomatous polyps and colorectal cancer. The abnormalities demonstrated most frequently are alterations of DNA sequences at specific locations on chromosomes 5, 17, and 18 (37,40,46). Chromosome deletion affects cell growth function. Many of these molecular changes have been seen both in established genetic syndromes such as FAP and in sporadic adnomas and cancers. A theoretic sequence of molecular alterations has been proposed to explain the development of adenomas and the transformation to cancer (Fig. 4.16) (46) (See Chapter 3.)

Adenomatous Polyps

Individuals with adenomatous polyps are at increased risk for colorectal cancer (4,47). The hypothesis that the majority of colorectal cancers evolve from benign pre-existing adenomas, proposed in the medical literature for decades, is now widely accepted (48). The evidence includes epidemiologic data which have related adenoma and carcinoma prevalence, the association of adenomas and carcinomas in patients, and the frequent discovery of residual benign adenoma tissue in colorectal cancers. Support for the adenocarcinoma sequence is also found in inherited colorectal cancer syndromes FAP and HNPCC. Newer evidence of ras-oncogene mutations and chromosome deletions add additional biologic evidence.

Adenomas are extremely prevalent in Western countries, observed in autopsy studies in 30 to 40 percent of individuals over age 60 (49). They are strongly age-related and predominant in males. The risk for colorectal cancer is higher in patients who have had an adenoma removed and have not been under surveillance. These observations were made prior to the availability of colonoscopy (50). However, it is estimated that only 5 percent of all adenomas undergo malignant transformation (51,52). In patients with a large polyp identified radiologically that is not removed, the frequency of cancer was observed to be 8 percent after five years and 24 percent after 20 years (53). It has been theorized that removal of all adenomas in the colon with periodic follow-up surveillance would result in the prevention of colorectal cancer. This is currently being tested (54–56). (See Chapter 3 on polyps.)

Inflammatory Bowel Disease

Among all patients diagnosed with colorectal cancer, only about 1 percent report a history of inflammatory bowel disease. Although colorectal cancer occurs more commonly in patients with ulcerative colitis than in the general population, the magnitude of the risk is not clear (Fig. 4.17). The best estimates indicate a cumulative cancer incidence of 5 percent after 20 years, and 12 percent after 25 years. It is unusual to see cancer in patients having colitis for less than eight years. The risk for patients with only left-sided colitis is delayed until approximately 15 years after onset of their disease. There is no increase in risk in the presence of proctitis only (57–65).

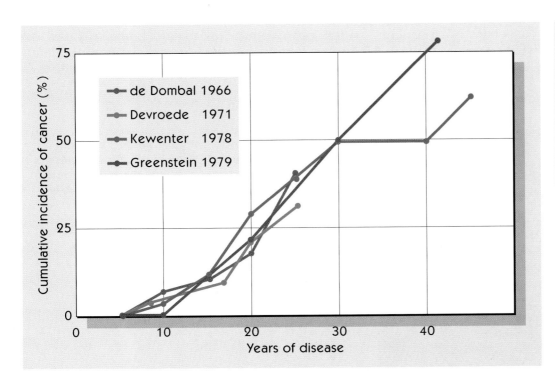

FIGURE 4.17 Frequency distribution of colorectal cancer in patients with ulcerative colitis. These observations may be high because of referral bias. See reference 61. (From Devroede G. Risk of cancer in inflammatory bowel disease. In: Winawer S, Schottenfeld D, Sherlock P, eds. *Colorectal Cancer: Prevention, Epidemiology, and Screening.* New York: Raven Press, 1980: 325–334.)

The pathogenesis of cancer in ulcerative colitis is the same as in adenomatous polyps. The mucosal surface of the colon in ulcerative colitis undergoes cytologic changes (dysplasia) and proliferative changes similar to those seen in adenomatous polyps. As these changes progress and become more severe, the probability that cancer will occur increases.

The risk of colorectal cancer in Crohn's disease is greater than in the general population, although it is still not well defined. Individuals with extensive colonic involvement and long duration of symptoms are at increased risk.

PATHOLOGY

Gross Pathology

Carcinomas of the large bowel generally assume one of four shapes: exophytic, ulcerative, infiltrative, or annular (Figs. 4.18 and 4.19). Rarely does site influence configuration. Exceptions include the cecum, where large polypoid carcinomas are common and may become big enough to obstruct the ileocecal junction by size alone.

Sessile or infiltrative lesions carry a poorer prognosis than do exophytic lesions. Infiltrating or annular carcinomas cause obstruction, change in bowel habit, and bleeding. Prognosis in such tumors is poor, with an overall five-year survival rate of less than 30 percent. Ulcerating carcinomas may originate as polypoid tumors, but with continued infection and necrosis the luminal component is gradually eroded. Such cancers occasionally perforate, and free perforation with peritonitis is life-threatening.

In virtually every major surgical series, carcinomas of the abdominal colon generally have better prognosis than cancers of the rectum. This poor outlook is almost entirely associated with cancers of the low or distal rectum (within 5 cm of the anal verge). Cancers of the mid- or upper rectum have a prognosis similar to that of sigmoid lesions. There are several reasons for this difference in survival. From the standpoint of natural history, cancers of the lower rectum tend to spread both to hypogastric lymph nodes along the pelvic side walls and to mesorectal lymph nodes along the superior hemorrhoidal artery. Surgically, the pelvic dissection required to extirpate all lymph nodes associated with the potential spread of rectal cancer is a difficult and seldom successful procedure. In addition, resultant treatment failures and the recurrent pelvic disease that frequently complicates the course of rectal cancer after resection combine to produce a poor outlook for rectal cancers. Newer adjuvant approaches, however, are improving this previously gloomy prognosis.

Histology

Important histologic features include degree of differentiation (histologic or cytologic grade); degree of mural penetration; presence or absence of lymph node involvement; character of leading tumor margin; lymphatic, venous, or perineural infiltration; presence of an associated inflammatory response; extranodal mesenteric implants; extramesenteric nodal involvement; presence or absence of involved surgical margins; and adjacent organ involvement (Fig. 4.20).

Histologic grading as a tool for assessing tumor differentiation is a useful diagnostic indicator. Most pathologists use either a numbering system (1–3 or 1–4) such as Broders' classification or a series of descriptive terms such as "well differentiated," "moderately differentiated," "poorly differentiated," and "undifferentiated" or "anaplastic." These systems are generally interchangeable. Well-differentiated tumors are those that are mostly or fully composed of gland-forming structures, with nuclei showing polarity and basal orientation. Moderately differentiated tumors are predominantly glandular but may demonstrate some loss of

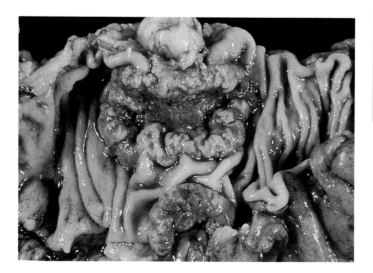

FIGURE 4.18 The central irregular eroded area and everted rolled edge are hallmarks of adenocarcinoma of the colon seen grossly. Although the tumor is relatively small, obliteration of the muscle and puckering of the wall indicate transmural extension. (From reference 66.)

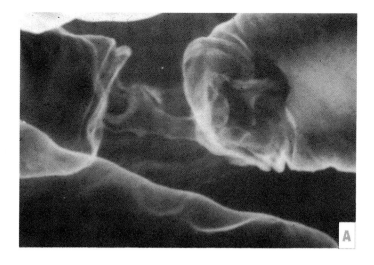
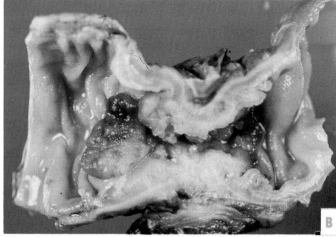

FIGURE 4.19 (A) This circumferential lesion of the sigmoid colon has resulted in significant narrowing of the lumen with the consequent apple-core configuration. **(B)** A longitudinal section through this circumferential carcinoma in the sigmoid colon demonstrates readily how the growth pattern of the tumor imparts the apple-core appearance. (From reference 66.)

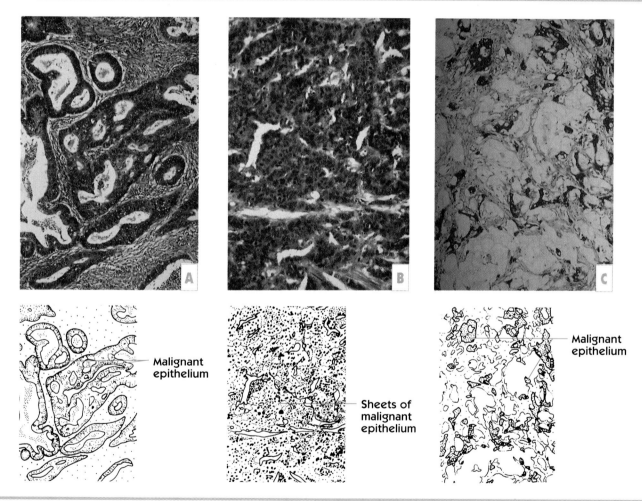

Malignant epithelium

Sheets of malignant epithelium

Malignant epithelium

FIGURE 4.20 Histologic appearances of colonic cancer. In the moderately differentiated pattern **(A)**, malignant epithelium forms obvious acini, but considerable nuclear pleomorphism remains within individual cells. The poorly differentiated pattern **(B)** consists of sheets of malignant epithelial cells with little acinar formation. Finally, in the mucinous adenocarcinoma **(C)**, nests of malignant epithelium lie in pools of mucin. H&E stain, x50. (From reference 5.)

polarity and nuclear orientation. There may be some tendency for tumor cells to form solid nests. Poorly differentiated tumors are those in which the tendency to form sheets and nests predominates over the formation of glandular elements. When glandular structures are not apparent, the tumor is considered undifferentiated. The majority of colorectal tumors fit into such a grading scheme.

Variants of undifferentiated carcinoma such as signet-ring cell carcinoma or mucinous carcinoma carry a particularly poor prognosis. The five-year survival rate of patients with undifferentiated carcinomas varies from 31 percent to 74 percent. "Mucinous carcinoma" is defined in terms of mucus occupying at least 60 percent of the tumor volume. The frequency of mucinous adenocarcinomas in young patients is usually high, especially in adoles-

cents. The role of mucin in the poor prognosis of rectal lesions is unknown. Tumor cell DNA content may be a better reflection of tumor grade and is associated more closely with prognosis in some but not all series (65). Aneuploidy (having other than an exact multiple of the basic diploid number of chromosomes) or heteroploidy are associated with a poor prognosis independent of the stage.

Carcinomas, which are epithelial in origin, spread directly into and through the bowel wall. Because of this, the degree of transmural spread is recorded as one of the two prime features of all large bowel cancer staging methods. "Severe epithelial dysplasia," "carcinoma in situ," "intramucosal carcinoma," and "severe atypia" are all terms indicating restriction of the cancer to the epithelial layer of origin. The term

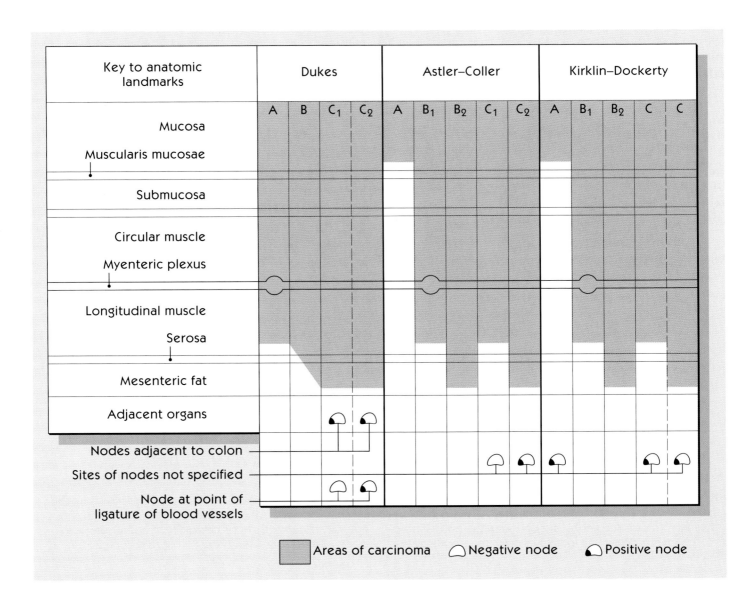

FIGURE 4.21 Staging of colorectal cancer. Three of the more popular systems currently in use for staging carcinoma of the colon are depicted; adjacent to these systems, survival data are given relative to the key factors (Fig. 4.22). When any one system is employed, the modification used should be specified. (From reference 66.)

"high-grade dysplasia" is used increasingly to cover all of these terms. The lack of systemic or nodal spread from carcinoma in situ is attributable to the absence of lymphatic vessels in the epithelial stroma. Invasive carcinoma is defined as cancer that has penetrated the muscularis mucosae. Invasion of the submucosa, muscularis propria, serosa, or perirectal fat constitutes varying degrees of penetration that are recognized in the classic staging methods. Further degrees of direct extension include adherence, invasion, and fistula formation into or involving an adjacent organ. The prognostic significance of nodal metastases is critical. In general, the survival of patients with nodal metastases is reduced to half that of patients without nodal disease. Correlations regarding survival have been made with the level of nodal involvement as well as with the number of involved lymph nodes.

Three other histologic features merit additional mention: the presence of neoplastic cells at the surgical margin of resection, adjacent organ involvement, and intramural or longitudinal spread of tumor. Positive surgical margins are rarely found in adequately resected specimens. Further resection is indicated if any conventional margin is positive or even questionable. While previous surgical and pathologic studies stressed proximal and distal margins, more recently the adequacy of the radial margins has become the important focus (67).

The involvement of adjacent organs is in and of itself not a limitation to curative en bloc resection.

Given an en bloc resection without violation of tumor, adhesions, abscess, or fistulous involvement, a cure is still possible with an appropriate resection.

Staging Methods

The original Dukes' classification of pathologic staging was designed to correlate survival after different types of treatment with the preoperative assessment of tumor stage (68). The validity of this staging method was borne out in the 1958 report of Dukes and Bussey (69); each stage correlated with a significant difference in five-year survival, such as 41 percent for stage C_1 vs. 14 percent for C_2. In 1939, the original Dukes' classification was extended for use in cases of colonic as well as rectal cancers (70). In 1949 Kirklin and co-workers (71) and in 1954 Astler and Coller (72) offered modifications of the Dukes' classification that combined the prognostic significance of the degree of mural penetration with the involvement of lymph nodes. Kirklin and associates proposed the Dukes' classification for lesions limited to the mucosa. Five-year survival figures for the Astler–Coller modification of the Dukes' classification were: A (one patient), 100 percent; B_1 (48 patients), 66.6 percent; B_2 (164 patients), 53.9 percent; C_1 (14 patients), 42.8 percent; and C_2 (125 patients), 22.4 percent. No D category for distant disease was suggested by either group (Figs. 4.21 and 4.22).

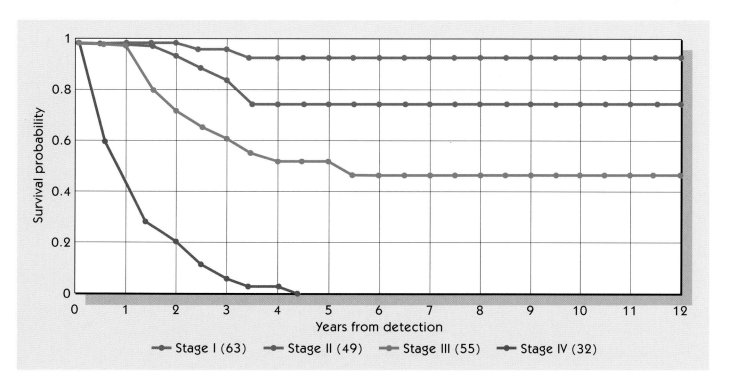

FIGURE 4.22 An illustration of the correlation of five-year survival with stage of cancer. See Figure 4.23 on page 4.16 for stage designations.

These staging methods indicated that mural penetration had a prognostic significance independent of nodal metastases. Since that time, the Gastrointestinal Tumor Study Group (GITSG) of the National Cancer Institute has put into use a further modification of the Dukes' classification that independently recognizes the values of both the degree of mural penetration and the number of involved lymph nodes (73,74).

More recent efforts to consolidate the numerous modifications of the Dukes' classification and provide a uniform method for staging large bowel cancer have led to the organization of the American Joint Committee (AJC) Task Force on Colon and Rectum Cancer (75). This task force has developed a single postsurgical pathologic assessment staging system for colon and rectum cancer by an analysis of 1826 cases (924 colon and 902 rectum cancers from several institutions). Using the TNM (Tumor-Node-Metastasis) classification as described by the UICC (Union International Contre le Cancer), the task force confirmed the importance of postsurgical staging (pTNM) (Fig. 4.23). A recent National Institutes of Health (NIH) Consensus Conference strongly supported use of the TNM system.

CLINICAL PRESENTATION

Cancers of the rectum and colon grow and obstruct, ulcerate and bleed, invade, cause pain, and sometimes perforate into either an adjacent organ, the serosa, or the peritoneal space. The clinical features in an individual patient are determined by the cancer's biologic growth characteristics and by its location in the colon.

Rectal bleeding is a symptom most often associated with cancers of the left side of the colon and the rectum. The passage of red blood, sometimes mixed with darker blood clots, is commonly seen, but bleeding is usually not massive. Bleeding may also be intermittent and hence the patient may attribute it to hemorrhoids. With cancers of the right side of the colon, bleeding is more apt to be slow, and mixing of blood and bowel contents is more likely to be occult. Patients with cancer in this region gradually become anemic because of blood loss and often present with weakness, dizziness, congestive heart failure, angina, or claudication. When right-sided colon cancers bleed more rapidly, a reddish-maroon stool may be noted.

Cancers that occur in the more voluminous and distensible cecum and right colon, where bowel contents are liquid, usually do not cause obstruction until they grow to a very large size. Cancers in the ascending colon are more likely to block the lumen. In such cases, if the ileocecal valve is competent, the cecum becomes painfully dilated with gas, creating a tender right-lower-quadrant mass. Patients may note relief when they massage this area and force the trapped gas past the obstruction. Cecal masses that invade the ileocecal valve may produce the clinical picture of small bowel obstruction with generalized abdominal distention, nausea, and bilious vomiting.

In the left colon, where the lumen is narrower and less distensible and the fecal stream is solid, cancers

FIGURE 4.23:
COMPARISON OF TNM AND DUKES STAGING SYSTEMS FOR COLONIC AND RECTAL CANCERS

STAGE	TNM DESIGNATION			DUKES' DESIGNATION
0	Tis	N0	M0	
I	T1	N0	M0	A
	T2	N0	M0	
II	T3	N0	M0	B
	T4	N0	M0	
III	Any T	N1	M0	C
	Any T	N2, N3	M0	
IV	Any T	Any N	M1	

commonly obstruct the passage of feces. This is a major cause of a change in bowel habit; the gradual narrowing of the lumen slows the fecal stream to produce constipation. Cramping abdominal pain occurs when the colon is intermittently distended proximal to the lesion. Some patients may develop a paradoxic diarrhea as colonic contents are forced past a partially obstructing cancer. Cramping may be particularly aggravated after meals as a result of increased peristaltic activity. Cramping may also be induced by laxatives used to treat constipation caused by the malignant obstruction.

Rectal cancers characteristically produce increase in frequency of stools, change in stool consistency and caliber, small amounts of bright red bleeding, fecal urgency, tenesmus, and incontinence. With advanced cancers, local invasion may be a source of perianal pain, hematuria, urinary frequency, and vaginal fistula. Perforation of colon cancers into the peritoneal cavity or into the retroperitoneum usually results in localized abscess. This can be a cause of fever and intermittent sepsis. Abdominal pain and signs of localized perineal irritation will usually be present.

Anorexia and weight loss are common in advanced colon cancer. Weakness and malaise may be related to anemia but are often an indication of advanced metastatic disease. Metastases from colon cancer will produce various symptoms, depending on the areas affected. Local invasion of the peritoneum or retroperitoneum may produce localized abdominal or back pain. Pelvic and sciatic pain, attended by neurologic signs, may result from invasion of the lumbosacral plexus, spine, and pelvis. Ascites, bowel obstruction, and ileus may develop from intra-abdominal tumor spread. Right-upper-quadrant pain, a large mass, or jaundice signal liver metastases. Pulmonary metastases may be a cause of cough and dyspnea. Late features may include changes in eating habits or even pica.

DIAGNOSIS

While bright red rectal bleeding can be due to a variety of benign lesions (hemorrhoids, diverticulosis, angiodysplasia, colitis, and adenomatous polyps), bleeding always should arouse suspicion of bowel cancer. The character and severity of rectal bleeding do not distinguish benign from malignant disease.

Changes in bowel habits, with constipation, cramping pain, and narrowed stool caliber, may result from diverticular disease as well as from cancer involving the left colon. It is often difficult to determine if a localized peritoneal abscess is due to a perforated diverticulum or a cancer. Inflammatory bowel disease or infectious colitis may cause bleeding, tenesmus, urgency, and diarrhea, but colorectal

cancer must still be considered. Alternating constipation and diarrhea with left-lower-quadrant pain suggest an irritable bowel syndrome, but cancer of the left colon can produce the same symptoms. In most patients with an irritable bowel syndrome, on the other hand, a careful history will document long-standing symptoms. While patients with irritable bowel syndrome do not have a higher frequency of colon cancer, they are still as susceptible to malignancy as anyone else. Hence, a sudden worsening or change in nature of the symptoms in a patient with a known irritable bowel should suggest the possibility of a supervening colon cancer. Other considerations include a variety of uncommon colorectal primary benign and malignant tumors, metastases from a noncolon primary, and benign conditions such as endometriosis.

Digital rectal examination is a crucial part of the physical examination and should not be omitted without good reason. This examination may detect an unsuspected mass lesion. Colon cancers that become large and bulky, usually on the right side, may be palpable. Metastatic spread to the liver may cause hepatomegaly, and the liver may be hard, nodular, and slightly tender. Peritoneal metastases may cause ascites, and peripheral lymphadenopathy may represent metastatic spread. Evidence of weight loss, cachexia, pallor, and jaundice suggests advanced disease.

Sigmoidoscopy, Colonoscopy, and Barium Enema

Patients who present with symptoms of neoplastic disease can be examined either by flexible sigmoidoscopy and barium enema or by colonoscopy. If a lesion is found by sigmoidoscopy or barium enema, colonoscopy is needed to ascertain the nature of the lesion, to remove it if it is a benign-appearing adenoma, to obtain a tissue sample if it is a malignant lesion, and to make certain that there are no other synchronous lesions elsewhere in the colon. When a cancer has been detected by sigmoidoscopy or barium enema, the colonoscopic approach will vary, depending on the nature and location of the lesion. Colonoscopy can usually be done safely in patients with small- to moderate-sized polypoid adenocarcinomas anywhere in the colon, the neoplasm being gently bypassed while looking for synchronous lesions. If colonoscopy requires difficult manipulation, the procedure is usually terminated. If the lesion obstructs the lumen, the colonoscope should not be passed beyond the lesion because of the risk of perforation.

Asymptomatic patients who have a positive fecal occult blood test or a positive finding on sigmoidoscopic or barium enema examination should undergo colonoscopy. About 50 percent of patients showing a positive fecal occult blood test for the first time will have a neoplastic lesion; about 38 percent of these lesions will be adenomas and 12 percent will be cancers. The predictive value of the fecal occult blood test for neoplastic lesions increases with the patient's age. Studies from around the world using the fecal occult blood test for screening have demonstrated that the yield for neoplastic lesions is much higher when colonoscopy is used in the diagnostic work-up. When single-column barium enema studies are used, approximately half the cancers and a majority of adenomas are missed, but they can be detected on colonoscopy. Double-contrast barium enema is almost as sensitive as colonoscopy for lesions over 2 cm in size, but small adenomas (<8 mm) can be difficult or impossible to demonstrate. In patients having an abnormal sigmoidoscopic examination, colonoscopy is advisable to check for additional lesions. Synchronous adenomas have been observed in about 50 percent of patients with cancer. When a cancer has been found, complete colonoscopy will disclose an additional synchronous cancer elsewhere in the colon in 1.5 percent to 5 percent of cases (Figs. 4.24–4.26) (77). Many physicians now prefer colonoscopy over barium enema because of these reasons.

Laboratory Tests

Tests that document iron-deficiency anemia and the presence of occult blood in the stool should prompt consideration of colon cancer. Hypoalbuminemia suggests malnutrition and advanced disease. Abnormal liver enzymes may indicate hepatic metastases, and elevated urea nitrogen or creatinine levels in the serum may be due to blockage of the ureters by expanding metastases from rectal cancers. Carcinoembryonic antigen (CEA) levels determined by commercially available radioimmunoassays are reproducible with some interlaboratory variations. Most asymptomatic patients with early stages of colon cancer have normal CEA values in their blood, and patients with elevated CEA tend to be those with more advanced cancer. Preoperative CEA has prognostic significance, with higher recurrence rates (90 percent) seen in patients having over 5 ng/ml as compared to those under 5 ng/ml (40 percent) (78).

APPROACH TO THE PATIENT

The present approach to management of colorectal cancer is multidisciplinary, involving the gastroenterologist, surgeon, medical oncologist, radiation therapist, stomal therapist, and others. Management can be divided into prevention, curative surgery, adjuvant treatment, and palliation of advanced or recurrent disease, usually with radiation, chemotherapy, cytokine therapy, endoscopic laser, or reoperation.

Prevention of colorectal cancer can be defined as primary or secondary (79,80). Primary prevention is the identification and eradication of factors responsible for colorectal cancer. At present, this approach is directed toward dietary nutrients. Secondary prevention may be defined as early detection of colorectal cancer prior to its more advanced, fatal consequences, as well as detection and eradication of premalignant disease before its transformation into cancer. The goal in secondary prevention is to reduce mortality in the entire targeted group. For colorectal cancer, this includes screening for early-stage cancer as well as identification and removal of the precursor lesion, adenomatous polyp, or adenoma.

Primary Prevention

DIETARY RECOMMENDATIONS

With the increasing recognition of the role of diet in the pathogenesis of various diseases, the concept that proper diet can promote health is now prevalent, both in the medical community and in the public. Consequently, in various countries there have been numerous nutritional recommendations to the public aimed at preventing of diseases in which diet is thought to play an important role. Some of the recommendations have been aimed at formulating a general healthy diet while others have focused on prevention of certain diseases, such as cardiovascular diseases or cancer.

The benefit of most nutritional recommendations has not been proven by rigorous clinical trials. Therefore, there is controversy as to whether such recommendations should be made to the public. It is possible, nevertheless, to formulate interim guidelines based on the large amount of current data and on basic nutritional principles:

1. Reduce consumption of both animal and vegetable fats. Fat should constitute no more than 25 percent of total calories.
2. Increase intake of high-fiber foods such as vegetables, legumes, fruits, whole grain cereals, and cruciferous vegetables (such as cauliflower, broccoli, cabbage, and Brussels sprouts). Dietary fiber intake should amount to at least 25 g/day.
3. Consume at least 800 mg of calcium a day (1200 mg/day for children and young adults). Select calcium-containing foods with a low fat content.
4. Balance energy intake and expenditure. Avoid excess body weight.
5. Reduce alcohol intake.

Secondary Prevention

Early detection of cancer is a general term that includes case-finding and screening. Case-finding is an approach taken by physicians in the clinic and office and usually includes patient history, physical examination results, various laboratory tests, and special tests to detect colonic neoplasia. Screening refers strictly to the testing of healthy volunteers from the general population for purposes of separating them into groups with high and low probability for having the disease. The objective of screening is the early detection of those diseases whose treatment is either easier or more effective when undertaken before the disease is established. The terms *early detection, case-finding,* and *screening* have been used interchangedly here, although the concept of each is quite different (80).

Colonoscopy was introduced in the early 1970s. It soon became clear that for the first time an accurate diagnostic assessment could be made of the colon. Colorectal cancer could be found and biopsied with a high degree of sensitivity. In addition, polypectomy through the colonoscope was introduced. It then became possible not only to find small colorectal cancers but also to find and remove premalignant lesions anywhere in the colon without the need for exploratory laparotomy and colotomy (81). These developments were key to the effective use of the new stool blood test slide, first researched by Greegor in the late 1960s. Individuals with positive tests could then have their colon searched for early cancer and for adenomatous polyps (82,83).

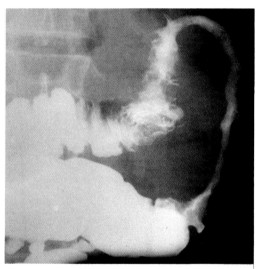

FIGURE 4.24 Carcinoma of the colon: scirrhous pattern. A spot film of a barium enema in a 48-year-old man with guaiac-positive stools shows a tubular narrowing of the splenic flexure. The narrowed segment, which measures 20 cm in length, was rigid and unchanging on fluoroscopy. (From reference 76.)

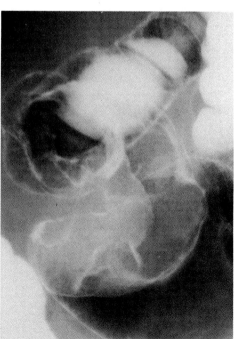

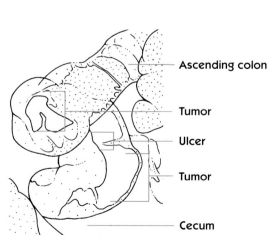

Ascending colon

Tumor

Ulcer

Tumor

Cecum

FIGURE 4.25 The voluminous capacity of the proximal ascending colon may allow for development of the bulky exophytic lesions seen more commonly there. (From reference 66.)

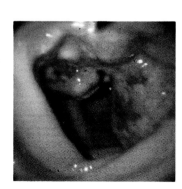

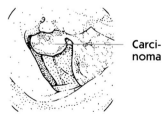

Carcinoma

FIGURE 4.26 Endoscopic view of carcinoma of the ascending colon.

SCREENING TESTS

Diagnosis of cancer by digital rectal examination has diminished as a result of the proximal migration of colorectal cancer; less than 10 percent are now detectable by this means. Several sigmoidoscopes, however, are now available, such as rigid scopes 25 cm in length, 35 cm fiberoptic sigmoidoscopes, 60 cm fiberoptic sigmoidoscopes, and 40–60 cm video endoscopes. The flexible sigmoidoscope has a two to three times greater yield for adenomas and cancer than the rigid scope and can adequately examine the entire rectosigmoid, where about 50 percent of cancers and adenomas occur (84–88). The effectiveness of sigmoidoscopy in screening has not been well studied, but in one series, more than 26,000 asymptomatic patients had 58 cancers detected. Of these, 81 percent were Dukes' A and B, and the 15-year survival was 90 percent (89). Studies evaluating the efficacy of periodic multiphasic health checkups in the Northern California Kaiser–Permanente program indicated a reduced mortality from colorectal cancer. This mortality reduction was reconfirmed in a 16-year follow-up, and the role of sigmoidoscopy was clarified (90–92). Adenomas are detected by sigmoidoscopy at a higher frequency than carcinomas. Trials evaluating the long-term benefit of

the flexible scopes are currently being planned in the U.S. and Europe (93).

A common test for occult blood in the stool is based on the phenolic oxidation of the guaiac to blue compound by the peroxidase-like enzymatic action of hemoglobin (94). However, various compounds with peroxidase-like activity other than hemoglobin, mainly peroxidase in certain uncooked vegetables and fruits, can produce a positive test. Although dietary factors have not been fully studied, data indicate that diet (except for red meat) has a small effect on the standard guaiac slide tests and has a greater effect after hydration of the slides. Elimination of red meat and the small number of peroxidase-rich raw vegetables and fruit from the patient's diet will improve test specificity and reduce false-positives. Iron and laxatives also have an unpredictable effect on positives and negatives, while vitamin C inhibits the test reaction, causing a false-negative in the presence of bleeding. Positive stool blood tests can result from physiologic blood loss, benign bleeding lesions, and neoplastic bleeding lesions. Isotope studies document fluctuation of occult bleeding from colorectal adenomas as well as the overall amount of bleeding; cancer and large adenomas bleed more than smaller ones. Hydration of stool smears with water prior to adding the

FIGURE 4.27:
RESULTS OF FIVE CONTROLLED TRIALS OF SCREENING THAT HAVE USED THE FECAL OCCULT BLOOD TEST

	COHORT SIZE	POSITIVITY RATE (%)	PREDICTIVE VALUE (%) (ADENOMAS & CANCERS)	DUKES' A&B CANCERS (%)	
				SCREENED GROUP	CONTROL GROUP
Göteborg, Sweden	27,000	1.9	22	65	33
Nottingham, England	150,000	2.1	53	90	40
New York, USA	22,000	1.7	30	65	33
Minnesota, USA	48,000	2.4	31	78	35
Fühnen, Denmark	62,000	1.0	58	81	55

This table is derived from multiple sources and summarizes mainly nonhydrated slide data, although hydrated slides have also been used in a phase of some programs. The data are primarily from initial screening. The Dukes' A cancers in the screened groups were 34–65 percent as compared to 8.24 percent in the control groups. See text and references for details.

reagent causes a higher number of positives and hence more cancers are detected, but there are also a larger number of false positives.

Other stool blood tests have been introduced, including immunochemical tests that are specific for human hemoglobin, a quantitative test for blood (Hemoquant) based on the fluorescence of heme-derived porphyrins, and more sensitive guaiac slide tests. The immunochemic tests are not affected by diet, vitamin C, or iron.

Nonheme peroxidase, vitamin C, and iron do not interfere with the Hemoquant tests; nor is the test influenced by degradation of hemoglobin in the intestine or by storage. However, the test specificity is adversely influenced by meat in the diet and by ingestion of aspirin and other drugs that could increase blood loss, making it unsuitable for screening. Maintenance of high specificity together with high sensitivity looks more promising with the new immunochemical tests (80).

AVERAGE-RISK PATIENTS

Studies were initiated worldwide to evaluate whether stool blood testing had potential value for colorectal cancer screening in average-risk patients (80). There are five controlled trials studying the possible usefulness of the stool blood test in screening for colorectal cancer (95–99). The five trials thus far show positive nonhydrated slide test rates of 1.0 percent to 4.0 percent, predictive values for adenoma and cancer of 22 percent to 58 percent, and a shift in the screened group to earlier Dukes' staging (65 percent to 90 percent Dukes' A and B) (Figs. 4.27 and 4.28). All data indicate an improved sensitivity for cancers but loss of specificity when slides are hydrated. The sensitivity of the nonhydrated slide is

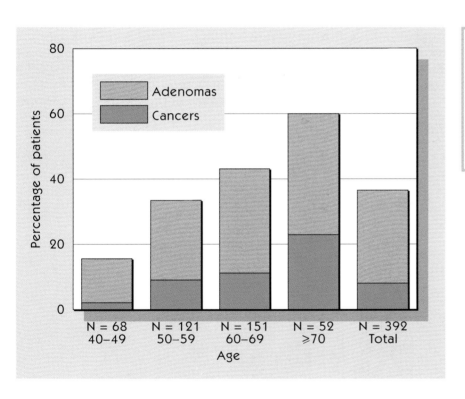

FIGURE 4.28 Rate of neoplastic findings in patients with positive hemoccult tests by age. (From Winawer SJ, Baldwin M, Herbert E, Sherlock P. Screening experience with fecal occult blood testing as a function of age. In: Yancik R, et al. *Perspectives on Prevention and Treatment of Cancer in the Elderly.* New York: Raven Press, 1983:265–274.)

reported to be 50–90 percent (Fig. 4.29). Complete evaluation of the colon is clearly necessary and colonoscopy is now being used for the diagnostic work-up. As yet survival data are available only in one program, but they can be expected to be favorable given the stage improvement (Fig. 4.30). Mortality data will be forthcoming within the next few years, provided complete follow-up and mortality review can be accomplished. It will be important to see whether identification of colonic adenomas and their removal will be associated with a reduced incidence of colon cancer in these patients.

HIGH-RISK PATIENTS

Screening has also been suggested for individuals at increased risk. Individuals with ulcerative colitis of more than eight years' duration involving the entire bowel or of more than 15 years with only distal colitis can have their colons examined every year or two, using dysplasia as an indicator of early cancer (57,100). Biopsies are taken from each segment of the colon during these examinations. There is about 50 percent probability that cancer will be found in individuals having low-grade dysplasia on biopsy, and about a 30 percent probability in the presence of high-grade dysplasia. The likelihood of having low-grade or high-grade dysplasia, however, is quite small. The precise sensitivity and specificity of dysplasia has

not been well established, and expert pathologic interpretation is required. Newer assessment techniques include flow cytometry to detect the presence of abnormal amounts of cellular DNA and lectin and mucin histochemistry. Early cancer in ulcerative colitis can be missed because of the absence of dysplasia and because these cancers can be flat and difficult to see. The barium enema is not sensitive for the detection of early cancer in ulcerative colitis.

Patients who have had adenomas removed are at increased risk for future adenomas and for colorectal cancer if new adenomas are not removed (47). The precise strategy for follow-up surveillance of those individuals has not been established. In the past, frequent follow-up colonoscopies were performed. Reports such as the National Polyp Study indicate that adenomas found at the follow-up examination are small and have unimportant pathology (54). The data also suggest that the earliest a follow-up colonoscopy needs to be done is three years. Individuals with numerous adenomas, with malignant adenomas, or with incomplete removal or incomplete examination of the colon may require more frequent individualized follow-up (52). It would be expected that appropriate follow-up of these cases could prevent most if not all cancers from developing in such patients. Individuals with a family history of col-

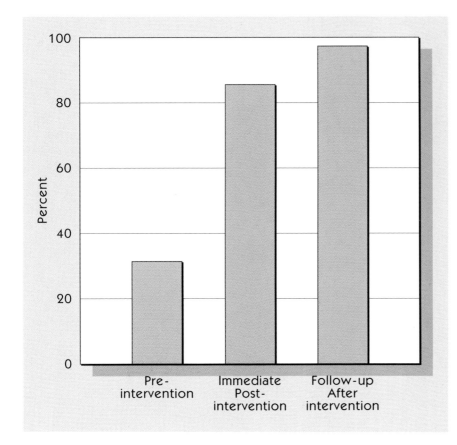

FIGURE 4.29 Accuracy of fecal occult blood test interpretation. Note the improved accuracy following an instructional intervention.

orectal cancer or adenomas and individuals in families with FAP, GS, or HNPCC also require surveillance (37).

RECOMMENDED GUIDELINES

Individuals should be encouraged to enter the health care system and advised not to use over-the-counter tests without medical guidance (Fig. 4.31). Symptomatic patients will need appropriate diagnostic evaluation and treatment. Those without symptoms should be categorized as either at average (standard) risk or at increased risk. Men and women at average risk should be offered stool blood tests annually beginning at age 50, with flexi-ble sigmoidoscopy every three to five years also beginning at age 50. A positive stool test or an ade-nomatous polyp at biopsy by sigmoidoscopy requires full colonoscopy for detecting possible colorectal cancer and for removing any polyps detected (80).

People at increased risk require individualized strategies. Those who have longstanding ulcera-tive colitis require colonoscopy with biopsy for dysplasia every year or two years, beginning with eight years or 15 years after onset of the disease, depending on whether universal or distal colitis is present. Individuals in families that are at risk for FAP and GS require sigmoidoscopy every six

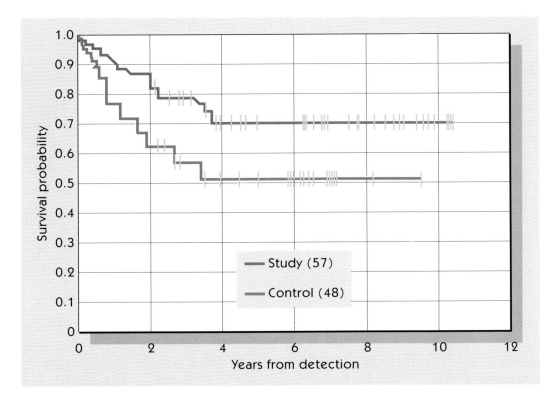

FIGURE 4.30 Survival from colorectal cancer in patients screened with fecal occult blood tests (study) and in patients presenting with symptoms (controls). (From reference 69.)

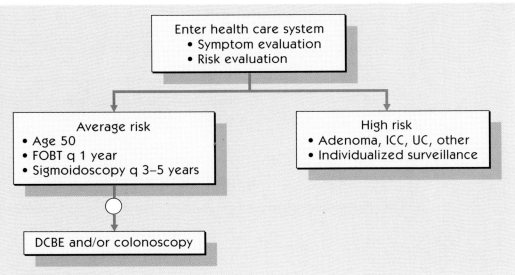

FIGURE 4.31 Recommended screening approach for the early detection of colorectal cancer. Colonoscopy is now being used as the preferred diagnostic approach in patients with a positive screening test. High-risk individuals include those with: ICC—inherited colon cancer (Lynch syndromes, familial adenomatous polyposis syndromes); UC—ulcerative colitis; and patients with a history of adenomas.

months beginning in adolescence if APC gene-positive. Those at risk for HNPCC should be given a colonoscopy every year or two beginning at age 21, and those having one first-degree relative with colorectal cancer should undergo colonoscopy every three to five years beginning at age 35 to 40 (Figs. 4.32 and 4.33) (101–105). (See Chapter 3.)

At present, only a small proportion of those destined to develop colorectal cancer can be identified as having an inherited genetic predisposition, but these individuals, along with other high-risk groups, could be placed under individualized surveillance. It is expected that in the future, the majority of those at risk for colorectal cancer will be identified by genetic markers. Periodic colonoscopy could be performed in these individuals, hence keeping their colons adenoma-free and leading to a dramatic reduction in colorectal cancer incidence.

Curative Surgery of the Primary Lesion

The majority of patients present with mural penetration or nodal involvement. The surgeon's goal must be to cure these patients (106). Nodal spread is relatively orderly and follows the lymph nodes along the named arterial blood supply (in sigmoid cancers, the inferior mesenteric artery) to the affected segment of the colon or rectum (107). Nodal spread rarely takes place before the cancer has penetrated the bowel wall and affects first the epicolic, then paracolic, then intermediate, and finally proximal nodes along the main arterial

trunk. By ligation of the total arterial blood supply at its origin, wide resection of the mesentery with the appropriate lymph nodes is assured. This ligation of the total arterial blood supply is essential to the appropriate operative treatment for curable colorectal cancers (108). For each site there are individual considerations, as described below.

The large bowel derives its blood supply from three major vessels: the superior mesenteric artery, the inferior mesenteric artery, and the hypogastric or internal iliac arteries. The primary lymph nodes for any given segment of bowel are found along the named arteries and veins that are regionally related to the primary tumor site. The design of any given resection is based upon the anatomic site of the primary tumor and the presence or absence of adjacent organ involvement (109).

Cecum and Ascending Colon

The appropriate operation is a right anatomic hemicolectomy. The right colic, ileocolic, and right branches of the middle colic arteries and veins are sacrificed at their origins. The mesentery is divided to the right of the mid-transverse colon. Posteriorly, the transverse mesocolon is dissected away from the right ureter, duodenum, and pancreas. An end-to-side or end-to-end ileocolostomy may then be performed (Fig. 4.34).

Hepatic Flexure

A potentially curable tumor spread may involve lymph nodes along the right and middle colic vessels. These vessels are taken at their origin. This

---

Figure 4.32:
Early Detection Strategies in Hereditary Nonpolyposis Colorectal Cancer

HNPCC familial risk
    ascertained
Colonoscopy every 2 yrs:
    age 25
Colonoscopy every year:
    age 35

From Burt RN, Bishop DT, Lynch HT, Rozen P, Winawer SJ. Risk and surveillance of individuals with hereditable factors for colorectal cancer. *WHO Bulletin,* 1991 (in press).

Figure 4.33:
Early Detection Strategies in Relatives of Patients with Colorectal Cancer

NO. OF PRIMARY RELATIVES WITH COLORECTAL CANCER	STRATEGIES
1–2	Colonoscopy every 3 to 5 yrs: ages 35 to 40
3	HNPCC
1 < age 30	Suspect HNPCC

resection sacrifices all of the right colon and most of the transverse colon. The operation is referred to as an extended right radical hemicolectomy. After its completion, the ileum may be anastomosed to the distal transverse colon.

TRANSVERSE COLON

The resection is based entirely on the middle colic arteries according to their origins. The middle colic vessels may form a vascular arcade occupying the entire transverse mesocolon. The gastrocolic ligament is divided along the gastroepiploic vessels, and the transverse mesocolon is resected along its entire length at the base of the pancreas, avoiding injury to the duodenum. The right colon is generally sacrificed, and an ileocolic anastomosis is performed in the descending colon.

SPLENIC FLEXURE

This operation incorporates features of both the transverse colectomy and the left hemicolectomy. Both the middle colic arteries and the left colic artery are at risk for nodal metastases. The left colic artery is divided, sparing the inferior mesenteric artery and its sigmoidal branches. The left branch of the middle colic artery or the origin of the entire middle colic artery is taken. While some surgeons might want to anastomose the right colon to the distal descending or sigmoid colon, the resulting tension would suggest that an ileodescending or ileosigmoid anastomosis is safer. There is no evidence to suggest that splenectomy enhances survival in patients with cancer of the splenic flexure. Some authors advocate left hemicolectomy, but this does not take into account potential spread along the middle colic route.

DESCENDING COLON

Lesions situated in the descending colon below the splenic flexure are treated by left anatomic hemicolectomy. The entire regional mesentery is resected, from the origin of the inferior mesenteric artery at the aorta to the inferior mesenteric vein above the duodenum at the inferior border of the pancreas. The proximal line of resection is the left transverse colon. The distal margin of resection is

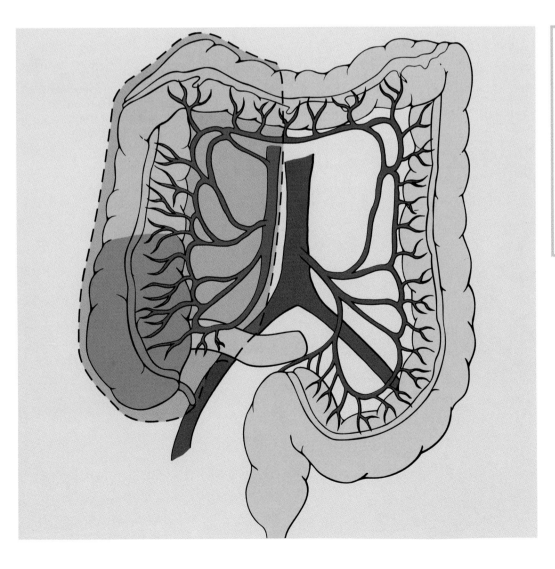

FIGURE 4.34 The anatomic limits of the right radical hemicolectomy. The site of the tumor is indicated by the solid area. The related resection surrounds the designated primary tumor. All vascular ligations are indicated at the true origin. Sufficient ileum is resected to encompass the tumor clearly and the entire ileocolic distribution.

in the sigmoid colon. Anastomosis of the transverse colon to the upper rectosigmoid or distal sigmoid is usually performed in end-to-end fashion. Care must be taken to prevent injury to the left ureter and to the spleen, since the entire left-sided mesocolon is dissected away from the retroperitoneum up to the duodenum or to the aorta (Fig. 4.35).

SIGMOID COLON

Resection is based upon the origin of the inferior mesenteric artery. The procedure is tailored to the location of the lesion; lesions of the proximal sigmoid may require treatment as if they were left colon lesions, while cancers of the distal sigmoid may require dissection of the iliac and aortic bifurcation nodes along with the specimen. Ideally located lesions of the middle sigmoid are dealt with by radical sigmoid resection. The inferior mesenteric vein is again divided inferior to the pancreas. The splenic flexure is usually mobilized, allowing anastomosis of the mid descending colon to the rectum without any tension. The remaining left colon need not be removed since the lymphatic drainage is along the inferior mesenteric vessels and not along the marginal vessels (Fig. 4.36).

RECTUM

The rectum may be defined as the distal 11 to 12 cm of the large bowel. Above this area, large bowel cancers are closer in behavior to colonic lesions in their local recurrence rates and distant metastases (110). Blood supply to the rectum is derived from three sources: the superior hemorrhoidal branches of the inferior mesenteric artery, the middle hemorrhoidal branches of the internal iliac, and hypogastric vessels by the inferior hemorrhoidal branches of the pudendal vessels. The principles guiding resection for cancer of the rectum are:

1. The resection of all regional spread of disease (i.e., mural penetration, nodal involvement in the mesentery, or adjacent involvement of pelvic or abdominal organs).
2. Sphincter preservation wherever possible and appropriate.
3. Awareness and reduction of treatment-related morbidities (70).

Rectal cancers mainly penetrate the wall of the rectum and spread to lymph nodes within the rectal mesentery along the superior hemorrhoidal artery. The spread may be proximal or lateral with-

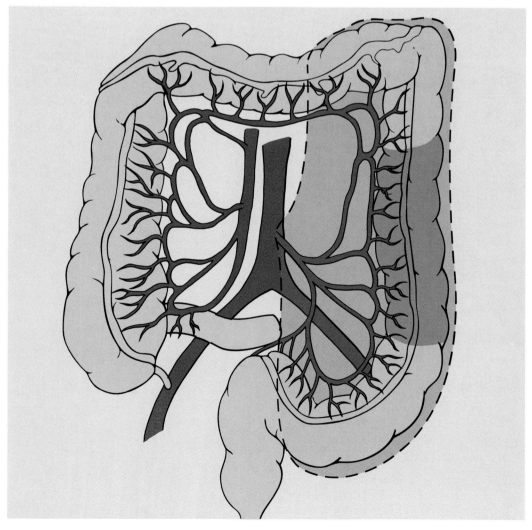

FIGURE 4.35 The left radical hemicolectomy is classically performed for lesions of the descending colon.

in the immediately adjacent mesorectum. Such findings are present in 65 to 80 percent of all curable patients. The avoidance of local recurrence depends on the complete resection of this regional disease (106).

Virtually all cancers of the mid-rectum (6 to 11 cm from the anal verge) are resectable with sphincter preservation. To accomplish such resections the surgeon must achieve good surgical margins and complete mobilization of the rectum (111). The mobilized rectum can be safely transected and anastomosed in this fashion. Current standards involve the use of circular stapling devices, which allow for anastomoses closer to the anal canal than were formerly possible by hand-sewn techniques. Anastomotic leak rates are in the range of 2 to 5 percent (112). The reduction in septic complications allows for fewer diverting colostomies. These are restricted to patients at high risk if septic complications were to take place, such as severe cardiac disease, obvious problems with the anastomosis at the time of operation, extensive or therapeutic prior radiation therapy, contamination, perforation, and so on. Some patients with very low anastomosis should have a diverting colostomy to avoid severe early postoperative dysfunction until the operative trauma has passed, allowing the return of resting and of voluntary continence (113).

Male patients suffer long-term or permanent impotence and female patients suffer bladder dysfunction if the lateral dissections for rectal cancer damage the sacral parasympathetic nerve supply (i.e., the S_3 or S_4 nerve roots). Recent efforts to identify these nerves have evolved into a current innovation, the nerve-preserving pelvic side-wall dissection. This operation accomplishes the goals of wide pelvic dissection while simultaneously reducing the sexual or urinary morbidity and the long-term consequences associated with prior pelvic procedures. Success in preserving potency has been observed in association with any but the most advanced tumors, which require extensive resection (114). Factors that influence the selection of elective treatment include the distance of the cancer from the anal verge, the size and configuration of the tumor (i.e., ulcerative vs. polypoid, sessile, or circumferential), the presence or absence of adjacent organ invasion, suspected pelvic side wall involvement, location (anterior or posterior), sex (wide or narrow pelvis), available means for

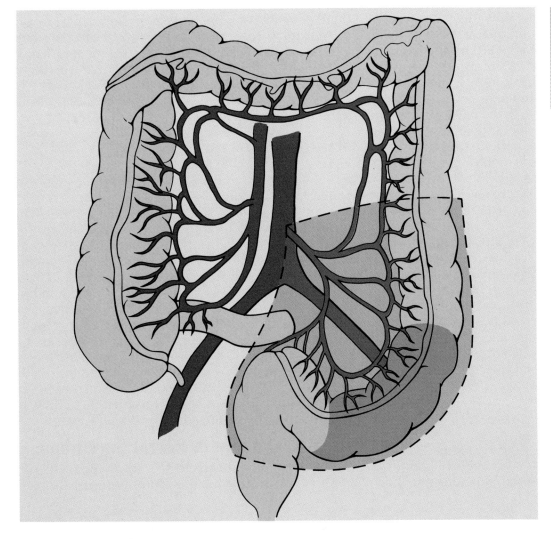

FIGURE 4.36 Tumors of the sigmoid can be resected by high ligations of the inferior mesenteric artery and wide sigmoid resection.

restoring colorectal continuity, and degree of differentiation.

For most cancers of the distal 5 cm of rectum, abdominoperineal resection is the accepted and appropriate operation. Margins of resection are intended to eradicate all recurrent regional disease, such as mural penetration and nodal (or extranodal) mesenteric spread. Dissection of the rectum is accomplished as far as the levators from within the abdomen. The lateral ligaments are divided at the pelvic side walls, while the middle hemorrhoidal arteries may be occluded without compromising the lateral dissection. The procedure is completed with the perineal phase (67).

Coloanal anastomoses are being used more frequently to restore continuity in patients with very low mid-rectal cancers or selected cases of low rectal cancers, but such procedures are still under scrutiny. Success of the coloanal anastomosis is directly related to the surgeon's experience. The complete resection of the rectum, combined with the common use of irradiation, makes postoperative anorectal function problematic in these patients with low rectal cancers. Functional results and cure rates remain under scrutiny (115).

ADJACENT ORGAN INVASION
Approximately 10 percent of large bowel cancers, especially rectal and rectosigmoid lesions, will be found adherent to or actually invading an adjacent organ. Although the most common sites of invasion include the male and female genitourinary systems and the female genitalia, many other organs in the abdominal cavity may be affected by a cancer of the large bowel. Sites of adherence or invasion should be treated by resection to achieve negative margins rather than by dissection along possibly involved planes (116). Many of these patients will have locally extensive tumors without nodal metastases. In general, 50 percent or more of these "unresectable" patients may be cured if the resection eradicates regional manifestations of the disease.

"UNRESECTABLE" CANCER OF THE LARGE BOWEL
Few cancers of the large bowel are really either inoperable or unresectable. Preoperative irradiation may convert such lesions to an operable form (117). A high proportion of lesions declared inoperable after a previous laparotomy may still be resectable by experienced surgeons who are familiar with management of this disease as well as adjacent organ resection and reconstruction. Multidisciplinary surgical efforts are often very rewarding.

Palliative Surgery
Preoperative staging, while detecting some cases of advanced disease, will fail to detect a significant number of cases with visceral metastases or peritoneal involvement. Thus, treatment decisions must still be made at the time of operation. For those patients found to have distant metastases at laparotomy, a resection of the primary tumor should be accomplished. An attempt should be made to avoid long-term morbidity or additional operations, such as colostomy closure after resection with colostomy. In rare cases of advanced disease, a bypass may prove to be a better option than resection. This is especially true when encountering widespread carcinomatosis or tumor that has infiltrated the mesentery in such a way that resection would necessitate transecting obviously neoplastic tissue, or when adjacent organs with a high resection morbidity (e.g., the duodenum) are involved. Also, a colostomy should not be performed in the presence of carcinomatosis in order to avoid exteriorizing the tumor or creating an ascites leak.

In rectal cancer, bulky tumors should be resected despite the presence of metastatic disease so as to avoid the symptoms of persistent pelvic disease such as tenesmus, pain, mucorrhea, burning, and bleeding. Resection and radiation therapy are of incalculable value to the patient with a bulky tumor who might otherwise suffer needlessly. Exclusion of the small bowel from the pelvis using omental pedicles or a mesh sling can be useful in such cases (118).

When the risk of local recurrence is deemed high, permanent colostomy is preferable to reconstruction. If resection and primary anastomosis are possible in smaller upper rectal lesions, it remains the procedure of choice. For lower rectal lesions that are small enough to be amenable to local control, repeated fulguration is an acceptable substitute for colostomy in selected cases.

MANAGEMENT OF THE PATIENT WITH A COLOSTOMY
Rehabilitation therapy for a patient suffering from cancer of the colon or rectum resulting in a colostomy must be tailored to that particular patient. The measures taken are appreciably influenced by the location of the colostomy, whether or not the patient is free of cancer, and the physical and mental ability of the patient to cope with the mechanics of colostomy care. These factors are compounded by the attitudes of the patients and their families. The vast majority of patients who have had a colostomy performed in the course of a curative resection for rectal cancer can lead normal lives. They must, however, receive competent, knowledgeable, and sympathetic instruction in the management of their colostomy and must have the support of their family, physician, and stoma therapist.

Local Treatment of Rectal Carcinoma
Certain early, carefully selected, low-lying rectal carcinomas do not require abdominoperineal resec-

tion. Early cancers of the rectum, as distinguished by a criteria such as small size (≤3 cm) and extreme mobility, are preferred lesions for local treatment. Most such cancers represent only early and localized invasion of the submucosa or superficial penetration of the muscularis propria, and have only about a 10 percent chance of lymph node metastases. Surgeons at the Memorial Sloan–Kettering Cancer Center in New York and at St. Mark's Hospital in London have practiced local excision in toto of selected rectal cancers for decades. This procedure has been considered applicable to about 3 percent of the cases treated at most major centers (119,120). The choice of local excision over fulguration is favored because excision is not only associated with fewer recurrences but it also provides the pathologist with an intact specimen for histologic examination. Criteria such as full thickness penetration, poor differentiation, a positive margin, venous or lymphatic vessel invasion, or a significant mucinous component should be evaluated carefully. A decision can then be made whether to extend resection in those cases where local excision would be inadequate treatment. Using this stepped resectional approach, most authors describe cure rates in the range of 80 to 90 percent, versus 40 to 50 percent for fulguration (121). Local excision requires a careful operation and an experienced pathologist with whom subsequent treatment decisions can be discussed.

In Morson's 1966 review of factors influencing prognosis, the rare occurrence of lymph node metastases preceding mural penetration (10.9 percent to 12.9 percent) was mainly associated with the presence of poorly differentiated tumors (122). In 1977, Morson and associates again reviewed the histologic findings in association with local excision at St. Mark's Hospital (123). Of 91 tumors that were considered completely excised, only three recurred, while 11 of these patients had a major resection after local excision. Of 18 patients in whom the completeness of the excision was in doubt, two patients had tumor recurrence. Of 23 patients in whom the excision was clearly incomplete, 14 had no further surgery because the excision was considered palliative. Locke and associates (119) have reported on the local treatment of rectal cancer at St. Mark's Hospital between 1948 and 1972. Of 22 patients with sessile rectal cancers treated for cure, 15 underwent local excision and only one died of cancer. In selecting cases for local treatment, most lesions larger than 3 cm should be excluded; tumors of this size should be treated by definitive resection.

Morson and co-workers probably have put local excision into its proper perspective. Local excision should be considered "a form of total biopsy" after which a thorough histologic examination can help determine whether the excision was complete or whether aggressive tumor characteristics indicate a further radical operation. The combined clinical and pathologic selection of patients for local treatment offers the best chance of continued success. In recent years, the role of whole pelvic external radiation therapy has been proposed as a means of halting potential spread in certain high-risk cancers that have been excised locally (124).

Treatment of Obstructing and Perforated Carcinomas

The clinical management of obstructing colonic carcinoma is a matter of continuing debate. Obstructing cancers have classically been handled by a staged series of three operations: colostomy, resection, and colostomy closure. Modern advocates propose, however, that obstructing lesions be handled by primary resection and reconstruction. They base their claim on two main premises: 1) the long-term survival after primary resection is better, and 2) the cumulative mortality inherent in the three-stage procedure is prohibitive. The problem remains, however, as to how the surgeon selects patients for colostomy only, for resection, for primary anastomosis, or for delay in reconstruction. A third alternative is resection with end colostomy and later colonic anastomosis, a two-stage procedure. This prevents the septic complications of an anastomosis performed under less than ideal circumstances (contamination, edema, etc.). It is clinically difficult to define which patients should be managed by laparotomy and resection instead of a diverting colostomy alone, but the two-stage procedure accomplishes immediate resection in the safest climate.

The management of colonic perforation generally parallels that of obstruction (125). The five-year survival rate is very poor and is generally associated with the presence of either distant metastases or widespread lymphatic disease, peritoneal seeding, or retroperitoneal invasion. In the patient without obvious tumor spread and in whom perforation has prompted laparotomy, the best policy is, if possible, immediate radical resection. Cancers of the rectosigmoid (i.e., 12 to 18 cm from the anal verge) are best considered as a unique group of "pelvic inlet tumors." They represent the most common site of disease associated with adjacent organ involvement (commonly, the bladder, uterus, etc.). They require special preparation, including the selective use of ureteral catheters and margins of resection. Reconstruction may be more difficult than in standard sigmoid cancers, and some of these patients can benefit from undergoing resection in the lithotomy position, with the planned use of circular stapling devices.

Follow-up After Surgery

Many different strategies have been advocated after curative surgery for colorectal cancer. The follow-up goals should encompass several concepts: 1) initial evaluation for possible adjuvant treatment; 2) surveillance to detect recurrent cancer; and 3) surveillance to detect and remove new colonic adenomas. Adjuvant treatment of colon and rectal cancer is discussed later. A reasonable surveillance program for detecting recurrent cancer should include office visits every three months for the first three years and then every six months, including CEA determination at each visit and a CBC and liver profile every six months. A CT scan of the abdomen and pelvis, and a chest x-ray are advisable annually for five years. Surveillance for new adenomas should include colonoscopy six months and one year after surgery and then every three years if normal.

Treatment of Recurrent Metastatic Disease

LOCAL RECURRENCE

In the abdominal colon, perianastomotic recurrence rarely occurs when adequate resection is performed. Such local recurrences may be amenable to further resection if they are not part of carcinomatosis. In this setting, the five-year survival rate of patients with resectable recurrence of course depends on the extent of residual disease after operation. Patients undergoing resection have been reported to have a five-year survival rate of 49 percent; in those with microscopic residual disease the survival rate was 12 percent (126). The vast majority of patients developing recurrent disease after adequate anatomic resections cannot undergo re-resection.

In patients who have had limited or segmental resections and who present with recurrence, a careful evaluation should be conducted to exclude distant disease. The carcinoembryonic antigen (CEA) level may be elevated and may occasionally be the sole indicator of recurrence. In patients with recurrent or metastatic colorectal cancer, CEA levels in the blood may rise before symptoms appear or laboratory tests show abnormalities, or even before radiographs become abnormal. Some authorities favor periodic CEA determinations (e.g., every three months) after colorectal cancer resection, but this is expensive and may only help in a minority of patients. However, a rising CEA may occasionally reveal a localized, surgically resectable metastasis (127). In conjunction with conventional radiologic techniques (computed tomographic scan or magnetic resonance imaging), radiolabeled monoclonal antibodies to CEA may be helpful in localizing such metastases (128). In the absence of defined lesions, a "second look"

laparotomy based on a rising CEA has not been shown to prolong survival (127). Ultrasonography, computed tomography (of the abdomen and pelvis), liver enzyme studies, chest radiography, and colonoscopy should be performed in the absence of obvious metastatic disease and when resection is considered a possibility. If all tests prove negative for metastases, the feasibility of exploratory surgery for resection can be discussed with the patient. Even then, the majority of patients will turn out to have distant metastases in addition to the local recurrence, preventing the possibility of cure. For this reason, candidates for surgery must be carefully selected.

PELVIC RECURRENCE

Pelvic recurrence frequently follows conventional surgery for rectal cancer. Isolated anastomotic recurrence is rare (129). More often than not, recurrence at the anastomosis is an index of pelvic disease with broad side wall or sacral involvement. From 4500 to 5000 rads of external beam radiation therapy should be administered when the diagnosis of pelvic recurrence is established. In the course of management, patients will frequently present with small bowel obstruction due to a combination of recurrent tumor and radiation enteritis. When recurrent rectal cancer is complicated by small bowel obstruction, especially in the presence of irradiated intestine, single or multiple enteroenterostomy bypasses achieve satisfactory palliation.

PERINEAL RECURRENCE

Perineal recurrence generally develops under one of four conditions: 1) inadequate margins of resection following abdominoperineal resection; 2) low rectal cancer that is poorly differentiated and widely infiltrating, with separate nests of tumor in the perirectal fat; 3) delay in management of a known cancer; and 4) repeated use of fulguration technique.

When visible tumor protrudes through the perineum, relief of pain and infection is the immediate obvious treatment followed by electrocoagulation to promote tumor necrosis. This technique differs significantly from fulguration and creates a gradual slough of tumor that is not likely to bleed extensively. Topical antiseptics such as povidone-iodine and potassium permanganate solution are helpful adjuncts. For cases in which perineal recurrence is resectable, careful assessment will invariably demonstrate that the visible tumor is only a fraction of the actual mass. Brachytherapy (interstitial implants or afterloading catheters containing radioactive substances) may be of value as an adjunct to treatment when a margin of resection proves positive (130).

LIVER METASTASES

Approximately 20 percent of patients at laparotomy for resection of large bowel cancer will be found to have liver metastases. This may escape detection when the common left-lower-quadrant paramedian incision is employed; the entire liver must be felt and seen. The extent of liver involvement should be described systematically. Metastases may be single or multiple, unilobar or multilobar, and may occupy as much as 75 percent of the liver substance. A histologic diagnosis of liver metastases is mandatory. The lack of such documentation in a previously operated patient may necessitate another laparotomy just for biopsy, or may prevent or delay therapy.

For the last three decades, surgeons have elected to remove even solitary hepatic metastases when such a procedure would render the patient clinically free of disease. Cure is possible because some primary tumors (i.e., Dukes' B lesion) may show no residual local disease and may have a single focus of hematogenous spread to the liver. Such an aggressive surgical approach has been shown to be successful at several institutions. The Mayo Clinic has reported a five-year survival rate of 42 percent in 40 patients who underwent resection of apparent solitary metastases; the ten-year survival rate was 28 percent (131). At the Memorial Sloan–Kettering Cancer Center, of 137 patients undergoing liver resections, 43 have been in patients with colorectal metastases. In the stage 1 cases (no vascular or biliary invasion), the survival rates in 39 survivors was 96 percent at one year, 79 percent at two years, and 71 percent at three years (132). When the value of liver resection was first undergoing scrutiny at the Memorial Hospital, 25 patients with resected solitary metastases were compared with 12 patients in whom solitary tumors were identified but left unresected. The five-year survival rates were 28 percent and zero, respectively (133).

In a nationwide survey, Foster (134) documented 46 five-year survivors (22 percent) among 206 patients who underwent a liver resection. Similar results have been reported by Hughes (135) in a nationwide registry involving over 800 cases encompassing numerous institutions and surgeons. Today, when liver resection is being considered but laparotomy demonstrates the presence of multifocal bilobar disease, the use of regional infusion chemotherapy to deliver therapeutic agents makes the overall operative effort more effective (136). The identification of patients with early liver disease (e.g., by markers such as CEA) remains one of the many critical and unsolved problems in this field.

CHEMOTHERAPY FOR RECURRENT DISEASE

The goal of treatment for metastatic disease is to destroy metastases and to improve both quality and duration of survival. Chemotherapy for colorectal cancer has developed very slowly because of the lack of effective drugs (137). During the last 30 years, oncologists have relied principally on a single agent, 5-fluorouracil (5-FU). Recent studies have shown that the true objective response rate with intermittent intravenous injections is approximately 10 percent. A variety of dosage schedules and methods have been tried, including bolus, intravenous, continuous intravenous, and oral routes. More intensive regimens have been compared to less intensive ones, but no significant survival advantage has been found. Other chemotherapeutic and immunotherapeutic compounds have been evaluated in advanced disease, but very few have any appreciable therapeutic value (Fig. 4.37).

There have been several different approaches to the biochemical modulation of 5-FU in an attempt to increase its effectiveness. 5-FU is thought to affect cellular metabolism in the following way: 5-fluoro-2-deoxyuridine-5′-monophosphate (5 – FdUMP), a metabolite of 5-FU, inhibits the cellular

---

FIGURE 4.37:
DEFINITIONS

Complete response: complete disappearance of measurable disease >1 month

Partial response: ≥50% decrease in measurable disease >1 month

Progression: >25% increase in measurable disease

Phase I: maximum tolerable dose, toxicities, starting dose

Phase II: efficacy

Phase III: comparison with other agents

Multimodality: radiation therapy/surgery/chemotherapy

Neoadjuvant: before surgery

Adjuvant: after surgery

enzyme thymidylate synthase. This results in a reduction in the de novo production of thymidylate (dTMP) from dUMP which, in turn, interferes with DNA synthesis. The intracellular concentration of the reduced folate 5,10-methylenetetrahydrofolate ($5\text{-}10\text{-}CH_2\text{-}FH_4$) will affect the ability of FdUMP to inhibit thymidylate synthase. Coadministration of folinic acid with 5-FU has been found in a number of controlled and uncontrolled studies to result in a modest improvement in survival (138). Powerful recombinant DNA technology has made available for clinical trials a variety of biologic response modifiers such as interferons (α, β, γ), and tumor necrosis factor. Interleukin-2 (IL-2) has been administered with or without lymphokine-activated killer cells. The combination of 5-FU plus interferon-α has been found to be active and is currently under study.

Metastases to intra-abdominal viscera (local-regional, peritoneal, and hepatic) are a major cause of death in colorectal cancer. Regional therapy may, therefore, be the best treatment. Both hepatic arterial infusion and intraperitoneal therapy have also been studied. While normal hepatocytes are nourished predominantly by the portal circulation, hepatic metastases derive most of their blood supply from the hepatic artery. Theoretically, hepatic arterial infusion chemotherapy may maximize tumor exposure to the drug, thereby minimizing systemic toxicity (Fig. 4.38). Using infusion pumps for the intra-arterial administration of floxuridine (FUDP) has been studied in several recent randomized trials, but to date, despite a significantly increased rate of partial response of liver metastases, a significant improvement in patient survival has not been demonstrated (139). Hepatobiliary and gastroduodenal mucosal toxicity have been significant in some reports, including sclerosis of intrahepatic bile ducts and ulceration of the stomach and duodenum (140). Concurrent administration of H_2 blockers, cytoprotective agents, or adrenocortical steroids have not prevented these side effects. Newer approaches under study include the use of programmable infusion pumps which allow for greater flexibility of drug administration, as well as biochemical modulation of 5-FU and FUDR by the coadministration of leucovorin (141).

Attempts have been made to enhance the therapeutic activity of drugs by administering them intraperitoneally. Theoretically, treatment of colorectal cancer by intraperitoneal administration would distribute the drug to the most common sites of metastatic spread, namely the liver (through portal circulation) and peritoneum.

Postoperative Adjuvant Therapy for Large Bowel Cancer

Considerable controversy exists about the value of perioperative or immediate postoperative adjuvant therapy in the management of patients with large bowel cancer. For colon cancer new data and current large-scale trials offer, for the first time, the possibility that some benefit may result from such therapy. For rectal cancer, convincing data have existed for several years that support the use of radiation plus chemotherapy.

COLON CANCER

The North Central Cancer Treatment Group reported the results of a study in which patients were randomized among three groups: levamisole only, 5-FU plus levamisole, and no chemotherapy following resection. Levamisole is an antihelminthic drug with possible immunomodulatory activity, but the mechanism of action is poorly understood. It may conceivably also act as a biochemical modulator of 5-FU. Preliminary results in 401 patients demonstrated that 5-FU plus levamisole improved disease-free survival over surgical resection alone, especially in patients with Dukes' C disease. Cancer recurrence was decreased 31 percent (142). A larger national (intergroup) study of levamisole plus 5-FU which included 1301 patients has demonstrated a 41 percent decrease in recurrence and a reduction in death rate by 33 percent in patients with Dukes' C colon cancers (143). Other trials still in progress are studying the combination of 5-FU plus leucovorin in Dukes' B_2 and C colon cancers. Based on a recent consensus conference, 5-FU plus levamisole is now the recommended therapy of choice in Dukes' C colon cancers and will be the control agent in future studies of adjuvant therapy (144). Adjuvant treatment with bacille Calmette-Guérin (BCG) or portal vein infusion has been less impressive.

RECTAL CANCER

Carcinomas of the rectum have a local recurrence rate which is considerably higher than that of colonic tumors; approximately 15 percent to 25 percent of patients with Stage B_2 rectal cancer and approximately 30 percent to 50 percent of those with Stage C tumors will develop pelvic recurrence after conventional surgical resection. The areas at greatest risk are the presacral space, the pelvic side walls, and the soft tissue anterior to the rectum. Several clinical pathologic features are predictive for local recurrence of rectal carcinoma;

extension of the tumor through the bowel wall and nodal involvement are the most important. The location within the rectum also has an influence, since there is a lower failure rate for tumors located in the high rectum or rectosigmoid (above the peritoneal reflection) than for those located in the low rectum, probably because of the technical difficulty of obtaining an adequate margin there (117). Because of the probability of local-regional recurrence, radiation therapy has been evaluated as adjuvant therapy for rectal cancer. Preoperative radiation therapy has been shown to decrease local recurrence, but overall survival is not influenced. The disadvantage of preoperative radiation therapy, however, is that patients with early-stage or unsuspected metastatic disease may be treated unnecessarily (67).

Several recent clinical trials have demonstrated the benefit of postoperative adjuvant therapy (chemotherapy plus radiation therapy). Chemotherapy (5-FU/methyl-CCNU with or without vincristine) alone or combined with radiation therapy has been prospectively compared to surgical resec-

tion or radiation therapy in patients with Dukes' B_2 and C rectal cancer. The studies of the GITSG and the North Central Cancer Treatment Group (NCCTG) demonstrated that the combination of chemotherapy and radiation was more effective than radiation therapy alone, chemotherapy alone, or postoperative observation in reducing the local-regional recurrence rate and prolonging disease-free and overall survival. The recent NCI consensus conference concluded that postoperative radiation chemotherapy plus radiation therapy were effective in Dukes' B_2 and C rectal cancers (143).

EPIDERMOID CARCINOMA OF THE ANUS

Squamous carcinomas and basaloid or transitional cancers are very likely all variants of the same tumors. These tumors arise in the anal canal at or above the dentate line (145) (Fig. 4.39). Many of them have combined histologic features, hence names such as "basaloid." The overall prevalence of these tumors is about 3.9 percent of all rectum and rectosigmoid cancers, but if only the anal

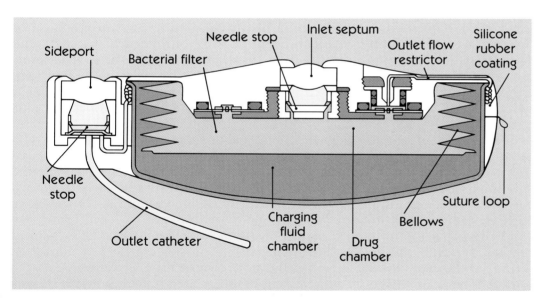

FIGURE 4.38 Cross-sectional diagram of Infusaid Model 400 hepatic arterial infusion device.

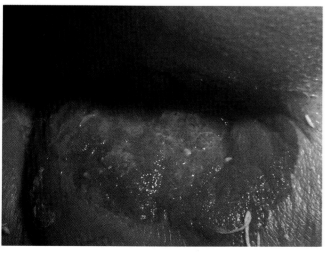

FIGURE 4.39 Anal carcinoma. This spreading lesion, contrary to its appearance, is a squamous carcinoma and is often incorrectly diagnosed initially. Symptoms may include pain and bleeding, or pruritus. Biopsy is very important whenever suspicions about perianal lesions are aroused. Management depends on the size and spread of the carcinoma. (From McNeil NI. *PPG: gastroenterology.* London: Gower Medical Publishing, 1987.)

canal and distal rectum (2 cm) are considered, epidermoid cancers constitute 30 percent of all malignant tumors.

In general, patients with this variety of cancer are slightly younger (average age, 58 years) than those with adenocarcinoma of the rectum (average age, 63 years). Females outnumber males two to one, whereas in adenocarcinoma, incidence is split evenly. Symptoms are similar to those of benign anorectal disease, with bleeding, mass or lump, or "hemorrhoids." Not infrequently, squamous cancer is diagnosed after hemorrhoidectomy when histologic examination is made of excised tissue. The pattern of lymph node spread differs from rectal adenocarcinoma. Inguinal, obturator, hypogastric, and mesenteric nodes are all vulnerable to metastases. The modern therapeutic approach is primarily a combination of external beam radiation therapy and chemotherapy, partly to enhance the value of radiation therapy, and partly to reduce the morbidity of high-dose external-beam therapy (146). Nigro and associates have introduced combined chemotherapy and radiation in the preoperative treatment of squamous carcinoma (147). They have reported on their initial experience with a small group of patients receiving systemic 5-FU (15 mg/m^2) and mitomycin-C (15 mg/m^2), together with 3000 rads of external beam radiation. Favorable tumor shrinkage was observed, suggesting that the combination might be used in place of radical surgery. Quan and co-workers have reported on the Memorial Hospital experience with the first 21 patients treated by this preoperative protocol (148). In contrast to Nigro and colleagues, who began chemotherapy and radiation simultaneously, chemotherapy and radiation were given sequentially at Memorial Hospital. In the first 21 patients, the immediate effects have been striking; eight patients had such dramatic response that no microscopically detectable disease was found in the resected specimens. In view of these findings, 13 other patients were initially treated by local excision rather than by abdominoperineal resection. In a follow-up study of 37 patients, 31 patients with measurable lesions had major clinical responses to combined preoperative treatment. Seventeen of 32 (53 percent) had no evidence of residual tumor in subsequently resected specimens. Of those who had a local excision only, four of 17 (24 percent) developed local recurrence compared with three of 18 (17 percent) of those treated by abdominoperineal resection. The ultimate effects on survival remain to be seen, but this treatment program has now been employed in the management of over 100 patients, and the early dramatic results have been borne out (148).

Prophylactic groin dissection in patients with an epidermoid carcinoma of the anus failed to cure any patient with positive nodes. The current policy, therefore, is to perform only therapeutic and not prophylactic lymph node dissection. Also, the benefit accruing from local surgery after complete tumor regression has saved or delayed the need for radical surgery and colostomy in many patients.

ANORECTAL MELANOMA

Malignant melanoma of the anal canal is an extremely aggressive tumor. Fortunately, it is also rare, with fewer than 250 cases documented in the English language literature. Quinn and Selah in 1977, having culled the literature, reported on nine patients who survived five years among the 107 patients whose case reports they have collected (149). At the Memorial Sloan–Kettering Cancer Center, 59 patients (31 women and 28 men) were seen through 1978. The average age was 55 years. Almost all patients are white, but a few cases have been reported among blacks. Symptoms are those associated with squamous carcinoma or benign anorectal disorders. Masses are nearly always attributed to hemorrhoids, as is intermittent minor bleeding. Melanin is normally present within the anal epithelium, but there is no adequate explanation for melanoma originating in rectal mucosa. Spread is similar to that of epidermoid carcinoma of the anal canal, with extension to inguinal, pelvic (obturator, hypogastric, iliac), and mesorectal sites. Distant metastases to liver, lung, long bones, spine, and skin have also been noted (38).

Treatment has evolved since the 1930s from local treatment together with irradiation, through the addition of colostomy to abdominoperineal resection, to augmentation by abdominopelvic and inguinal lymph node dissection. Since survival seems more related to stage than to treatment, it has been suggested that the primary lesion should always be excised. However, there is currently no support for one form of surgical procedure over another. A local complete excision of the primary melanoma may be as valid, in an individual case, as a radical resection. Radiation therapy does not seem to have any effective role in the treatment of the primary tumor, but may be useful in the management of brain or bone metastases. Chemotherapy is still investigative at this time. Immunotherapy of melanoma has received much interest and attention, and local tumor immunotherapy may cause regression of local disease. There are no data, however, to support the use of nonspecific immunotherapy in preventing systemic disease.

LYMPHOMA

Primary lymphoma of the colon is extremely rare (Figs. 4.40 and 4.41). Of the 4234 adult patients with non-Hodgkin's lymphoma registered at Memorial Hospital before 1979, only 104 had primary lymphomas of the gastrointestinal tract, and of these only 13 tumors were considered to have originated in the large bowel (150). Unlike small bowel lymphoma, there does not appear to be any known precursor of lymphoma in the colon. Presenting signs and symptoms are those observed in other large bowel neoplasms. Except for seven cases of sigmoid and rectal primary lesions, most of the lymphomas were first diagnosed at laparotomy. This situation should change radically with the use of flexible fiberoptic endoscopy. Of the 13 colorectal lymphomas seen at Memorial Hospital, the mean age of the patients was 61 (31 years to 79 years) and, in contrast to other gastrointestinal sites, there was a male-to-female ratio of 2.3 to 1. Surgery and radiotherapy provided good local control in most patients. Nevertheless, 68 percent of patients with gastrointestinal lesions were later found with lymphomas at distant sites, thus strongly suggesting the need for systemic therapy. Survival was significantly related to the stage and to the involvement of adjacent structures. Age, sex, site, depth of mural penetration, and number of foci involved had no bearing on survival. Stage 3 and 4 disease was of major significance, since no patient survived past one year. Because there is a distinct possibility for a second, third, or even fourth malignant lesion to appear, post-treatment surveillance is crucial.

TUMORS OF THE SMALL BOWEL

Benign and malignant tumors of the small bowel are clinically uncommon, representing less than 5 percent of gastrointestinal tract tumors (151–153). The most common small bowel tumors are adenocarcinoma, lymphoma, sarcoma, and carcinoid. Also involving the small intestine are metastatic

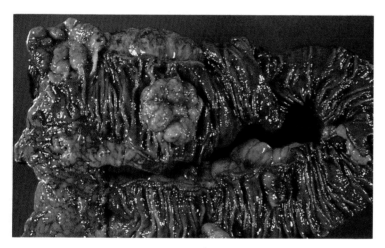

FIGURE 4.40 These multiple polypoid masses of a well-differentiated lymphocytic lymphoma have large areas of intact mucosa, though some ulceration may occur in larger lesions. (From reference 66.)

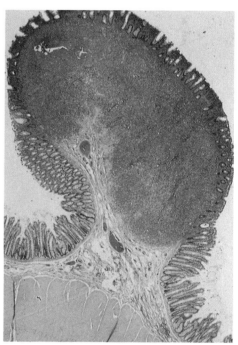

FIGURE 4.41 The mature-appearing lymphocytes comprising one of the smaller nodules of this lymphoma proved to be monoclonal. Mucosal and muscular architecture can still be recognized through the tumor infiltrate (x4). (From reference 66.)

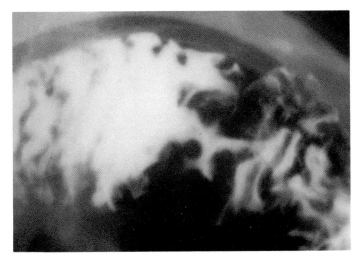

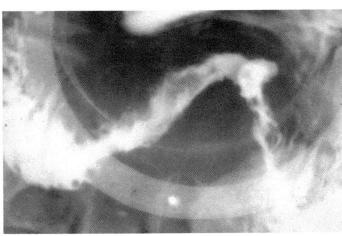

FIGURE 4.42 The concentric and markedly narrowed lumen affecting a very short segment of jejunum is the hallmark of adenocarcinoma. (From reference 66.)

FIGURE 4.43 The irregular narrowing and uneven nodular surface imparted by this lymphoma involving the distal duodenum and proximal jejunum reflect the variable manner in which lymphoma can involve the bowel wall. (From reference 66.)

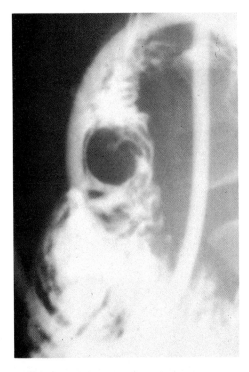

FIGURE 4.44 This loop of jejunum contains a solitary, round intramural mass with central umbilication; this combination is diagnostic of smooth muscle tumors. (From reference 66.)

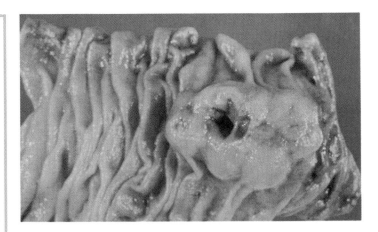

FIGURE 4.45 Characteristic central ulcer of a smooth muscle tumor of small bowel. This patient presented with massive blood loss. The mucosa adjacent to the ulcer is intact. (From reference 66.)

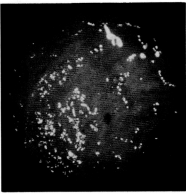

FIGURE 4.46 A reddish-brown lesion, characteristic of Kaposi's sarcoma of the duodenum. (From reference 157.)

tumors such as metastatic melanoma, breast and ovarian cancer, sarcoma, and others.

The most common malignant tumor of the small intestine is adenocarcinoma (Fig. 4.42). The duodenum is the most common site except in patients with Crohn's disease, in whom the distal bowel is the most common site (154). Adenocarcinoma of the proximal duodenum has been associated with familial polyposis and Gardner's syndrome, and Peutz–Jeghers syndrome (155). These cancers tend to be infiltrative and are usually well advanced, with regional or distant metastases, at the time of diagnosis. Clinical presentation usually includes symptoms of partial chronic intestinal obstruction, which is often associated with mild chronic blood loss anemia. The diagnosis is often suggested by upper gastrointestinal and small bowel series, but a definitive diagnosis is usually made at surgical exploration. Proximal duodenal cancers can present with biliary tract obstruction (see Chapter 5) or as atypical peptic ulcers. Surgical resection is the treatment of choice but is usually not curative. Chemotherapy may be needed for follow-up palliative treatment, but the response is usually poor.

Other primary tumors of the small bowel are less common than adenocarcinoma. Carcinoids are discussed in Chapter 6. Sarcomas primarily involve the stomach (see Chapter 2) but can uncommonly involve the small bowel. Obstruction and bleeding are the most frequent clinical presentations. Lymphomas of the small intestines are usually part of disseminated process but can less commonly be primary in the small bowel, especially in patients with a longstanding history of gluten enteropathology or AIDS (156). The ileum is the most common site and the majority are non-Hodgkin's lymphoma. The configuration of these tumors vary from polypoid to infiltrating. Small bowel obstruction, weight loss, and chronic occult bleeding are the usual clinical manifestations. The diagnosis of most small bowel tumors is suspected on small bowel series and confirmed histologically at surgical exploration. Localized tumors can be treated by surgical resection followed by radiation therapy, while disseminated tumors or those with regional node involvement require follow-up chemotherapy. The primary tumor needs to be resected in most patients, even in the presence of extraintestinal spread, as long as the clinical status of the patient is not advanced because of obstruction, bleeding, or perforation, spontaneously or during radiation and chemotherapy (Figs. 4.43–4.46).

REFERENCES

1. Morson BC, Sobin LH. Histological typing of intestinal tumors. In: *International Histological Classification of Tumors,* No. 15. Geneva: World Health Organization, 1976.

2. Parkin DM, et al. Estimates of the worldwide frequency of sixteen major cancers in 1980. *Int J Cancer* 41:184–197, 1988.

3. National Cancer Institute. *Annual cancer statistics review including cancer trends: 1950–1985.* Bethesda, MD: ACI, 1988.

4. Schottenfeld D, Winawer SJ. Large intestine. In: Schottenfeld D, Fraumeni J Jr, eds. *Cancer Epidemiology and Prevention.* Philadelphia: W.B. Saunders, 1982:703–727.

5. Misiewicz JJ, Bartram PB, Cotton PB, et al. *Atlas of clinical gastroenterology.* London: Gower Medical Publishing, 1985.

6. National Research Council, Committee on Diet, Nutrition and Cancer. *Diet, nutrition and cancer.* Washington, DC: National Academy Press, 1982.

7. Wynder EL. The epidemiology of large bowel cancer. *Cancer Res* 35:3388–3393, 1975.

8. Berg JW, Howel MA. The geographic pathology of bowel cancer. *Cancer* 34:807–814, 1974.

9. MacLennan R, et al. Diet, transit time, stool weight and colon cancer in two Scandinavian populations. *Am J Clin Nutr* 31:S239, 1978.

10. Martinez IR, et al. Factors associated with adenocarcinomas of the large bowel in Puerto Rico. In: Birch JM, ed. *Advances in Medical Oncology, Research and Education,* Vol. 3. New York: Pergamon Press, 1979:45–52.

11. Armstrong B, Doll R. Environmental factors and cancer incidence and mortality in different countries with special reference to dietary practices. *Int J Cancer* 15:617–631, 1975.

12. Reddy BS, et al. Metabolic epidemiology of large bowel cancer: fecal mutagens in high and low risk populations for colon cancer: a preliminary report. *Mutat Res* 72:511–522, 1980.

13. Haenszel W, et al. Large bowel cancer in Hawaiian Japanese. *J Natl Cancer Inst* 51:1765–1779, 1973.

14. Modan B, et al. Low fiber intake as an etiologic factor in cancer of the colon. *J Natl Cancer Inst* 55:15–18, 1975.

15. Lyon JL, et al. Energy intake: its relationship to colon cancer risk. *J Natl Cancer Inst* 78:853–861, 1987.

16. Potter JB, McMichael AJ. Diet and cancer of the colon and rectum: a case control study. *J Natl Cancer Inst* 76:569, 1986.

17. Graham S, et al. Diet in the epidemiology of cancer of the colon and rectum. *J Natl Cancer Inst* 61:709–714, 1978.

18. Jain M, et al. A case-control study of diet and colorectal cancer. *Int J Cancer* 26:757–768, 1980.

19. Carroll KK. Experimental studies on dietary fat and cancer in relation to epidemiological data. In: Ip C, et al., eds. *Dietary Fat and Cancer.* New York: Alan R. Liss, 1986.

20. Reddy B, et al. Effect of type and amount of dietary fat and 1,2-dimethylhydrazine on biliary bile acids, fecal bile and neutral sterols in rats. *Cancer Res* 37:2132, 1977.

21. Nauss KM, et al. Dietary fat and fiber: relationship to caloric intake, body growth and colon tumorigenesis. *Am J Clin Nutr* 45:243–245, 1987.

22. Broitman S, et al. Polyunsaturated fat, cholesterol and large bowel tumorigenesis. *Cancer* 40:2455, 1977.

23. Carroll KK, Khor HT. Dietary fat in relation to tumorigenesis. *Prog Biochem Pharmacol* 10:308–353, 1975.

24. Rose DP, et al. International comparison of mortality rates in cancer of the breast, ovary, prostate and colon and per capita food consumption. *Cancer* 58:2364–2371, 1988.

25. Kolonel LN, et al. Multiethnic studies of diet, nutrition and cancer in Hawaii. In: Huyashi Y, ed. *Diet, Nutrition and Cancer.* Tokyo: Science Society Press, 1986:29–40.

26. Burkitt DP, Trowel HC, eds. *Refined carbohydrate foods and disease.* London: Academic Press, 1975:333–345.

27. Kunes S, et al. Cancer control study of dietary etiological factors. The Melbourne Colorectal Cancer Study. *Nutr Cancer* 9:21–42, 1987.

28. U.S. Department of Health and Human Services. *The*

Surgeon General's report on nutrition and health. PHS Publication No. 88-50210. Washington, DC: DHHS, 1988.

29. Hill MJ. Metabolic epidemiology of dietary factors in large bowel cancer. *Cancer Res* 35:3398–3402, 1975.

30. IARC Intestinal Microecology Group. Dietary fibre, transit-time, faecal bacteria, steroids and colon cancer in two Scandinavian populations. *Lancet* 2:207–211, 1977.

31. Miller AB, et al. Food items and food groups as risk factors in a case-control study of diet and colorectal cancer. *Int J Cancer* 32:155–161, 1983.

32. Walker ARP, et al. Fecal pH, dietary fibre intake and proneness to colon cancer in four South African populations. *Br J Cancer* 53:489–495, 1986.

33. *Physiological effects and health consequences of dietary fiber.* Bethesda, MD: Life Science Research Office, Federation of American Societies for Experimental Biology, 1987.

34. Reddy BS, et al. Effect of restricted caloric intake on azoxymethan-induced colon tumor incidence in male F344 rats. *Cancer Res* 47:1226–1228, 1987.

35. Lipkin M, Newmark H. Effect of added dietary calcium on colonic epithelial cell proliferation in subjects at high risk for familial colon cancer. *N Engl J Med* 313:1381–1384, 1985.

36. Shike M, Winawer SJ, Greenwald PH, et al. Primary prevention of colorectal cancer. *Bulletin of the World Health Organization* (3):377–385, 1990.

37. Burt RW, Bishop DT, Lynch HT, et al. Risk and surveillance of individuals with heritable factors for colorectal cancer. *Bulletin of the World Health Organization* 68(5):655–665, 1990.

38. Bussey HJR, Veale AMO, Morson BC. Genetics of gastrointestinal polyposis. *Gastroenterology* 74:1325–1330, 1978.

39. Gardner EJ, Burt RW, Freston JW. Gastrointestinal polyposis: syndromes and genetic mechanisms. *West J Med* 132:488–499, 1980.

40. Bodmer WF, Bailey CJ, Bodmer J, et al. Localization of the gene for familial adenomatous polyposis on chromosome 5. *Nature* 328:614–616, 1987.

41. Woolf CM. A genetic study of carcinoma of the large intestine. *Am J Hum Genet* 10:42–47, 1958.

42. Macklin MT. Inheritance of cancer of the stomach and large intestine in man. *J Natl Cancer Inst* 24:551–571, 1960.

43. Lovett E. Familial factors in the etiology of carcinoma of the large bowel. *Proc R Soc Med* 67:21–22, 1974.

44. Burt RW, Bishop DT, Cannon LA, et al. Dominant inheritance of adenomatous colonic polyps and colorectal cancer. *N Engl J Med* 312:1540–1544, 1985.

45. Cannon-Albright LA, Skolnick MH, Bishhop T, et al. Common inheritance of susceptibility to colonic adenomatous polyps and associated colorectal cancers. *N Engl J Med* 319:533–537, 1988.

46. Vogelstein B, Fearon ER, Hamilton SR, et al. Genetic alterations during colorectal tumor development. *N Engl J Med* 319:525–532, 1988.

47. Winawer SJ, O'Brien MJ, Waye JD, et al. Risk and surveillance of individuals with colorectal polyps. *Bulletin of the World Health Organization* (in press).

48. Morson BC. The polyp cancer sequence in the large bowel. *Proc R Soc Med* 67:451–457, 1974.

49. Williams AR, Balasooriya BAW, Day DW. Polyps and cancer of the large bowel: a necropsy study in Liverpool. *Gut* 23:835–842, 1982.

50. Morson BC. The evolution of colorectal carcinoma. *Clin Radiol* 35:425–431, 1984.

51. O'Brien MJ, Winawer SJ, Zauber AG, et al. The national polyp study: patient and polyp characteristics associated with high-grade dysplasia in colorectal adenomas. *Gastroenterology* 98:371–379, 1990.

52. Lambert R, Sobin LH, Waye JD, Stadler GA. The management of patients with colorectal adenomas. In: Holleb A, ed. *Third International Symposium on Colorectal Cancer.* New York: American Cancer Society, 1984: 43–52.

53. Stryker SJ, Wolff BG, Culp CE, et al. Natural history of untreated colonic polyps. *Gastroenterology* 93:1009–1013, 1987.

54. Winawer SJ, Zauber A, Diaz B, O'Brien MJ, et al. The national polyp study: overview of program and preliminary report of patient and polyp characteristics. In: Steele G, Winawer SJ, Burt R, Karr JP, eds. *Basic and Clinical Perspectives of Colorectal Polyps and Cancer.* New York: Alan R. Liss, Inc. 1988: 35–49.

55. Waye JD, Braunfeld SF. Surveillance intervals after colonoscopic polypectomy. *Endoscopy* 14:79–81, 1982.

56. Kronborg O, Fenger C. Prognostic evaluation of planned follow-up in patients with colorectal adenomas. (An interim report). *Int J Color Dis* 2:203–207, 1987.

57. Levin B, Lennard-Jones J, Riddell RH, et al. Surveillance of patients with chronic ulcerative colitis. *Bulletin of the World Health Organization.* Geneva, Switzerland: WHO, 1991.

58. Sachar DB. Cancer in inflammatory bowel disease In: Goebell H, Peskar BM, Malchow H, eds. *Inflammatory Bowel Disease—Basic Research and Clinical Implications.* MTP Press Ltd. 1988:289–294.

59. Butt J, Lennard-Jones J, Ritchie J. A practical approach to the cancer risk in inflammatory bowel disease. *Med Clin N Am* 64:1203–1220, 1980.

60. Gyde SN, Prior P, Allan PN, et al. Colorectal cancer in ulcerative colitis: a cohort study of primary referrals from three centers. *Gut* 29:206–217, 1988.

61. Katzka I, Brody R, Morris E, Katz J. Assessment of colorectal cancer risk in patients with ulcerative colitis: experience from a private practice. *Gastroenterology* 85:22–29, 1983.

62. Brostran O, Lofberg R, Nordenvall B, et al. The risk of colorectal cancer in ulcerative colitis: an epidemiologic study. *Scand J Gastroenterol* 221:1193–1199, 1987.

63. Gilat T, Fireman Z, Grossman A, et al. Colorectal cancer in patients with ulcerative colitis: a population study in Central Israel. *Gastroenterology* 94:870–877, 1988.

64. Lennard-Jones JE. Cancer risk in ulcerative colitis. surveillance or surgery. *Br J Surg* 72:584–586, 1985.

65. Enker WE. Flow cytometric determination of tumor cell DNA content and proliferative index as prognostic variables in colorectal cancer. *Perspect Colon Rectal Surg* 3(1):1–33, 1990.

66. Mitros, FA. *Atlas of gastrointestinal pathology.* New York: Gower Medical Publishing, 1988.

67. Enker WE. Cancer of the rectum. Operative management and adjuvant therapy. In: Fazio VW, ed. *Current Therapy in Colon and Rectal Surgery.* Toronto: B.C. Decker, Inc., 1990: 120–130.

68. Dukes CE. The classification of cancer of the rectum. *J Pathol Bacteriol* 35:323, 1932.

69. Dukes, CE, Bussey HJR. The spread of rectal cancer and its effect on prognosis. *BRJ Cancer* 12:309, 1958.

70. Simpson WC, Mayo CW. The mural penetration of the carcinoma cell in the colon. Anatomical and clinical study. *Surg Gynecol Obstet* 68:872, 1989.

71. Kirklin JW, Dockerty MB, Waugh JM. The role of the peritoneal reflection in the prognosis of carcinoma of the rectum and sigmoid colon. *Surg Gynecol Obstet* 88:326, 1949.

72. Astler VB, Coller FA. The prognostic significance of direct extension of carcinoma of the colon and rectum. *Ann Surg* 139:846, 1954.

73. Holyoke ED, Lokich J, Wright H. Adjuvant therapy for adenocarcinoma of the colon following clinically curative resection. In: *Proceedings, Gastrointestinal Tumor Study Group, National Cancer Institute.* Bethesda: NIH, 1975.

74. Enker WE, Laffer U Th, Block GE. Enhanced survival of patients with colon and rectal cancer is based upon wide anatomic resection. *Ann Surg* 190:350–360, 1979.

75. Wood DA, Robbins GF, Lippin C, Lum D, Stearns MW Jr. Staging cancer of the colon and rectum. *Cancer* 43:961–968, 1979.

76. Kassner EG. *Atlas of radiologic imaging.* New York: Gower Medical Publishing, 1989.

77. Schottenfeld D, Winawer SJ. Large intestine. In: Schottenfeld D, Fraumeni JF, eds. *Cancer Epidemiology and Prevention*. Philadelphia: W.B. Saunders, Inc., 1982:703–727.

78. Zamcheck N, Liu P, Thomas P, Steele G. Search for useful biomarkers of pre or early malignant colon tumors. In: Steele G, Burt RW, Winawer SJ, Karr JP, eds. *Basic and Clinical Perspectives of Colorectal Polyps and Cancer*. New York: Alan R. Liss, Inc., 1988:251–275.

79. Winawer SJ, Prorok P, Macrae F, Bralow SP. Surveillance and early diagnosis of colorectal cancer. *Cancer Detect Prev* 8:373–392, 1985.

80. Winawer SJ, Schottenfeld D, Flehinger BJ. Colorectal cancer screening. (Review). *JNCI* 84 (4): 243–253, 1991.

81. Hunt RH, Waye JD, eds. *Colonoscopy techniques, clinical practice and colour atlas*. Great Britain: Chapman and Hall Ltd. (Yearbook Medical Publishers, Inc.), 1981.

82. Greegor DH. Diagnosis of large bowel cancer in the asymptomatic patient. *JAMA* 201:943–945, 1967.

83. Greegor DH. Occult blood testing for detection of asymptomatic colon cancer. *Cancer* 28:131–134, 1971.

84. Crespi M, Weissman GS, Gilbertsen VA, et al. The role of proctosigmoidoscopy in screening for colorectal neoplasia. *CA* 34(3):158–166, 1984.

85. Bohlman TW, Katon RM, Lipshutz GR, et al. Fiberoptic pansigmoidoscopy. An evaluation and comparison with rigid sigmoidoscopy. *Gastroenterology* 72:644–649, 1977.

86. Zucker GM, Medusa MJ, Chonez JS, et al. The advantages of the 30 cm flexible sigmoidoscope over the 60 cm flexible sigmoidoscope. *Gastrointest Endosc* 30:59–64, 1984.

87. Groverman HS, Sanowski RA, Klaube M. Training primary care physicians in flexible sigmoidoscopy: performance evaluation of 17,167 procedures. *West J Med* 148:221–224, 1988.

88. Gilbert DA, Shaneyfelt SL, Silverstain FE, Mahler AK, Hallstrom AP, 674 members of the ASGE. The national ASGE colonoscopic survey—analysis of colonoscopic practices and yields. (Abstract). *Gastrointest Endosc* 30:143, 1984.

89. Hertz RE, Deddish MR, Day E. Value of periodic examinations in detecting cancer of the rectum and colon. *Postgrad Med* 27:290–294, 1960.

90. Dales LG, Friedman GD, Ramcharan S, et al. Multiphasic checkup evaluation study. 3 outpatient clinic utilization, hospitalization and mortality experience after seven years. *Prev Med* 2:221–235, 1973.

91. Friedman GD, Collen MF, Fireman BH. Multiphasic health checkup evaluation: a 16 year follow-up. *J Chron Dis* 39(6):453–463, 1986.

92. Selby JV, Friedman GD, Quesenberry CP Jr, Weiss NS. A case-control study of screening sigmoidoscopy and mortality from colorectal cancer. *N Eng J Med* 326 (10): 653–657, 1992.

93. Selby JV, Friedman GD. Sigmoidoscopy in the periodic health examination of asymptomatic adults. *JAMA* 261(4):595–600, 1989.

94. Gnauck R, Macrae FA, Fleisher M. How to perform the fecal occult blood test. *CA* 34:134–147, 1984.

95. Flehinger BJ, Herbert E, Winawer SJ, Miller DG. Screening for colorectal cancer with fecal occult blood test and sigmoidoscopy: preliminary report of the colon project of Memorial Sloan-Kettering Cancer Center and PMI Strang Clinic. In: Chamberlain J, Miller AB, eds. *Screening for Gastrointestinal Cancer*. Toronto: Hans Huber Publishers, 1988:9–16.

96. Kronborg O, Fenger C, et al. Initial mass screening for colorectal cancer with fecal occult blood test. *Scand J Gastroenterol* 22:677–686, 1977.

97. Gilbertsen VA, McHugh R, Schuman L, William SE. The early detection of colorectal cancers: a preliminary report of the results of the occult blood study. *Cancer* 45:2899–2901, 1980.

98. Hardcastle JD, Thomas WM, Chamberlain J, et al. Randomized controlled trial of fecal occult blood screening for colorectal cancer. The results of the first 107,349 subjects.

Lancet 1:1160–1164, 1989.

99. Kewenter J, Bjork S, Haglind E, et al. Screening and rescreening for colorectal cancer: a controlled trial of fecal occult blood testing in 27,700 subjects. *Cancer* 62(3):645–651, 1988.

100. Lofberg N, Brostrom O, Karlen P, et al. Colonoscopic surveillance in long standing total ulcerative colitis—a 15 year follow-up study. *Gastroenterology* 99(4):1021–1031, 1990.

101. Canadian Periodic Health Examination Task Force. The periodic health examination. *Can Med Assoc J* 121(9):1193–1254, 1979.

102. National Cancer Institute. Early Detection Branch, Division of Cancer Prevention and Control. *Working guidelines for early cancer detection*. Washington, DC: NCI, 1987.

103. Knight KK, Fielding JE, Battista RN. Occult blood screening for colorectal cancer. *JAMA* 261(4):587–593, 1989.

104. American Cancer Society. Guidelines for the cancer-related checkup: recommendations and rationale. *Cancer* 30: 194–240, 1980.

105. U.S. Congress, Office of Technology Assessment. *Costs and effectiveness of colorectal cancer screening in the elderly*. (Background paper). OTA-BP-H-74. Washington, DC: US Government Printing Office, September 1990.

106. Enker WE. Surgical treatment of large bowel cancer. In: Enker WE, ed. *Carcinoma of the Colon and Rectum*. Chicago: Year Book Medical Publishers, Inc., 1978:73–106.

107. Herter FP, Slanetz CA. Patterns and significance of lymphatic spread from cancer of the colon and rectum. In: Weiss L, Gilbert HA, Ballon SC, eds. *Lymphatic System Metastases*. Boston: G.K. Hall Medical Publishers, 1980:275.

108. Enker WE, Laffer U, Block GE. Enhanced survival of patients with colon and rectal cancer is based upon wide anatomic resection. *Ann Surg* 190:350–360, 1979.

109. Enker WE. Operative management of colonic carcinomas. In: Block GE, Moosa AR, eds. *Operative Colorectal Surgery*. Philadelphia: W.B. Saunders, 1991 (in press).

110. Pilipshen SJ, Heilweil M, Quan SHQ, Sternberg SS, Enker WE. Patterns of pelvic recurrence following definitive resections of rectal cancer. *Cancer* 53:1354–1362, 1984.

111. Heald RJ, Ryall RDH. Recurrence and survival after total meso-rectal excision for rectal cancer. *Lancet* 1:1479–1482, 1986.

112. Beart RW Jr, Kelly KA. Randomized prospective evaluation of the EEA stapler for colorectal anastomoses. *Am J Surg* 141:143–147, 1981.

113. Parks AG, Peray JP. Resection and sutured colo-anal anastomosis for rectal carcinoma. *Br J Surg* 69:301–304, 1982.

114. Enker WE. Nerve preserving pelvic side wall dissection in the operative treatment of rectal cancer. American Surgical Association (Abstract). (Submitted).

115. Paty PB, Enker WE. Colo-anal reconstruction following low anterior resection for rectal carcinoma. *Hepatogastroenterology* 1991 (in press).

116. Hunter JA, Ryan JA Jr, Schultz P. En bloc resection of colon cancer adherent to other organs. *Am J Surg* 154:67–71, 1987.

117. Doseretz DE, Gunderson LL, Hedberg S, et al. Pre-operative irradiation for unresectable rectal and rectosigmoid carcinomas. *Cancer* 52:814–818, 1983.

118. Devereux DF, Kavanah MT, Feldman MI, et al. Small bowel exclusion from the pelvic by a polyglycolic acid mesh sling. *Surg Oncol* 26:107–112, 1984.

119. Locke MR, Cavins DW, Ritchie JK, Lockhart-Mummery HE. The treatment of early colorectal cancer by local excision. *Br J Surg* 65:346–349, 1978.

120. Baron PB, Enker WE, Zakowski M, et al. Immediate versus salvage resection after local treatment for early rectal cancer. *Am J Surg* (Submitted).

121. Biggers OR, Beart RW Jr, Ilstrup DM. Local excision of rectal cancer. *Dis Colon Rectum* 29:374–377, 1976.

122. Morson BC. Factors influencing the prognosis of early cancer of the rectum. *Proc R Soc Med* 59:607–608, 1966.

123. Morson BC, Whiteway JE, Jones EA, Macrae FA, Williams CB. Histopathology and prognosis of malignant colorectal polyps treated by endoscopic polypectomy. *Gut* 5:437–444, 1984.

124. Rich TA, Weiss DR, Mies C, et al. Sphincter preservation in patients with low rectal cancer treated with radiation therapy with or without local excision or fulguration. *Radiology* 156:527–531, 1985.

125. Glenn F, McSherry CK. Obstruction and perforation in colorectal cancer. *Ann Surg* 173:983–992, 1971.

126. Vassilopoulos PP, Yoon JM, Ledesma E. Treatment of recurrence of adenocarcinoma of the colon and rectum at the anastomatic site. *Surg Gynecol Obstet* 152:777–780, 1981.

127. Steele G Jr, Zamcheck N, Mayer R, et al. Results of CEA initiated second look surgery for recurrent colorectal cancer. *Am J Surg* 139:544–548, 1980.

128. Lyden MH, Thompson CH, Liechtenstein M, et al. Visualization of metastases from colon carcinoma using an iodine 121-radio-labeled monoclonal antibody. *Cancer* 57:1135–1139, 1986.

129. Beart RW Jr, Martin JK Jr, Gunderson LL. Management of recurrent rectal cancer. *Mayo Clinic Proc* 61:448–450, 1986.

130. Fourquet A, Enker WE, Shank B, et al. The value of interstitial radiation in advanced and recurrent colorectal cancer. *Endo Hypertherm Oncol* 1:113–117, 1985.

131. Wilson SM, Adson M. Surgical treatment of hepatic metastases from colorectal cancer. *Arch Surg* 111:330–334, 1976.

132. Fortner JG, Silva JS, Golbey RB, et al. Multivariate analysis of a personal series of 247 consecutive patients with liver metastases from colorectal cancer. *Ann Surg* 199:306–316, 1984.

133. Attiyeh FF, Wanebo HJ, Stearns MW Jr. Hepatic resection for metastases from colorectal cancer. *Dis Colon Rectum* 21:160–162, 1978.

134. Foster JH, Berman MM. *Solid liver tumors.* Philadelphia: W.B. Saunders, 1977.

135. Hughes K. Hepatic metastases registry: resection of the liver for colorectal metastases: a multi-institutional study of patterns of recurrence. *Surgery* 100:178–284, 1986.

136. Cohen AM, Kaufman SD, Wood WC, Greenfield AJ. Regional hepatic chemotherapy using an implantable drug infusion pump. *Am J Surg* 145:529–533, 1983.

137. Abbruzzese JL, Levin B. Treatment of advanced colorectal cancer. *Hematol Oncol Clin North Am* 3:135–153, 1989.

138. Arbuck SG. Overview of clinical trials using 5-fluorouracil and leucovorin for the treatment of colorectal cancer. *Cancer* 63(Suppl):1036–1044, 1989.

139. Hohn DC, Stagg RJ, Friedman MD, et al. A randomized trial of continuous intravenous versus hepatic intra-arterial floxuridine in patients with colorectal cancer metastatic to the liver: the Northern California Oncology Group Trial. *J Clin Oncol* 7:1646–1654, 1989.

140. Kemeny N, Daly J, Reichman B, et al. Intrahepatic or systemic infusion of fluorodeoxyuridine in patients with liver metastases from colorectal carcinoma. *Ann Intern Med* 107:459 465, 1987.

141. Patt YZ, Roh M, Chase J, Levin B, Hohn D. A phase I trial of hepatic arterial infusion (HAI) of floxuridine (FUDR) and folinic acid (FA) for colorectal cancer (CRC) metastatic to the liver. *Proc 26th Annual Meeting Amer Soc Clin Oncol* (459):118, 1990.

142. Laurie JA, Moertel CG, Fleming TR, et al. Surgical adjuvant therapy for large bowel carcinoma: an evaluation of levamisole and the combination of levamisole and fluorouracil. *J Clin Oncol* 7:1447–1456, 1989.

143. Moertel CG, Fleming TR, MacDonald JS, et al. Levamisole and fluorouracil for adjuvant therapy of resected colon carcinoma. *N Engl J Med* 322:352–358, 1990.

144. National Institute of Health Consensus Conference. Adjuvant therapy for patients with colon and rectal cancer. *JAMA* 264(11):1444–1450, 1990.

145. Sternberg SS. Pathological aspects of colon and anorectal cancer. In: Stearns MW Jr, ed. *Neoplasms of the Colon, Rectum, and Anus.* New York: John Wiley, 1980: 37–62.

146. Stearns MW Jr, Urmacher C, Sternberg SS, Woodruff J, Attiyeh F. Cancer of the anal canal. *Curr Probl Surg* 4:1–44, 1980.

147. Nigro N, Vaitkevicius VK, Considine BJ. Combined therapy for cancer of the anal canal. A preliminary report. *Dis Colon Rectum* 17:354, 1974.

148. Quan SH, Magill GB, Leaming RH, Hajdu SI. Multidisciplinary preoperative approach to the management of epidermoid carcinoma of the anus and anorectum. *Dis Colon Rectum* 21:89, 1978.

149. Quinn D, Selah C. Malignant melanoma of the anus in a Negro: report of a case and review of the literature. *Dis Colon Rectum* 20:627, 1977.

150. Weingrad D, DeCosse JJ, Sherlock P, et al. Primary gastrointestinal lymphoma. *Cancer* 49:1258–1265, 1982.

151. Ebert PA, Zuidema GD. Primary tumors of the small intestine. *Arch Surg* 91:452, 1965.

152. Wilson JM, Melvin DB, Gray GF, Thorbjarnarson B. Primary malignancies of the small bowel: a report of 96 cases and a review of the literature. *Ann Surg* 180:175, 1974.

153. Williamson RC, Welch CE, Malt RA. Adenocarcinoma and lymphoma of the small intestine: distribution and etiologic associations. *Ann Surg* 197:172, 1983.

154. Lightdale CJ, Sternberg SS, Posner G, Sherlock P. Carcinoma complicating Crohn's disease: report of seven cases and review of the literature. *Am J Med* 590:262, 1975.

155. Guyton D, Schreiber H. Intestinal polyposis and periampullary carcinoma—changing concepts. *J Surg Oncol* 29:158, 1985.

156. Al-Bahrani ZR, Al-Mondhiry H, Bakir H, Al-Saleem T. Clinical and pathologic subtypes of primary intestinal lymphoma. Experience with 132 patients over a 14-year period. *Cancer* 52:1666–1672, 1983.

157. Silverstein FE, Tytgat GNJ. *Atlas of gastrointestinal endoscopy.* New York and London: Gower Medical Publishing, 1987.

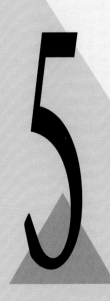

Cancer of the
Pancreas and
Biliary Tract

Eugene P. DiMagno

Pancreatic ductal adenocarcinoma remains equivalent to a death sentence. It is an insidious, aggressive, and rapidly growing tumor that has a multifocal origin within the pancreas. Inroads have been made, though, in identifying risk factors, in developing diagnostic methods (including an algorithm that has 90 percent sensitivity and specificity), and in palliating these patients with both surgical and nonoperative approaches. This chapter discusses these subjects as well as more unusual tumors of the pancreas, and cancers of the ampulla and biliary tract that may have a similar clinical presentation as ductal adenocarcinoma of the pancreas.

CANCER OF THE PANCREAS
Epidemiology

Pancreatic cancer is the fourth most common cause of cancer-related mortality in men and the fifth most common in women. The five-year survival rate for pancreatic cancer in the United States from 1979 to 1984 was 3 percent and 5 percent, respectively, for whites and blacks. The age-adjusted death rate has continued to rise over the past five decades (Fig. 5.1). In females, it has increased from four to eight deaths per 100,000 population, and in males from five to 12 (1). For women the rate appears to be quite linear, whereas for men it has apparently reached a plateau. In fact, for men it may have decreased slightly over the past decade.

RISK FACTORS AND PREVENTION
AGE AND SEX   Pancreatic cancer is a disease of the elderly. More than 80 percent of patients affected are between the ages of 60 and 80 (2). Pancreatic cancer is unusual below the age of 40, but in women, there appears to be a small early peak of occurrence between the second and fourth decade of life (3). These tumors in women may be papillary cystic in type, which are associated with better survival (4).

Consistently, in all series, men slightly outnumber women, as the sex rates approximate 1.5:1 (2). The death rate in both white and nonwhite males appears to increase with age, whereas for all females the death rate plateaus at approximately 65 years.

OTHER RISK FACTORS   Risk for pancreatic cancer can be divided into high, moderate, and unconfirmed risk groups (Fig. 5.2). Patients with hereditary pancreatitis or hereditary nonpolyposis colon cancer syndrome (the Lynch II syndrome) are at high risk for developing pancreatic cancer. Five percent to 20 percent of persons with hereditary pancreatitis develop pancreatic cancer (5,6). Similarly, families with type II Lynch syndrome have an increased

incidence of pancreatic cancer, as well as neoplasms of the breast and gynecologic organs (7).

Moderate-risk groups include chemical workers, cigarette smokers, and people with high-fat diets and diabetes mellitus. Industrial carcinogens implicated as a risk factor for pancreatic cancer include coal tar derivative (8), coke (9), methylnitrosourethane, acetominofluorene, methylcolanthrene, paradimethylaminobenzene, benzidine, and β-naphthylamine (10). Chemical workers have an increased incidence of cancer, and 50 percent of cancer deaths in chemical workers are from pancreatic cancer (11). On the other hand, in one study, no excess pancreatic cancer was found among chemists (12), and in two other studies, there was no increased risk of cancer in relation to a specific occupation (13,14). There have been at least six prospective studies in which the mortality ratio of pancreatic cancer in cigarette smokers was increased to ranges between 1.6 and 3.1 (2). These studies were conducted among male British physicians (15), two groups of males in the U.S. (ages 45–64 and 65–79) (16), U.S. veterans (17), Japanese males and females (2), Canadian veterans (2), and Swedish males and females (2).

Diet has also been reported to be significantly associated with pancreatic cancer. In 1973 Wynder and associates (18) conducted a survey of the daily fat intake and the incidence rate of pancreatic cancer mortality in a variety of countries (Fig. 5.3). These investigators found a positive correlation (r = 0.67) between the amount of fat ingested per day and the incidence of pancreatic cancer. They (18,19) and others (20) have also noted an association between cholesterol ingestion and pancreatic cancer. The fatty acid content of the diet may be important. Linoleic acid (corn, safflower, sunflower oils) acts as a promoter of pancreatic cancer, whereas oleic acid (olive oil) and eicosaptaenoaic acid (derived from fish and marine mammals) do not (21).

The relation between diabetes mellitus and pancreatic cancer is somewhat complicated. Carbohydrate intolerance is present in up to 80 percent of patients with pancreatic cancer (22). Diabetes mellitus, however, usually occurs secondary to pancreatic cancer and does not precede its onset. However, in patients with well-established diabetes mellitus for more than two years there is a two- to threefold increased risk for pancreatic cancer (21,22,23); in this situation diabetes mellitus is likely a risk factor, a risk more prevalent in females.

In contrast to hereditary pancreatitis, the association between nonhereditary chronic pancreatitis and pancreatic cancer is unconvincing; a zero to 9.4 percent incidence of pancreatic cancer has been reported to develop in patients with nonhereditary chronic pancreatitis (24).

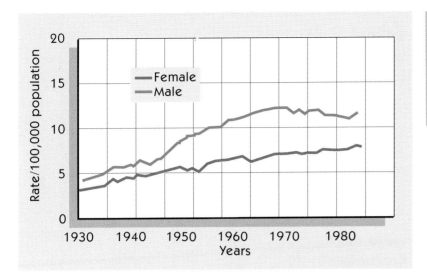

FIGURE 5.1 Age-adjusted death rate for pancreatic cancer in the United States, 1930–1984. The overall estimated annual mortality rate for 1982–1986, adjusted to the age distribution of the 1970 U.S. census, is 8.6 per 100,000 population. (Adapted from reference 1.)

FIGURE 5.2:
RISK FACTORS FOR PANCREATIC CANCER

HIGH RISK
Hereditary pancreatitis
Hereditary nonpolyposis
   syndrome

MODERATE RISK
Chemical workers
Cigarette smokers
Ingestion of high-fat diet
Diabetes mellitus

UNCONFIRMED RISK
Nonhereditary calcific
   pancreatitis
Coffee
Alcohol
Anatomy (lack of prominent
   channel between bile and
   pancreatic ducts)
Previous cholecystectomy or
   gastrectomy

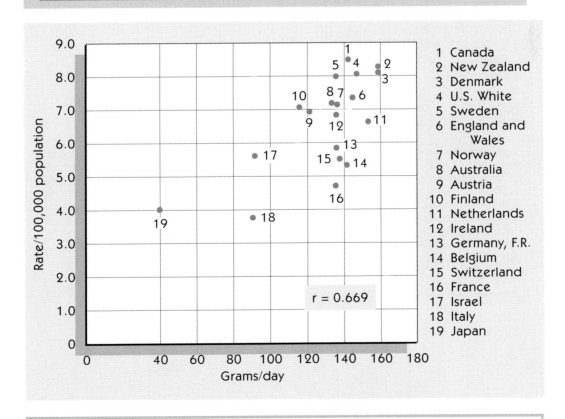

1 Canada
2 New Zealand
3 Denmark
4 U.S. White
5 Sweden
6 England and
   Wales
7 Norway
8 Australia
9 Austria
10 Finland
11 Netherlands
12 Ireland
13 Germany, F.R.
14 Belgium
15 Switzerland
16 France
17 Israel
18 Italy
19 Japan

r = 0.669

FIGURE 5.3 Relation between pancreatic cancer mortality and total fat intake among countries. (From reference 18.)

FIGURE 5.4:
PRIMARY MALIGNANT NEOPLASMS OF THE NONENDOCRINE PANCREAS*

	PATIENTS	
	NO.	%
DUCT (DUCTULE) CELL ORIGIN	573	88.8
Duct cell carcinoma (494)		
Giant cell carcinoma (27)		
Giant cell carcinoma (osteoclastoid type) (1)		
Adenosquamous carcinoma (20)		
Adenosquamous (spindle cell) carcinoma (0)		
Microadenocarcinoma (solid microglandular) (16)		
Mucinous ("colloid") carcinoma (9)		
Cystadenocarcinoma (mucinous) (5)		
Papillary cyst tumor (1)		
ACINAR CELL ORIGIN	8	1.2
Acinar cell carcinoma (7)		
Acinar cell cystadenocarcinoma (1)		
MIXED CELL TYPE	1	0.2
Duct-islet cell (1)		
CONNECTIVE TISSUE ORIGIN	4	0.6
Leiomyosarcoma (1)		
Malignant fibrous histiocytoma (1)		
Malignant hemangiopericytoma (1)		
"Osteogenic" sarcoma (1)		
UNCERTAIN HISTOGENESIS	59	9.2
Pancreaticoblastoma (1)		
Unclassified (58)		
Large cell (50)		
Small cell (7)		
Clear cell (1)		
TOTAL	645	

*Adapted from references 29 and 30. The authors obtained data from 500,000 surgical specimens and 13,882 autopsies performed at Memorial Hospital, New York, NY. In the study, 821 patients were listed as having pancreas (nonislet) cancer; adequate clinical and pathologic material was available for study in 645 patients. Other tumors that are rare and not reported in their series include: some duct tumors (mucinous-carcinoid carcinoma, carcinoid, oncocytic carcinoid, "oat-cell" carcinoma, ciliated cell carcinoma), mixed cell tumors (duct-islet-acinar cell, acinar-islet cell, carcinoid-islet cell), connective tissue tumors (fibrosarcoma, rhabdomyosarcoma malignant neurilemoma, liposarcoma), and malignant lymphoma (histocytic and plasmacytoma).

The relation between alcohol use and pancreatic cancer is weak and inconsistent. Similarly, it is unclear whether coffee is a significant risk factor for pancreatic cancer.

Reflux of duodenal contents into the pancreatic duct may be associated with pancreatic carcinogenesis. In an autopsy study we found a trend toward an increased incidence of abnormal ductal epithelium in patients who did not have a prominent common channel between the bile and pancreatic ducts (25). Papillary hyperplasia, pyloric glanduloplasia, squamous metaplasia, and carcinoma of the pancreas (in one patient) were significantly associated with a very short common channel, interposed septum between the bile duct and common bile duct, or separate openings of the two ducts. The cause of this association is unknown. In dogs, a species that has separate openings for the bile duct and the main pancreatic duct, a small amount of duodenal content refluxes into the pancreatic duct during phases II and III of the interdigestive period and during the first postprandial hour (26). At these times duodenal pressure may exceed pancreatic ductal pressure. The amount of reflux, however, is extremely small (less than 1 percent of duodenal content) and whether in humans duodenal content refluxes into the pancreatic duct is unknown. Thus, the relation between the anatomy of the pancreaticobiliary ducts, reflux of duodenal content into the pancreatic ducts, and pancreatic carcinogenesis remains uncertain.

It is also uncertain whether cholecystectomy or gastrectomy is related to the development of pancreatic cancer. In recent cohort studies, we found no association between these operations and the future development of pancreatic cancer (27,28).

Although many risk factors cannot be altered, it seems reasonable to expect that the incidence of pancreatic cancer could be decreased if smoking were eliminated, less cholesterol and fat were ingested, and the major sources of dietary fat were olive oil and fish.

Pathology of Pancreatic Ductal Adenocarcinoma (Fig. 5.4)

Primary malignant neoplasms of the nonendocrine pancreas have been divided into six major groups and 36 subtypes (4,29,30). Ninety percent of pancreatic carcinomas originate from ductal epithelium, and 75 percent of the total number of tumors are classically mucinous-producing ductal cell carcinomas. Most of the nonductal tumors arise from acinar cells or connective tissue or are of uncertain histogenesis. Two tumors are notable because they occur in specific populations. Papillary cystic tumors are responsible for the slight increase in pancreatic tumors in young women (4), whereas the rare pancreaticoblastoma occurs primarily in children (31). Sixty percent to 70 percent of ductal cell adenocarcinomas arise in the part of the pancreatic head which is derived from the dorsal pancreas anlage and contains the common bile duct within its substance (30) (Fig. 5.5). The remaining tumors arise from the central portion of the pancreatic head behind the ampulla of Vater or in the

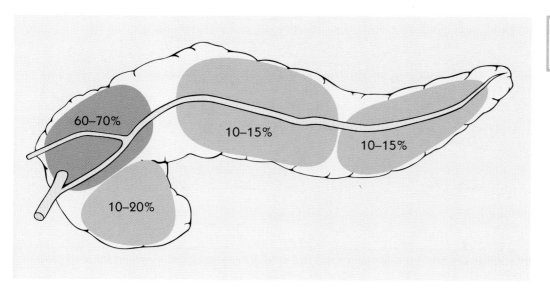

FIGURE 5.5 Sites of origin of pancreatic ductal adenocarcinoma.

60–70%

10–15%

10–15%

10–20%

uncinate process close to the ventral pancreatic duct. These latter tumors commonly are detected late, because in their course they are not associated with jaundice and the tumors may not be easily detectable with computed tomography (CT).

When first diagnosed, tumors vary in size according to their site of origin. Tumors of the head of the pancreas have a median diameter of 2.6 cm to 3.5 cm whereas tumors of the body and tail are 5 cm to 7 cm in diameter. Carcinomas of the body and tail are probably larger at the time of diagno-

sis because they are detected later (4), a hypothesis supported because most tumors of the head at autopsy are 2.5 cm to 3.5 cm larger than at the time of diagnosis.

The most common and earliest extension of the tumors is to the retroperitoneal space. Later, cancers of the head may invade the stomach, duodenum (Figs. 5.6–5.8), gallbladder, and peritoneum. Tumors of the body and tail (see Figs. 5.6 and 5.7) may spread to the stomach, liver, spleen, left adrenal gland, and peritoneum. Because the tumor is

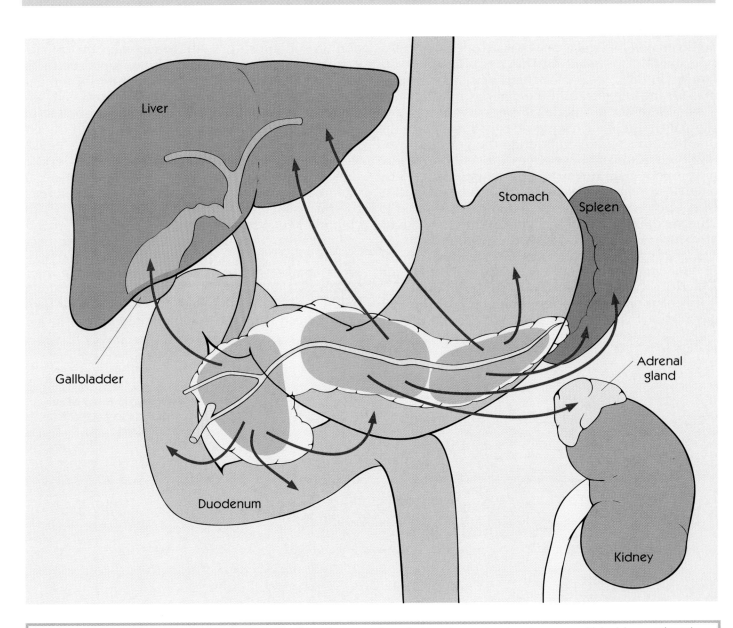

FIGURE 5.6 Extension of pancreatic tumors arising from the head, body, and tail of the pancreas to regional structures. The earliest extension of tumors from any site is to the retroperitoneum. Later, tumors of the head invade the stomach, duodenum, gallbladder, and peritoneum, whereas tumors of the body and tail spread to the spleen, stomach, liver, and left adrenal gland.

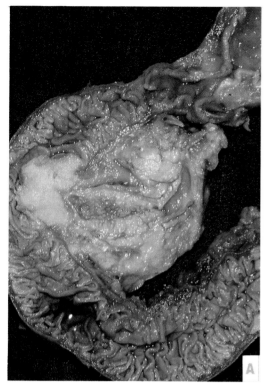

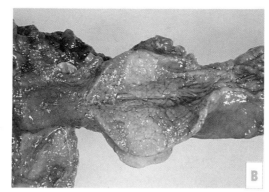

FIGURE 5.7 Macroscopic appearances of a carcinoma (A) invading the head of the pancreas, infiltrating the duodenum and destroying the pancreatic duct (courtesy of Mr. M. Knight), and **(B)** carcinoma of the body (courtesy of Dr. J. Newman), and **(C)** tail. (From Misiewicz JJ, et al. *Atlas of clinical gastroenterology.* London: Gower Medical Publishing, 1987.)

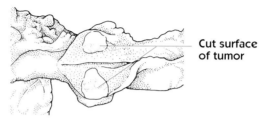

Cut surface of tumor

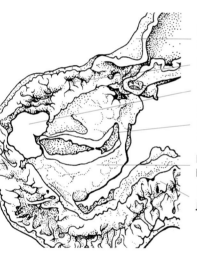

Pyloric canal

Duodenum

Tumor

Dilated pancreatic duct

Normal pancreas

Proximal jejunum

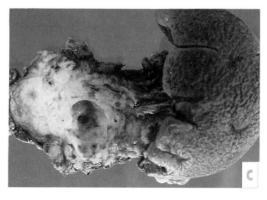

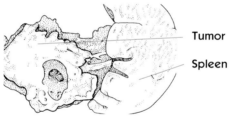

Tumor

Spleen

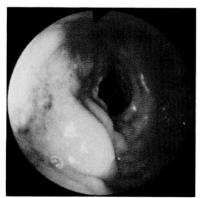

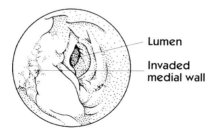

Lumen

Invaded medial wall

FIGURE 5.8 Invasion of the medial wall of the duodenum by pancreatic cancer. Note asymmetry of the duodenal lumen. (From Silverstein FE, Tytgat GNJ. *Atlas of gastrointestinal endoscopy.* New York: Gower Medical Publishing, 1987.)

characterized by well-differentiated to poorly differentiated duct glands embedded in a dense network of fibrous tissue (Fig. 5.9), as the tumor invades the pancreas and surrounding tissue it envelops and fixes vessels, and microscopically invades fat, lymph channels, and perineural areas.

Another characteristic of ductal cell carcinoma is the expression of a number of pancreatic cancer-associated antigens. By using immunocytochemistry, a number of antigens have been demonstrated within ductal adenocarcinoma cells, including carcinoembryonic antigen (CEA), pancreatic oncofetal antigen (POA), and the monoclonal antigens CA-19-9 and DA-PAN-2. Since benign pancreatic tumors (cystadenomas), acinar cell carcinomas, and endocrine tumors do not express these pancreatic-associated antigens, antibodies against them have been developed into tests to diagnose ductal pancreatic cancer. In general, these tests are unreliable because they lack tumor and pancreas specificity due to cross-activity with duct cells of other organs (see Diagnosis section).

Clinical Presentation

The presenting symptoms of pancreatic cancer are nonspecific because a variety of diseases present in a similar fashion. In a study of pancreatic cancer (32), we found that 40 percent of the 70 patients who had symptoms suggestive of pancreatic cancer had other diseases. The diagnoses of these patients were pancreatitis (n=7), nine nonpancreatic intra-abdominal neoplasms (three lymphomas, four carcinomas of the small intestine, one ovarian carcinoma, and one uterine cancer with retroperitoneal metastases), and 24 miscellaneous non-pancreatic, non-neoplastic diseases including a negative laparotomy (n=16), cholecystitis (two), and one each of celiac artery aneurysm, abdominal sarcoidosis, granuloma of the abdominal wall,

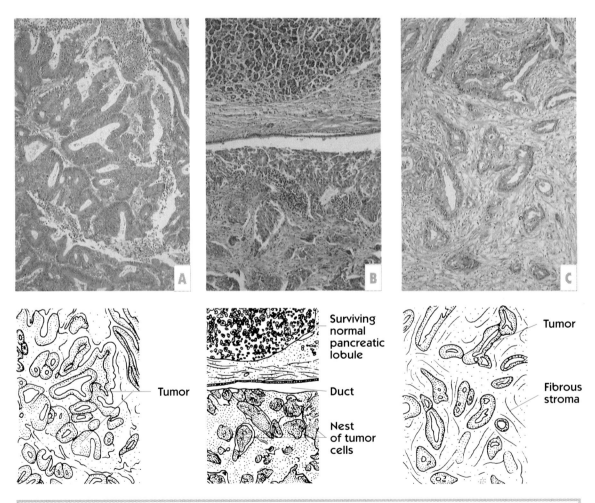

FIGURE 5.9 Three histologic patterns of pancreatic carcinoma: (A) a typical well-differentiated tumor; **(B)** a moderately differentiated lesion with nests of cells producing a squamoid configuration; and **(C)** an adenocarcinoma, but with a dense fibrous stroma. With the latter, it would be easy to biopsy mostly fibrous tissue that would then be difficult to differentiate from chronic pancreatitis. H&E stain, x50. (From Misiewicz et al., 1987.)

alcoholic hepatitis, small bowel ulcers, or duodenal ulcers.

PAIN

Pain is the presenting symptom in up to 79 percent of patients with pancreatic cancer (Fig. 5.10) and occurs in 90 percent of patients during the course of the disease (33). The most frequent sites of abdominal pain are the epigastrium (46 percent) and the left (13 percent) or right (18 percent) abdomen. Lower abdominal pain is less frequent, but it may occur in up to 11 percent of patients, and may be the only location of pain (3 percent) (34).

Initially, abdominal pain may be vague and rather nonspecific, and can occur up to three months before the onset of jaundice. Consequently, early in the course of the disease, it is commonly ignored by both patients and physicians. Even then, however, a careful history may elicit features suggestive of visceral, organic pain originating from the retroperitoneum. This pain is most often described as persistent, disagreeable, aching in character, and causing night awakening. Pain relief may occur by bending forward, lying on the side and drawing the knees up to the chest or chin, and sometimes by crouching forward on all four extremities on the bed or the floor. Pain may be increased by lying supine or eating. The cause of postprandial pain may be an abnormal rise in intraductal pressure behind a completely or partially obstructed pancreatic duct.

JAUNDICE

Jaundice is a presenting symptom in 80 to 90 percent of patients with cancer of the head of the pancreas and in 6 to 13 percent of patients with carcinomas of the tail (33,35). In cancer of the head of the pancreas, jaundice occurs secondary to compression or direct extension of the tumor into the bile duct, whereas in cancer of the tail of the pancreas, jaundice is usually the result of hepatic metastasis or obstruction of the extrahepatic bile duct at the porta hepatis by lymphadenopathy secondary to metastases. Painless jaundice rarely occurs in pancreatic cancer because a careful history will reveal pain in virtually all patients with pancreatic cancer.

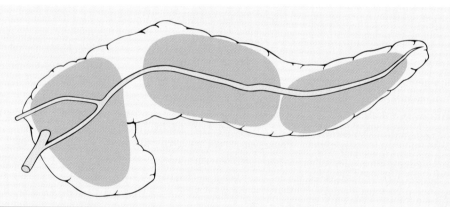

FIGURE 5.10 Frequency of the presenting symptoms of cancer of the pancreas arising in the head or body and tail.

Head		Body and tail	
Symptoms	% Patients	Symptoms	% Patients
Weight loss	92	Weight loss	100
Jaundice	82	Pain	87
Pain	72	Weakness	42
Anorexia	64	Nausea	43
Dark urine	63	Vomiting	37
Light stools	62	Anorexia	33
Nausea	45	Constipation	27
Vomiting	37	Food intolerance	7
Weakness	35	Jaundice	7

Weight Loss

Significant weight loss of more than 10 percent of ideal body weight is an almost universal finding in patients with pancreatic cancer. In two prospective studies (32,36) 41 of 42 patients with pancreatic cancer had weight loss exceeding 10 percent of ideal body weight, and mean weight loss was 18 percent of precancer body weight. Weight loss was only observed when patients had malabsorption, decreased calorie consumption, or both. In our experience, weight loss correlated with malabsorption, but not caloric consumption, and fat malabsorption was more frequent (75 percent) and more severe than protein malabsorption (50 percent) (Fig. 5.11). Carbohydrate malabsorption in patients with pancreatic cancer, to my knowledge, has not been investigated, but it probably occurs.

Malabsorption likely plays a major and more important role than food intake in weight loss in carcinomas of the head of the pancreas compared with cancers of the body and tail. But decreased food intake contributed to weight loss in some patients with carcinomas located in the head. If careful measurements are made, 50 percent of all patients with cancer of the pancreas will be found to have decreased consumption of calories (36), and in patients with cancers of the body and tail decreased food intake is a major contribution to weight loss.

Diabetes Mellitus

In carefully performed studies glucose intolerance is present in as many as 81 percent of patients with pancreatic cancer (22). An abnormal glucose tolerance test is due to either previously recognized or newly acquired diabetes mellitus, conditions that are significantly more frequent in pancreatic cancer patients compared with a control group of patients without pancreatic cancer who present with identical symptoms as the former. In other studies, carbohydrate intolerance has been reported to occur in 20 percent to 60 percent of patients with pancreatic cancer (37).

It is probable that the patients with pancreatic cancer and glucose intolerance are composed of two groups because the incidence of glucose intolerance in pancreatic cancer is higher than can be expected due to genetic factors. One group has hereditary diabetes, a known risk factor for pancreatic cancer. A second group of patients has glucose intolerance for less than two years and has developed hyperglycemia secondary to the pancreatic cancer. Usually, this group of patients has mild diabetes. Thus, it is rare that the presenting symptoms of pancreatic cancer are those of new onset brittle diabetes mellitus such as hyperphagia, polydipsia, and polyuria.

Other Symptoms

Alterations of stool character and habit occur commonly in patients with pancreatic cancer because of the high incidence of malabsorption. Light-colored stools occur in 62 percent of patients with cancer of the head of the pancreas (33). Diarrhea, however, is not a common symptom, and some patients with cancer of the head of the pancreas and up to 27 percent of patients with cancers of the tail (33) may complain of constipation. These findings should not be too surprising as we have found that patients with severe pancreatic insufficiency and gross steatorrhea (mean fecal fat = 70 g fat/24 h) have only slightly increased fecal weight (463 ± 75 g compared to a normal fecal weight of 200 g/24 h) and not all have diarrhea (38). Thus, patients with pancreatic cancer may have a relatively normal stool pattern (no diarrhea), or even constipation, and yet have significant malabsorption that requires treatment with pancreatic enzymes.

Other nonspecific symptoms such as nausea, vomiting, weakness, and anorexia occur in 30 to 36 percent of patients with cancers of the head or body and tail. Rare symptoms, which occur in less than 5 percent of patients, include superficial thrombophlebitis, gastrointestinal bleeding, psychiatric disturbances, and symptoms related to diabetes mellitus. Superficial thrombophlebitis was originally described in patients with pancreatic cancer by Trousseau in the 19th century, but nowadays it is more commonly associated with cancers originating from other sites such as the lung. Gastrointestinal bleeding may occur as a late complication secondary to direct invasion of the tumor into the stomach, duodenum, or colon, or from varices arising from occlusion of the splenic or portal vein by the tumor or pancreatitis secondary to the tumor.

Depression is not a common major clinical problem, but it and emotional liability as measured by the Minnesota Multiphasic Personality Inventory (MMPI) were reported in 76 percent of patients with pancreatic cancer, whereas these conditions occur in only 20 percent of patients with other intra-abdominal neoplasms (39). It is uncertain, however, whether these symptoms are directly associated with pancreatic cancer or occur secondary to chronic illness produced by the cancer (40).

Physical Findings (Fig. 5.12)

Patients with pancreatic cancer of the head, and patients with cancers of the body and tail, have different presenting signs. More than 80 percent of patients with cancer of the head of the pancreas have hepatomegaly and jaundice (33,35,41). In contrast, patients with cancer of the body and tail may have abdominal tenderness and pain, but hepatomegaly and jaundice are present less than 30 percent of the time. Jaundice begins as scleral icterus and progresses to include the skin. Some patients may have severe pruritus which leads to persistent scratching, excoriation, and lichenification of the skin.

A palpable gallbladder (Courvoisier's sign) is present in 30 percent of patients with a carcinoma of the head of the pancreas. An abdominal mass or ascites occurs in less than 20 percent of patients with carcinoma of any pancreatic region. Compres-

sion or occlusion of the portal or splenic vein by the tumor may cause portal hypertension and produce ascites, splenomegaly, and peripheral edema. If the tumor compresses the aorta or splenic artery, an abdominal bruit may be heard.

Diagnosis

Because the clinical presentation of pancreatic cancer is so nonspecific, patients frequently undergo a large battery of tests, including routine laboratory tests such as chemistry and hematology groups,

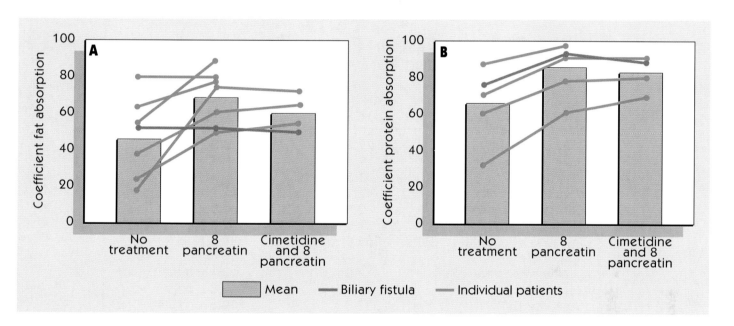

FIGURE 5.11 Coefficient of fat (A) and protein (B) absorption in pancreatic cancer patients with no treatment and when receiving pancreatic extract. A total of 14 patients were treated, but data are shown only for the six patients with severe steatorrhea (less than or equal to 80 percent coefficient in fat absorption) and the five patients with severe protein malabsorption (less than 85 percent coefficient protein absorption). A single patient who had severe steatorrhea and did not improve with pancreatin developed a biliary cutaneous fistula between no treatment and administration of pancreatin. All patients with severe protein malabsorption improved with pancreatin. Addition of an H₂ blocker did not affect malabsorption. (Adapted from reference 36.)

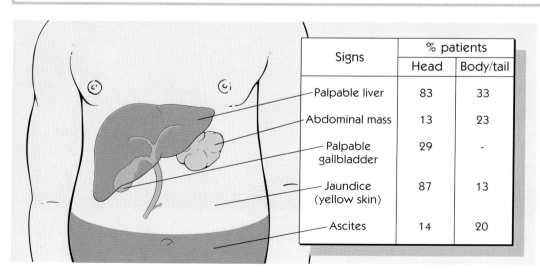

FIGURE 5.12 Presenting signs of pancreatic cancer.

Signs	% patients	
	Head	Body/tail
Palpable liver	83	33
Abdominal mass	13	23
Palpable gallbladder	29	-
Jaundice (yellow skin)	87	13
Ascites	14	20

gastrointestinal barium studies, and endoscopy. Some of them provide clues to the diagnosis of pancreatic cancer, but none establishes the diagnosis.

ROUTINE LABORATORY TESTS

Patients with pancreatic cancers have many routine laboratory tests that are within the range of values found in patients with pancreatitis or benign gastrointestinal disorders (see Fig. 5.13; calcium, phosphorus, and prothrombin time). In contrast, higher levels of plasma glucose, amylase, and lip-ase are found in patients with pancreatitis compared to benign gastrointestinal disorders, but these tests do not discriminate between pancreatic cancer and pancreatitis (42). Similarly, high values for alkaline phosphatase, bilirubin, and aspartate amino-transferase (AST) are found in patients with pancreatic cancer, but these tests do not distinguish between pancreatic cancer and hepatic disorders. Nevertheless, it is customary to obtain a routine battery of tests in patients who are suspected of having pancreatic cancer. This bat-

FIGURE 5.13:
SEROLOGIC TESTS IN PATIENTS SUSPECTED OF HAVING PANCREATIC CANCER

LABORATORY TESTS	PANCREATIC CANCER (n = 9)	PANCREATITIS (n = 9)
Glucose (mg/d)	122.5 ± 6.9	103.8 ± 8.2
Calcium (mg/d)	9.6 ± 0.1	9.5 ± 0.1
Phosphorus (mg/d)	3.5 ± 0.1	3.6 ± 0.2
Prothrombin time (sec)	12.2 ± 0.3	11.9 ± 0.2
Direct bilirubin (mg/d)	2.4 ± 0.6	0.0 ± 0.0
Indirect bilirubin (mg/d)	1.9 ± 0.4	0.5 ± 0.1
Alkaline phosphatase (U/l)	565.0 ± 71.8	239.0 ± 76.2
Aspartate aminotransferase (U/l)	47.6 ± 6.1	19.1 ± 3.8
Lipase (U/l)	95.8 ± 21.7	245.8 ± 55.2
Amylase (U/l)	337.3 ± 152.4	609.6 ± 113.4

Adapted from reference 42.

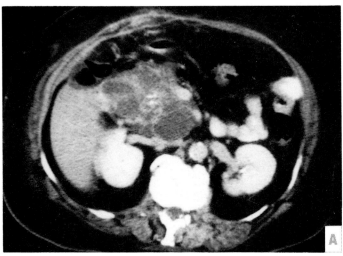
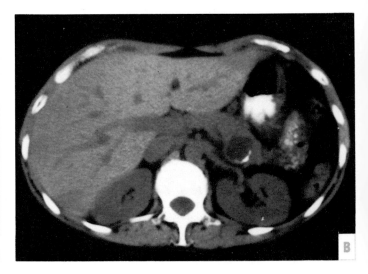

FIGURE 5.14 Calcification of serous microcystic cystadenomas (A), which are benign lesions, are characterized as central stellate "starburst or sunburst" lesions. The cysts are multiple and small, equal to or less than 2 cm. Calcifications of macrocystic lesions **(B)**, which are malignant mucous cystadenocarcinomas, are linear and in the wall of the cyst, greater than 4.5 cm in diameter.

tery includes pancreatic enzymes as well as x-rays of the chest and abdomen.

Elevated serum pancreatic enzymes indicate the presence of pancreatic disease, but do not differentiate between acute or chronic inflammation of the pancreas and pancreatic cancer. Bony lesions on the chest x-ray, pleural effusions, or ascites on the flat plate may be indicative of either pancreatic cancer or pancreatitis, but frank pulmonary or bony metastases are diagnostic of cancer. In my opinion, if metastases are found, no further diagnostic tests are needed. Some physicians, who believe that even metastatic disease should be treated aggressively, however, would obtain special tests to find the primary tumor.

Calcification of the pancreas has a 95 percent predictive value for the diagnosis of chronic pancreatitis because primary adenocarcinomas of the pancreas almost never calcify. It is wise, however, to keep in mind that patients with calcific chronic pancreatitis, particularly those with hereditary pancreatitis, may develop pancreatic cancer, and pancreatic calcifications may be present in 10 percent of patients with cystadenomas (43,44; Fig. 5.14) and can also occur in cavernous lymphangiomas (45) of the pancreas. In patients with chronic calcific pancreatitis, disappearing calcifi-

cations have been described as a rare sign of pancreatic cancer (46,47).

IMMUNOLOGIC TESTS

Because of the unsatisfactory diagnostic yield from common routine laboratory tests, there has been an intensive effort over the past decade to find sensitive and specific serologic markers for the diagnosis of pancreatic cancer (Fig. 5.15). Unfortunately, at this time, none of the available markers meets this standard sufficiently to be used routinely to screen or diagnose patients with pancreatic cancer (48). In our own experience, we found that total thyroxin, some gastrin parathyroid hormone calcitonin immunoglobins (IgA, IgG, IgM), and carcinoembryonic antigen (CEA) were not sensitive or specific (42). We and others have found that serum CEA is elevated in both nonpancreatic and pancreatic cancers compared to patients with nonpancreatic diseases. Although CEA levels are increased in up to 85 percent of patients with pancreatic cancer, they are also increased in 65 percent of patients with nonpancreatic cancers and 46 percent of patients with benign pancreatic diseases (49–52). Similarly, the other tumor markers listed in Figure 5.15, including galactosyltransferase (53), CA 19–9 (54), and CA 125 (55), have been investigated, but

FIGURE 5.15:
TUMOR MARKERS IN PANCREATIC CANCER

ONCOFETAL ANTIGENS
Carcinoembryonic
   antigen (CEA, CEA-S)
Alpha fetoprotein (AFP)
Pancreatic oncofetal
   antigen (POA)
Basic fetoprotein (BFP)
α-CAP 1

PROTEINS
Lactoferrin
Ferritin
B$_2$ microglobulin
Immunosuppressive
   acidic protein

PEPTIDE HORMONES
B human chorionic
   gonadotropin
Parathormone
Calcitonin
C-peptide
Gastrin
Glucagon
Insulin

ENZYMES
Trypsin
Trypsinogen
Chymotrypsin
Amylase
Pancreatic ribonuclease
   (RNase)
Galactosyltransferase II

MONOCLONAL ANTIBODIES
CA 19-9
DU-Pan-2

GLYCOPROTEINS
Non-cross-reacting antigen
   (NCA)
EDC 1
B$_2$ glycoprotein
Tennagen

OTHERS
Fucose
Leukocyte adherence
   inhibition assay

Note: This long list of tumor markers has been developed and most have been tested in patients with pancreatic cancer. At present, none of the available markers is sensitive or specific enough for the diagnosis of pancreatic cancer to be used as routine screening or for diagnostic tests.

thus far none has proven clinically useful in the diagnosis of pancreatic cancer.

IMAGING TESTS

The most direct, simple, and specific tests to diagnose pancreatic cancer are those that image the pancreas. Among them, ultrasonography (Fig. 5.16A), computed tomography (Fig. 5.16B), and endoscopic retrograde pancreatography (Fig. 5.17) are the only ones commonly available, with ultrasonography used most often. Thermography and radioselenium scanning of the pancreas are no longer in use because they lack sensitivity and specificity. In contrast, newer tests such as magnetic resonance imaging (MRI) and endoscopic ultrasonography (56) are available in some centers, but they are not widely used because their sensitivity and specificity at present are no better than the usual imaging tests.

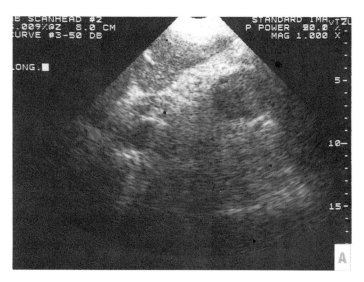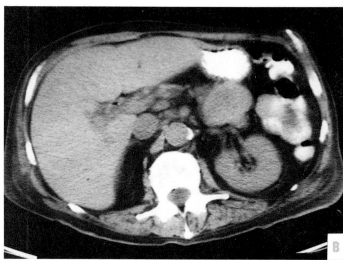

FIGURE 5.16 (A) Ultrasound and **(B)** CT of pancreatic cancer.

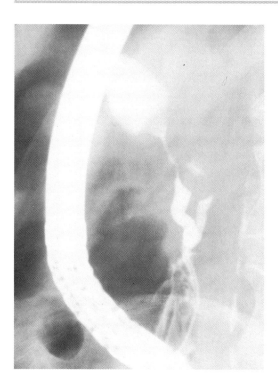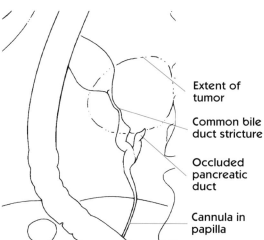

Extent of tumor

Common bile duct stricture

Occluded pancreatic duct

Cannula in papilla

FIGURE 5.17 ERCP demonstrating a blocked pancreatic duct, due to a carcinoma, which has caused stricturing of the common bile duct, leading to dilatation of the proximal biliary tree. (From Misiewicz et al., 1987.)

The sensitivity and specificity of ultrasonography and computed tomography are similar (80 percent) for detection of pancreatic cancer (32,57–60) (Fig. 5.18). Most authorities agree, however, that CT is slightly more sensitive. Because it is more expensive, however, we recommend ultrasonography as the first imaging test for diagnosing pancreatic cancer (Fig. 5.19).

Endoscopic pancreatography has a sensitivity and specificity of 90 percent for the diagnosis of pancreatic cancer (32,53). The usual abnormalities in pancreatic cancer are pancreatic duct obstruction, encasement of the pancreatic duct, and the "double duct sign" (see Fig. 5.17). The latter abnormality is produced by obstruction of the distal pancreatic and bile ducts by a cancer in the head of the pancreas. In pancreatic cancer, the common duct obstruction is abrupt and can be differentiated from obstruction secondary to chronic pancreatitis which produces a tapered narrowing. Parenchymal tumors may be detected by forcing contrast media into the entire collection system (acinarization), but this technique may cause acute pancreatitis. Rarely, a tumor cavity may be filled during ERP and represent a sign of pancreatic cancer.

In patients with pancreatic cancer it has become increasingly popular to obtain a pancreatic cytology (Fig. 5.20) during real time ultrasonography or CT scanning, which allows visualization of the tip of the aspiration needle so that it can be positioned within the tumor mass. Either technique is 90 percent sensitive for diagnosis of pancreatic cancer (61,62). These procedures should be performed in patients who have unresectable lesions or a cancer in the body or tail since there are no five-year survivors among patients who have a cancer in this location. Percutaneous needle aspiration is not indicated in patients who have resectable lesions of the head of the pancreas, defined as the absence of metastases and localization of the tumor within the borders of the pancreas.

FUNCTION TESTS

Formerly, invasive pancreatic function tests that require gastrointestinal intubation to obtain exocrine pancreatic secretion were commonly used in the diagnosis of pancreatic cancer. Secretin, cholecystokinin, or a combination of these hormones are given intravenously after intubation to stimulate the pancreas. These tests have a sensitivity and specificity between 80 percent and 90 percent (32). Low outputs of pancreatic enzymes occur in 90 percent of the patients with cancer of the pancreatic head and 70 percent of patients with cancer of the body and the tail of the pancreas (63). A few patients with malabsorption from causes other than chronic pancreatitis (mucosal small bowel disease), or who have another gastrointestinal cancer, may have an abnormal test. However, because of the invasiveness of these tests and the

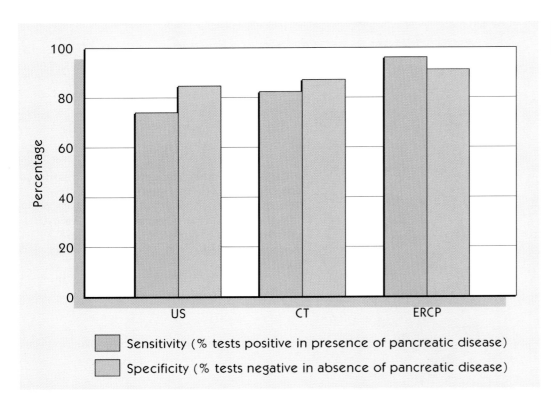

FIGURE 5.18 Sensitivity and specificity of ultrasonography (US), CT, and ERCP for diagnosis of pancreatic cancer.

Sensitivity (% tests positive in presence of pancreatic disease)
Specificity (% tests negative in absence of pancreatic disease)

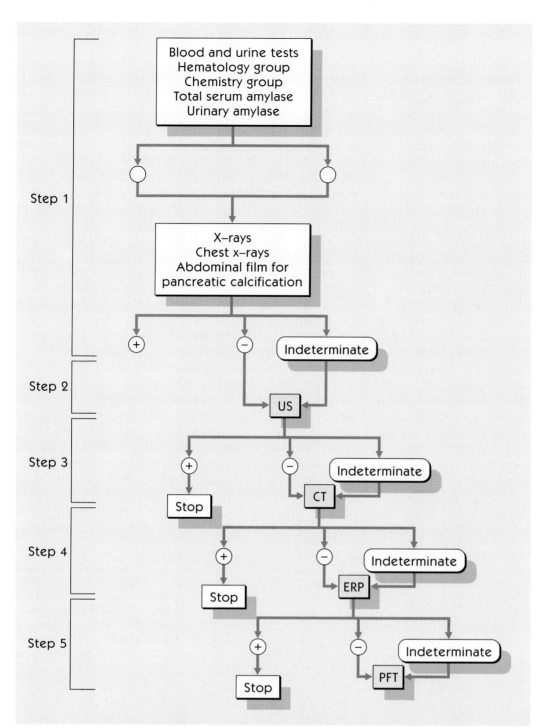

Step 1

Blood and urine tests
Hematology group
Chemistry group
Total serum amylase
Urinary amylase

X–rays
Chest x–rays
Abdominal film for
pancreatic calcification

(+) (−) Indeterminate

Step 2

US

Step 3

(+) (−) Indeterminate

Stop CT

Step 4

(+) (−) Indeterminate

Stop ERP

Step 5

(+) (−) Indeterminate

Stop PFT

FIGURE 5.19 Algorithm for the diagnosis of pancreatic cancer. None of the tests among the hematology or chemistry groups, or serum or urinary pancreatic enzymes, distinguishes among pancreatitis, hepatic disorders, or pancreatic cancer. Thus, finding a "positive" test at this point is not an indication for stopping investigation. The total serum amylase was chosen because it is routinely available. If lipase or pancreatic isoamylase is available, these tests may be preferable. Urinary amylase is included because it is elevated for longer periods of time than total serum amylase. By contrast, finding frank pulmonary or bony metastasis on chest x-ray, or calcification of the pancreas on the abdominal x-ray, is sufficient reason to stop investigation.

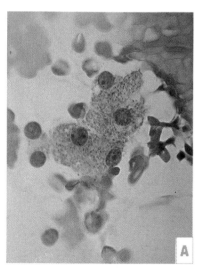
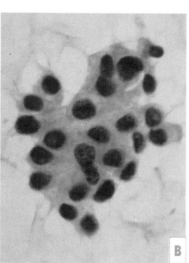

FIGURE 5.20 Pancreatic cytology contrasting (A) benign and **(B)** malignant exocrine cells. The latter possess the usual characteristics of malignant cells; that is, increased nuclear:cytoplasmic ratio and hyperchromatic nuclei. Papanicolau stain, x400. (From Misiewicz et al., 1987.)

emergence of sensitive and specific imaging tests, the use of invasive pancreatic function tests to detect pancreatic cancer has declined sharply.

Unfortunately, noninvasive tests of pancreatic function, although they are simpler and less expensive than invasive tests, are not as reproducible and too insensitive or nonspecific to diagnose pancreatic cancer (64). Noninvasive tests have been developed to measure: 1) undigested food in stool or diminished products of digestion in breath (quantitative fecal fat, triolein breath test, H_2 breath test); 2) products of synthetic compounds hydrolyzed by intraluminal pancreatic enzymes, which are absorbed by the gut and appear in blood and urine (NBT-PABA test, pancreolauryl test, dual-labeled Schilling test); and 3) hormones (human pancreatic polypeptide) which are either decreased in the fasting state and/or after stimulation with cholecystokinin.

ALGORITHM FOR DIAGNOSIS OF PANCREATIC CANCER

We recommend ultrasonography as the first test to diagnose pancreatic cancer (see Fig. 5.19). Computed tomography should be performed if ultrasonography fails for technical reasons (approximately 10 percent of examinations), or if it is negative and pancreatic cancer is still suspected. If computed tomography is negative and pancreatic cancer continues to be a consideration, we perform endoscopic retrograde pancreatography. Rarely, in our experience, is it necessary to perform an invasive pancreatic function test, the final test of the algorithm.

Approach to the Patient
SURGERY

Among all possible treatments, surgical resection of pancreatic cancer is the only one that offers any chance of cure. Unfortunately, the overall survival of patients with pancreatic cancer is 1 to 2 percent. Approximately 10 percent of patients have resectable tumors at the time of diagnosis, and the five-year survival rate, even after resection of pancreatic cancers, is only 10 percent (Fig. 5.21). In a series of 1300 patients referred to our institution over 34 years, only 13 percent of patients underwent a resection for cure (3).

The surgical procedure of choice continues to be the pancreaticoduodenectomy, or Whipple procedure (Fig. 5.22). Total pancreatectomy (Fig. 5.23) has been advocated by some surgeons because this operation eliminates the possibility that recurrence will be due to multiple foci of carcinoma, which are present in 16 percent to 30 percent of pancreases removed at pancreatectomy. Total pancreatectomy also abolishes the possibility of the spread of the tumor by direct extension, interductal seeding, lymphatic dissemination, and the danger of an anastomotic leak from a pancreatico-jejunostomy which may occur after a pancreaticoduodenectomy. Nevertheless, the Whipple procedure has remained the operation of choice because there is no definite evidence that total pancreatectomy is associated with less operative mortality or postoperative complications or improved survival.

Although pancreatoduodenectomy has been as-

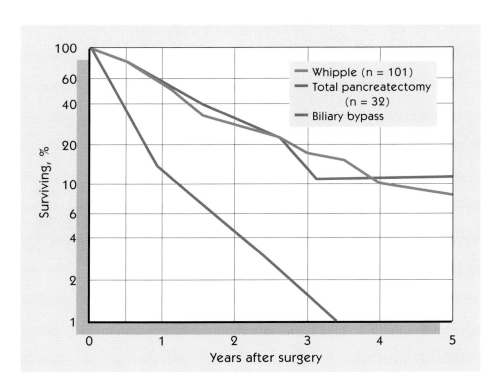

FIGURE 5.21 Survival after total pancreatectomy, pancreaticoduodenectomy (Whipple), and palliative surgical procedures (biliary bypass). (Adapted from reference 3 and van Heerden JA, Heath PM, Alden CR. Biliary bypass for ductal adenocarcinoma of the pancreas. Mayo Clinic experience, 1970–1975. *Mayo Clin Proc* 55:53,1980.)

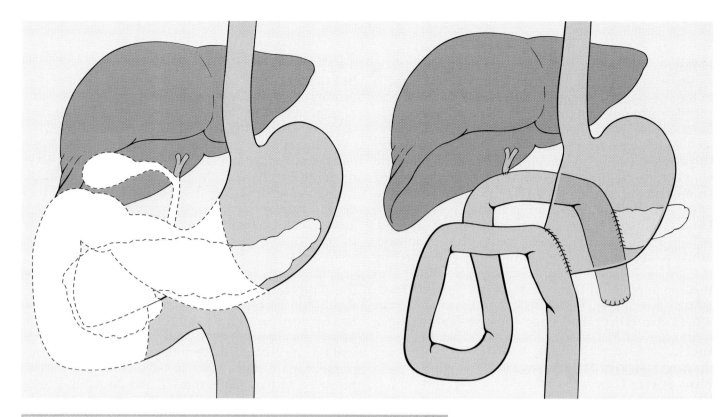

FIGURE 5.22 Pancreaticoduodenectomy. The shaded areas are removed. The reconstruction following resection is shown at right.

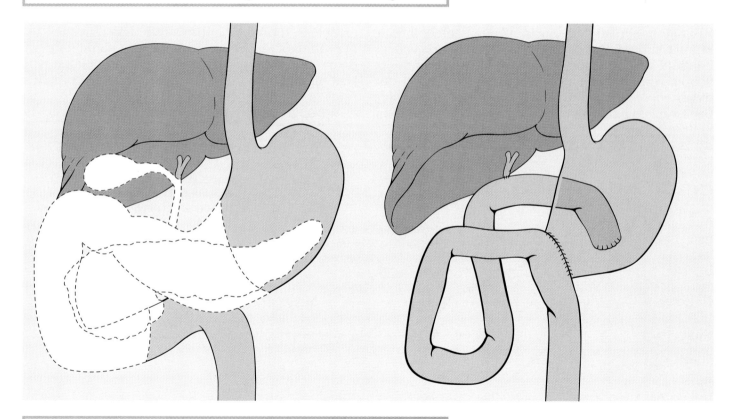

FIGURE 5.23 Reconstruction after total pancreatectomy.

sociated with operative mortality rates as high as 21 percent mainly due to anastomotic leakage and hemorrhage at the pancreaticojejunostomy (65), in experienced hands the mortality from this procedure has been reported to be as low as 2 percent to 5 percent (66–68). Furthermore, it is likely that the extent of lymph node involvement does not affect five-year survival (3,69). This issue, however, is controversial since others have found that five-year survival rates are adversely affected by lymph node involvement (70,71). Increasing evidence shows that the size of tumor at operation may affect surgical outcome. Tsuchiya and associates recently reported that Japanese patients with tumors less than or equal to 2 cm in diameter who underwent a Whipple operation had a 37 percent five-year and ten-year survival rate (72). These data are encouraging and support the hypothesis that "early" pancreatic cancer is curable by pancreatoduodenectomy. Unfortunately, at present most pancreatic cancers are larger than 2 cm at the time of diagnosis.

Other operations have been advocated for the surgical treatment of pancreatic cancer. The regional pancreatectomy proposed by Fortner (73) has been used when major vessels have been invaded by a tumor. In this operation, one or more vessels are reconstructed by resection of the involved portion of the vessel and direct reanastomosis or by using grafts. This radical operation has not gained acceptance because of its expense (long operating times and blood requirements), high operative mortality and morbidity, and its failure to be associated with an increase in survival compared to the conventional Whipple operation. The pylorus-preserving pancreaticoduodenal resection (74) is not frequently used as a surgical treatment of pancreatic cancer because it may compromise freedom from cancer at the surgical margins; it is used mainly in surgical treatment of patients with cancer of the lower duodenum and ampulla and benign pancreatic diseases.

PALLIATIVE SURGICAL PROCEDURES
Palliative procedures are performed to relieve symptoms of biliary or duodenal obstruction (or both) and pain.

BILIARY OBSTRUCTION   Cholecystojejunostomy is the biliary drainage procedure of choice unless the cystic duct enters the common duct close to the tumor. In this situation a choledochojejunostomy should be performed. An alternative to the surgical relief of jaundice is the placing of stents within the biliary tree. A variety of procedures have been described to stent the biliary tree including endoscopic, percutaneous, and combined endoscopic and radiologic methods. Clearly, the endoscopic method is better than the percutaneous method. In a control trial there was a greater relief of jaundice (81 percent vs. 61 percent) and a lower 30-day mortality rate (15 percent vs. 30 percent) when endoscopic and percutaneous stent methods were compared (75). The higher mortality rate with percutaneous stent placement was due to hemorrhage and bile leaks secondary to puncture of the liver.

Currently, it appears that endoscopic stenting may be superior to surgical drainage if life expectancy is one to two months. In contrast, if stents are required for a longer period of time, they are associated with increasing complications. For example, in a preliminary report of a prospective randomized trial in patients with malignant obstructive jaundice, endoscopic stenting and surgical bypass were equally successful in relieving jaundice (94 percent with each procedure) (76). Endoscopic stenting, however, was associated with a lower morbidity (23 percent vs. 43 percent), procedure-related mortality (zero percent vs. 10 percent), and 30-day mortality (6 percent vs. 15 percent). In this trial there was no statistical difference in overall survival (life table), but stenting was associated with increases in late morbidity such as duodenal obstruction (14 percent vs. 3 percent) and recurrent jaundice (17 percent vs. 3 percent). Interestingly, the size of the endoscopic stent (10 fg vs. 12 fg) is not associated with the rate of stent change or overall complication rates, but large stents are more difficult to place successfully (51 percent vs. 98 percent) (77). At present we advise endoscopic stent placement for patients who are at high surgical risk and who have a short life expectancy (one to three months). Conversely, double bypass surgery should be performed if patients are thought to have a resectable tumor and can withstand surgery but actually have an unresectable tumor at surgery, or if they are found to have an unresectable tumor by a diagnostic test and have a life expectancy of six to seven months.

DUODENAL OBSTRUCTION   Duodenal obstruction is common in patients with pancreatic cancer. Incomplete or functional obstruction occurs in 40 percent to 60 percent of patients, whereas complete duodenal obstruction occurs in 5 percent to 15 percent of patients—usually as a preterminal event (76,78). Organic obstruction is usually due to invasion of the third or fourth part of the duodenum. Recently, Barkin and associates found that 60 percent of patients with histologically proven carcinoma of the pancreas, and no gastric or duodenal organic obstruction, had delayed gastric emptying of solids; one-third of these patients had nausea and vomiting (79). Patients who undergo surgery and are found to have an unresectable tumor should have a gastrojejunostomy performed. At the initial operation, prophylactic gastrojejunostomy should be strongly considered if postoperative chemotherapy or radiation therapy is to be undertaken; as a second operation after such therapy, it is hazardous. The concept of prophylactic gastroenterostomy (80) has been challenged by many surgeons who advocate a gastrojejunostomy only when obstruction is present or imminent. It seems reasonable, however, to perform a prophylactic gastroenterostomy if patients are expected to survive more than a few weeks. In patients who develop symptoms of gastroparesis and have not had a gastroenterostomy, a combination of a cholinergic (bethanechol, 25 mg t.i.d.), and a prokinetic agent (metoclopramide, 10 mg q.i.d.) might enhance gastric emptying. Metoclopramide has been used successfully to alleviate symptoms of gastroparesis in patients with delayed gastric emptying due to neoplasms (81).

CHEMOTHERAPY (FIG. 5.24)
No single chemotherapeutic drug or combination of drugs has prolonged or enhanced the quality of life in patients with pancreatic cancer. Single drugs that reduce tumor size, but not survival, are 5-fluorouracil (5-FU), mitomycin-C, streptozotocin, doxorubicin hydrochloride (Adriamycin), epirubicin, ifosfamide, semustine (methyl-CCNU), and high-dose methotrexate. 5-FU produces a partial response rate in 10 percent to 15 percent of patients and a median survival time of less than 20 weeks (82). The other agents have either a similar effect (mitomycin-C) or less effect. Other drugs are totally ineffective (Actinomycin D [also known as Dactinomycin or cosmegen], doxorubicin, carmustine [BCNU] and standard dose methotrexate, Cis-platinum, melphalan, and L-asparaginase). High-dose methotrexate and ifosfamide are toxic and not used. In contrast to early reports, FAM (combination of 5-FU, Adriamycin, and mitomycin C) in a large study of 144 patients has been shown to be no better than 5-FU alone (83). Similarly, FAMM$_C$ (5-FU, doxorubicin, mitomycin, and semustine) and SMF (streptozotocin, mitomycin-C, and 5-FU) have not had significantly different results than 5-FU alone (84).

RADIATION TREATMENT
The Gastrointestinal Study Group has conducted randomized trials showing that the combination of 5-FU and radiation or SMF and radiation improves survival compared to radiation or chemotherapy alone (85) (Fig. 5.25). Recent improvements of radiation treatment are intraoperative electron beam radiation (4500–5500 cGy) (86) and 1251 implant (120–210 Gy) (87). Although these modalities may limit local progression of the tumor, there has been no significant change in survival compared to extended external beam alone, because of the inability to control liver and peritoneal metastases.

MANAGEMENT OF MALABSORPTION
Fat and protein malabsorption occurs in 75 percent and 50 percent of patients with pancreatic cancer, respectively (36). Fat malabsorption tends to be severe (mean coefficient of fat absorption = 67 percent), whereas protein malabsorption is of moderate severity (mean coefficient of absorption = 81 percent). Administration of standard doses of pancreatin (Viokase, eight tablets with meals) improves moderate or severe fat and protein malabsorption, but does not improve mild fat or protein malabsorption (see Fig. 5.11). Thus, in addition to pancreatic insufficiency, other as yet unidentified causes of malabsorption may be present in pancreatic cancer patients.

In our patients the gastrointestinal tract was intact, and symptoms of delayed gastric emptying were not present, but gastric emptying was not measured. Although not applicable to our patients, bypass operations of the stomach and biliary tract may be associated with mild malabsorption secondary to poor mixing of nutrients with pancreatic secretion and bile, and partial or complete obstruction of the biliary tree as in cholestatic liver disease (88) can lead to moderately severe steatorrhea. The increase in fat malabsorption in the patient who developed a biliary cutaneous fistula emphasizes the importance of bile for fat malabsorption. Whereas there are no appreciable back-up systems for lipolysis or bile-salt micellar solubilization of long-chain triglycerides, the main form of dietary fat, there are alternative mechanisms for protein digestion and absorption such as brush border amino-oligopeptidases, transport mechanisms for small peptides, and pinocytosis which may substitute for lack of pancreatic endo- and exopeptidases (89). There is no evidence that small intestinal morphologic abnormalities are present to explain malabsorption. In two studies, we have performed small intestinal biopsies on a few patients with pancreatic cancer and pancreatic insufficiency and have found normal small intestinal mucosa (36,90).

The regimen we used for pancreatic enzyme replacement consists of ingesting eight tablets of a preparation of pancreatin (Viokase) with meals containing 25 g of fat (37). We administer two tablets immediately after the patient eats a few bites of the meal, two tablets at the end of the meal, and the remaining four tablets interspersed during the meal (91–93). Common mistakes made in enzyme replacement therapy include not giving enough lipase, ingesting tablets before meals, and eating snacks without ingesting enzymes.

Enough lipase should be given to theoretically abolish steatorrhea. In patients with pancreatic insufficiency, steatorrhea does not occur unless

---

FIGURE 5.24:
CHEMOTHERAPY

SINGLE AGENTS NO MORE EFFECTIVE THAN 5-FU	COMBINATIONS OF AGENTS NO BETTER THAN 5-FU
Methotrexate	FAM (5-FU, doxorubicin, adriamycin, mitomycin C)
Doxorubicin	
Carmustine (BCNU)	FAMM (5-FU and semustine)
Actinomycin D	SMF (streptozotocin, mitomycin, and 5-FU)
Cisplatinum	
Melphalan	
L-asparaginase	
Semustine (methyl-CCNU)	

Note: No single agent or combination of agents prolongs or enhances the quality of life. 5-fluorouracil (5-FU) produces partial response rate in 10–15% and median survival of 20 weeks. Other single agents that have been tested and combinations of agents no better than 5-FU are listed.

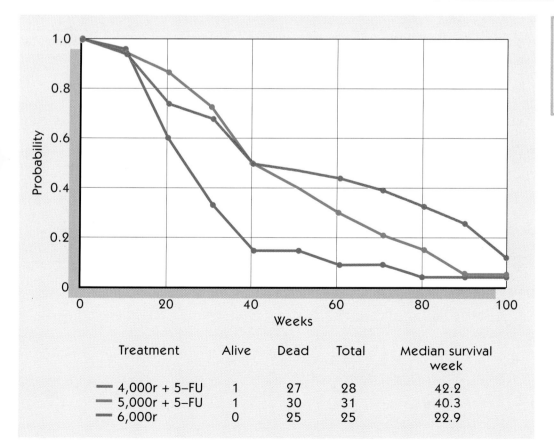

FIGURE 5.25 Effect of radiation and 5-FU on survival measured from date of surgery in pancreatic cancer. (From reference 85.)

Treatment	Alive	Dead	Total	Median survival week
4,000r + 5–FU	1	27	28	42.2
5,000r + 5–FU	1	30	31	40.3
6,000r	0	25	25	22.9

lipase secretion into the duodenum is below 10 percent of normal (94), and steatorrhea is not abolished unless peak postprandial lipase concentrations are greater than 5 percent of normal (87) (Fig. 5.26). At least 30,000 international units of lipase must be ingested to provide enough lipase to achieve these postprandial levels (91–93). This amount of lipase will abolish steatorrhea if no intragastric inactivation of lipase occurs, and at least 7500 units of lipase are emptied from the stomach per hour postprandially. In the usual clinical situation, these assumptions are not met and less lipase is delivered to the duodenum. Thus, in most patients steatorrhea is significantly decreased, but it is not abolished. Whether enteric-coated microencapsulated preparations alleviate steatorrhea more frequently than standard pancreatin (e.g., Viokase) has not been investigated, but are worthy of a trial if malabsorption is not improved by pancreatin. The addition of H_2 blockers (cimetidine) did not improve steatorrhea in a small number of patients with pancreatic cancer we tested (see Fig. 5.11).

MANAGEMENT OF PAIN

DRUG THERAPY (FIG. 5.27)   Most patients with pain due to pancreatic cancer can be successfully managed by drug therapy if analgesics are taken at regular intervals and if adequate doses of narcotic analgesics and adjuvant drugs are given when needed.

In patients with mild to moderate pain, the drugs of choice are aspirin, acetominophen, and nonsteroidal anti-inflammatory drugs (NSAIDs) (see Fig. 5.27). The major side effect of these drugs is their effect on the upper gastrointestinal mucosa (gastritis, ulceration), and they may produce gastrointestinal symptoms and hemorrhage. If one drug of this class does not provide significant relief, another can be tried. Eventually, if this group of drugs fails to relieve pain, opioid analgesics should be used. Most patients, however, can be successfully managed with aspirin or the combination of aspirin and codeine.

Opioid analgesics, in contrast to nonopioid analgesics, do not have a "ceiling" effect; the loss of pain is linear as the dose of the opioid is increased on a log scale until unconsciousness supervenes. Thus, the dose of opioid is governed by side effects and sensitivity to the drug. Unfortunately, elderly patients (the population of patients with pancreatic cancer) are more sensitive to loss of mental function and constipation. Thus, it is wise to begin treatment with one-half the recommended dose (Fig. 5.28) and the dosing schedule should be based on plasma half-life—generally, doses of most analgesics are given at intervals of four hours.

In patients with severe pain, if an opioid drug is no longer effective, even when given at appropriate doses and at regular intervals, or produces side effects, another opioid should be substituted at one-half the equianalgesic dose (see Fig. 5.28).

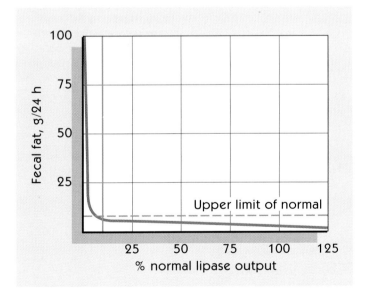

FIGURE 5.26 Relation of peak lipase concentration to steatorrhea in pancreatic insufficiency. (From reference 94.)

The amount of opioid most patients will require is quite stable. Escalation of the dose most commonly occurs in terminally ill patients and indicates disease progression. In this situation, enough drug must be given to keep patients comfortable. Concern regarding drug addiction and drug dependence in patients with progressive pancreatic cancer is inappropriate.

If an opioid does not provide pain relief, the combination of an opioid plus an antihistamine (100 mg hydroxyzine IM), or an opioid plus an amphetamine (10 mg Dexedrine IM), have been advised by some authorities (95). Combinations, such as an opioid plus a benzodiazepine or an opioid plus a phenothiazine, increase sedation but not analgesia (96).

Side effects limit giving increased doses of drugs. If sedation and drowsiness are not desirable, they can be reduced by decreasing the dose and giving the drug more frequently, or switching to another drug. Nausea and vomiting caused by an opioid are best treated by switching to another

FIGURE 5.27:
ANALGESICS COMMONLY USED ORALLY
FOR MILD TO MODERATE PAIN

DRUG	DOSE* (mg)	DOSE RANGE (mg)
NON-NARCOTICS		
Aspirin	650	650
Choline magnesium Trisalicybate (Trilisate)	1500	1500–3000
Acetaminophen	650	650
Ibuprofen (Motrin)	200	200–400
Fenoprofen (Nalfon)	200	200–400
Diflunisal (Dolobid)	500	500–1000
Naproxen (Naproxyn)	250	250–500
MORPHINE-LIKE AGONISTS		
Codeine	32–65	32–65
Oxycodone	5	5–10
Meperidine (Demerol)	50	50–100
Proxyphine HCl (Darvon)	65–130	65–130
Proxyphene mapsylate (Darvon-N)		
MIXED AGONIST-ANTAGONISTS		
Pentazocine (Talwin)	50	50–100

Adapted from reference 95.
For these equianalgesic doses the time of peak analgesia ranges from 1.5 to two hours and the duration from four to six hours. Oxycodone and meperidine are shorter-acting (three to five hours) and diflunisal and naproxen are longer-acting (eight to 12 hours).
* These are the recommended starting doses from which the optimal dose for each patient is determined by titration and the maximal dose limited by adverse effects.

FIGURE 5.28:
ORAL AND PARENTERAL OPIOID ANALGESICS FOR MODERATE TO SEVERE PAIN

	ROUTE*	EQUIANALGESIC DOSE (mg)†	DURATION (hr)	PLASMA HALF-LIFE (hr)
NARCOTIC AGONISTS				
Morphine	IM	10	4–6	2–3.5
	PO	60	4–7	
Codeine	IM	130	4–6	3
	PO	200	4–6	
Oxycodone	IM	15	3–5	—
	PO	30		
Heroin	IM	5	4–5	0.5
Levorphanol	IM	2	4–6	12–16
(Levodromoran)	PO	4	4–7	
Hydromorphone	IM	1.5	4–5	2–3
(Dilaudid)	PO	7.5	4–6	
Oxymorphone	IM	1	4–6	2–3
(Numorphan)	PO	10	4–6	
Meperidine	IM	75	4–5	3–4
(Demerol)	PO	300	4–6	12–16 **
Methadone	IM	10		15–30
(Dolophine)	PO	20		
MIXED AGONIST-ANTAGONISTS				
Pentezocine	IM	60	4–6	2–3
(Talwin)	PO	180	4–7	
Nalbuphine	IM	10	4–6	5
(Nubain)	PO	—		
Butorphanol	IM	2	4–6	2.5–3.5
(Stadol)	PO	—		
PARTIAL AGONISTS				
Buprenorphine	IM	0.4	4–6	?
(Temegesic)	SL	0.8	5–6	

Adapted from reference 95.

*IM denotes intramuscular, PO oral, and SL sublingual.
†Based on single-dose studies in which an intramuscular dose of each drug listed was compared with morphine to establish the relative potency. Oral doses are those recommended when changing from a parenteral to an oral route. For patients without prior narcotic exposure, the recommended oral starting dose is 30 mg for morphine, 5 mg for methadone, 2 mg for levorphanol, and 4 mg for hydromorphone.
**Normeperidine.

drug or using antiemetics such as chlorpromazine, haloperidol, cyclizine, or metoclopramide hydrochloride. Constipation caused by opioids may be managed by a regimen of anthraquinone derivatives, especially senna compounds (97). One-half of a Senokot tablet is alleged to reverse the constipating effect of 60 mg of codeine or the equivalent dose of another opioid. No controlled studies, however, have investigated the appropriate treatment of constipation arising from the use of opioids.

The vast majority of patients should be controlled by oral regimens, but inevitably a few patients will need to use a percutaneous or intramuscular route (Fig 5.29). The subcutaneous route is less painful and should be used if possible. The intravenous route should be avoided. A recent innovation has been the development of patient-controlled analgesia. With this method a small battery-operated pump is used to inject opiate subcutaneously. The patient obtains a dose by pressing a button. Pumps are programmed with safeguards to prevent overdose. An even newer innovation is the development of epidural administration, which produces analgesia with low doses of narcotics and, consequently, few side effects. While neither of these techniques has been approved for general use, they may be extremely beneficial in treating patients in severe pain secondary to advanced pancreatic cancer.

In our experience the use of neurolytic celiac plexus block has greatly simplified the treatment of pain in patients with pancreatic cancer. Injection of the ganglion either intraoperatively, or transcutaneously by using biplane x-rays or CT scans, affords pain relief in the majority of patients. In three small series composed of 20 (98), 28 (99), and 13 (100) patients, 92 percent had complete pain relief. In a single large series of 100 patients (101) (97 with pancreatic cancer and three with chronic pancreatitis), 60, 34, and six patients had marked, good, and ineffective analgesia, respectively. My personal experience parallels these reports; celiac plexus block is a very effective means to control pain, and the method is attended by few serious complications. In these four studies (with a total of 161 patients), two patients had serious neurologic complications, and two patients had transient radicular pain which improved. An additional patient has been reported to have developed paraplegia following a celiac plexus block with phenol (102).

Less Common Ductal Exocrine Pancreatic Tumors

MUCINOUS CYSTADENOCARCINOMA

Formerly, mucinous cystic pancreatic neoplasms (see Fig. 5.26) had been divided into mucinous cystadenoma and mucinous cystadenocarcinoma. All these lesions, however, should be considered malignant neoplasms because there have been numerous reports of "benign" mucinous cystadenomas recurring and metastasizing (103,104); when these tumors are carefully examined, foci of malignant transformation can be seen (Fig. 5.30).

FIGURE 5.29:
ETIOLOGY OF EXTRAHEPATIC DUCT CANCER

GALLSTONE

PROLONGED CHOLESTASIS AND INFECTION (ROLE UNCERTAIN)
Sclerosing cholangitis
Chronic suppurative cholangitis
Biliary parasites
Typhoid carriers
Ulcerative colitis
Congenital (choledochal cysts, microhemartomas of van Meyerberg, Caroli's disease)
Solitary adenoma, biliary papillomatosis–premalignant lesions

The tumors are large, bulky, unilobular or multi-lobulated cysts containing mucin. Curvilinear calcifications may occur within the fibrous capsule. The cysts are lined with mucinous columnar epithelium that form papillary projections and may contain foci of atypical or invasive adenocarcinoma.

Mucinous cystic neoplasms occur more commonly in women (6:1 female-to-male ratio) and present in patients from age of 40 to 60 as epigastric pain or discomfort. Because the pain may simulate chronic pancreatitis and cystic lesions are found on imaging tests, the latter may be considered pancreatic pseudocysts and fairly frequently are drained. Although differentiation of cystadenoma from a pancreatic pseudocyst secondary to chronic pancreatitis may be difficult with imaging tests, the absence of historic features that can lead to benign pancreatic disease (such as trauma, previous pancreatitis, alcohol, and biliary tract diseases) should raise suspicions of a cystic neoplasm. In a Mayo Clinic series of 45 patients with cystadenoma (105), the mean age of onset was 55 years. Pain, weight loss, nausea, and vomiting occurred in 56 percent, 40 percent, and 25 percent of patients, respectively. Jaundice was uncommon since most cystadenomas arise in the body and tail of the pancreas. Even a tumor that originates in the head may not be associated with jaundice because fistulas between the biliary tract, the cyst, and the gut may spontaneously arise and drain the biliary tract. Although the diagnosis of a cystic neoplasm can be suggested by CT or ultrasonography, a definite diagnosis can

only be made by pathologic confirmation. Because of the possible confusion between a pseudocyst and a cystic neoplasm, the wall of the suspected pseudocyst should be biopsied prior to a drainage procedure.

Even though mucinous cystic neoplasms may reach sizes as large as 30 cm in diameter, they should be resected because the outcome is very favorable. In comparison to usual ductal carcinomas, five-year survival rates may be as high as 50 percent.

Mucinous cystadenocarcinomas should be differentiated from microcystic cystadenomas which have no malignant potential and are characterized by multiple 1- to 2-cm diameter cysts containing a glycogen-rich fluid. One-third have a central "sunburst" calcification. Older females more commonly have microcystic adenomas; the mean age at diagnosis is 65 years.

GIANT CELL TUMORS

Giant cell tumors have a variety of morphologic features, but are characterized by the presence of bizarre giant cells and sarcomoid cells supported by minimal fibrous tissue. Four distinct histologic types have been identified: spindle cell, malignant giant cell, pleomorphic, and anaplastic tumors (106). All such patients have a poor prognosis. Most giant cell tumors have a worse prognosis (median survival, two months) than the common ductal carcinoma, and in one series (107) all pleomorphic cancers had metastases at the time of diagnosis.

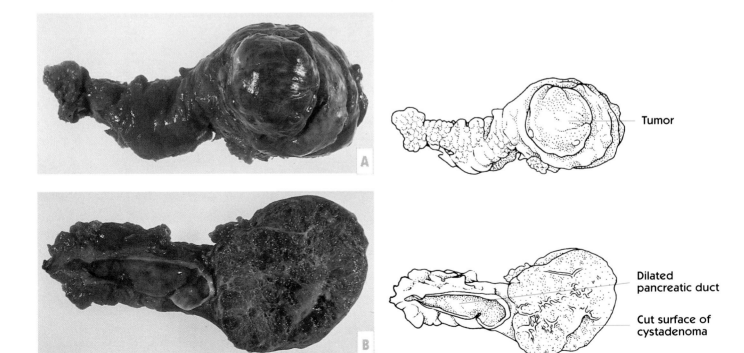

FIGURE 5.30 (A,B) Macroscopic appearances of a cystadenoma of the pancreas. The cut surface (**B**) reveals its trabecular pattern, and the accompanying duct obstruction and dilatation. (From Misiewicz et al., 1987.)

OTHER RARE TUMORS

Acinar cell carcinomas are uncommon and characterized by acinar arrangements supported by minimal fibrous stroma. Although the tumor cells contain no stainable amylase, zymogen granules are identifiable by electron microscopy (108), and some patients may have elevated serum lipase levels and associated nonsuppurative panniculitis of the extremities and bone marrow. They may also manifest subcutaneous nodules and polyarthritis (109). These tumors usually occur in the elderly and, rarely, in children (110).

Another rare tumor, pancreatoblastoma, occurs almost exclusively in children (from 15 months to 17 years old) (31). This tumor may be encapsulated and have a relatively benign course, or be a poorly defined nonencapsulated tumor with a bad prognosis because it spreads into adjacent organs and recurs after resection. This rare tumor is important because it may have a favorable outcome, and should be approached with aggressive surgery.

AMPULLARY CANCERS
Epidemiology

Ampullary cancers are very uncommon compared to pancreatic cancers. In a preliminary study of Olmsted County, Minnesota, residents for 1950 to 1988, 175 pancreatic cancers were diagnosed compared to only 12 ampullary cancers, a 14.6:1 ratio (111). The crude incidence rate of ampullary cancer is 0.4 compared to 5.9 per 100,000 person-years of the Olmsted County population.

Pathology

In comparison to pancreatic ductal cancer, ampullary tumors are small, rarely more than 3.5 cm in diameter, polypoid, and soft. Histologically they are usually low-grade adenocarcinomas with a papillary arrangement.

Clinical Presentation

Patients present with mild jaundice, which may fluctuate, and anemia. Both findings are presumably due to sporadic sloughing of the tumor and bleeding into the duodenum. The laboratory findings are consistent with the clinical findings, as the mean bilirubin concentration is 7 mg/dl, seldom exceeding 10 mg/dl. The hemoglobin may be reduced and occult blood may be present in stool.

Diagnosis

The diagnosis is usually suggested by finding dilatation of the bile ducts to the level of the duodenum, and the absence of a mass on abdominal CT or ultrasound examination. This finding mandates endoscopic visualization of the medial wall of the duodenum and biopsy of the lesion, but biopsy results in the diagnosis of malignancy only 50 percent of the time, as the tumor may be located within the papilla. Endoscopic retrograde cholangiopancreatography is also often performed prior to surgical exploration.

Treatment

Pancreaticoduodenectomy is the treatment of choice, and is associated with a 50 percent five-year survival rate (112). Of all cancers of the periampullary area, ampullary cancer has the best five-year survival rate and should be treated surgically unless there are formidable contraindications. If a patient is not a candidate for pancreaticoduodenectomy, a surgical ampullectomy or endoscopic papillotomy with or without a stent placement should be considered.

Because patients with benign villous adenomas of the ampulla of Vater have a similar clinical presentation (obstructive jaundice, biliary colic, or acute pancreatitis), it is often impossible to distinguish between these two entities until a frozen section is obtained at surgery. The treatment of a benign villous adenoma is submucosal excision.

CANCER OF THE BILE DUCTS
Epidemiology

Carcinomas of the extrahepatic ducts are far less common than pancreatic ductal cancer. It is difficult to obtain accurate information regarding the frequency of these tumors, which are therefore commonly discussed together with other rare carcinomas of this region such as gallbladder, ampullary, and hepatocellular cancers. In Rochester, Minnesota (113), the age-adjusted incidence rates of carcinoma of the extrahepatic ducts, including the ampulla of Vater and gallbladder, was 3.1 and 5.1 per 100,000 population, for men and women, respectively, from 1935 to 1971. Twenty of 52 (40 percent) tumors originated from the extrahepatic ducts and ampulla of Vater. In a recent preliminary study (111) of this same population, the crude incidence of cancer of the gallbladder, bile ducts, ampulla, and ductal pancreatic cancer per 100,000 person-years from 1950 through 1988 was 1.2, 0.7, 0.4, and 5.9, respectively. These data are similar to other populations where the age and sex-adjusted incidence approximated three per 100,000 population (114). In autopsies, the incidence ranges from 0.01 to 0.46 percent (115).

In most studies, the tumors are slightly more common in men. The male:female sex ratio of 1656 patients included in 23 studies was 1.3:1 (116). The male:female sex ratio of 2.2:1 in Rochester, Minnesota (113), was the second highest among all those reported (116).

Etiology

There is no single underlying recognized cause of cancers of the extrahepatic ducts, but prolonged cholestasis and infections, or both, seem to be common to the etiologies identified thus far (see Fig. 5.29). Gallstones are commonly listed as an etiology and are present in 30 percent of patients with extrahepatic duct cancers (117), but in a cohort study of more than 2400 persons with gallstones in Olmsted County, Minnesota, we found no increase in the incidence of any cancer except that of the gallbladder (27). Thus it is not clear that gallstones, although commonly present, play any etiologic role.

In contrast, sclerosing cholangitis (118) and chronic suppurative cholangitis, two conditions associated with cholestasis and infection, have been implicated in the etiology of extrahepatic cancers, as have been a variety of liver flukes (*Clonorchis sinensis, Opisthorchis viverrini*), particularly in the Far East (119,120) and among typhoid carriers. Ulcerative colitis also has been associated with cancer of the extrahepatic ducts (121,122). This association, however, may be due to the known connection between sclerosing cholangitis and chronic ulcerative colitis. Whereas few patients with ulcerative colitis have sclerosing cholangitis, the former is present in over 50 percent of patients with sclerosing cholangitis (118). Congenital anomalies such as choledochal cysts, microhemartomas of von Meyenberg, and congenital intrahepatic dilatation of the bile ducts (Caroli's disease) (123,124) are associated with extrahepatic biliary cancer and also cause cholestasis and infection. Anabolic steroids and the past use of thorium dioxide (Thorotrast) as an imaging dye have been implicated as carcinogens (125). Lastly, solitary adenomas of the bile duct and biliary papillomatosis are considered premalignant lesions (126).

Pathology

More than 95 percent of the tumors are sclerotic adenocarcinomas (Fig. 5.31) of variable differentiation (Fig. 5.32) whereas approximately 3 percent are anaplastic cancers (116). Rarer tumors are squamous cell carcinomas, rhabdomyosarcomas, granular cell tumors, and cystadenomas.

The location and dissemination of the tumor, particularly its local spread, are extremely important when considering treatment options. In a review of 19 studies, Sons and Borchard (116) determined that 30 percent of extrahepatic bile duct tumors were within the hepatic ducts or originated at the confluence of the hepatic duct or proximal hepatic duct (Fig. 5.33), 25 percent were located in the suprapancreatic common bile duct (Fig. 5.34), and 40 percent in the distal or intrapancreatic duct (Fig. 5.35). In 5 percent of cases, it was not possible to determine precisely the site origin. Extrahepatic ductal cancers are characterized by local contiguous spread. Most commonly, the tumor spreads to the liver (35 percent), pancreas (15 percent), gallbladder (11 percent), and duodenum (8 percent) (116). The tumor involves the portal vein and invades perineural tissue within or adjacent to the bile duct, a criterion of malignancy, in 75 percent and 90 percent of patients, respectively (127). Metastases to regional lymph nodes (choledochal, pancreaticoduodenal, or hepatic artery) and liver occur in 50 percent of patients, but distant spread to the lungs and skeletal system (10 percent) and kidney and brain (3 percent) are much less frequent (116).

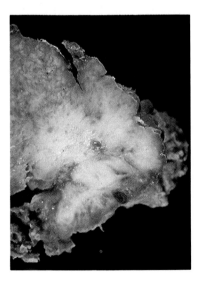
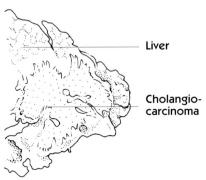

Liver

Cholangio-carcinoma

FIGURE 5.31 A typical cholangiocarcinoma with its sclerotic outline. (From Misiewicz et al., 1987.)

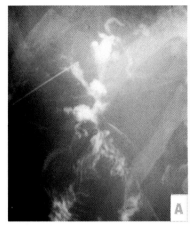
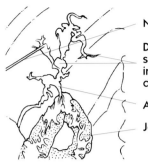
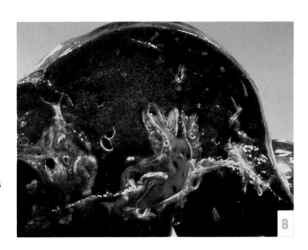

Needle

Dilated and strictured intrahepatic ducts

Anastomosis

Jejunum

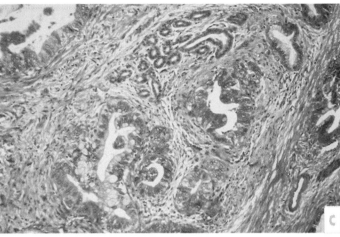
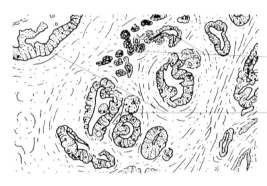

Residual nonmalignant glands

Malignant bile duct epithelium

FIGURE 5.32 (A) Percutaneous transhepatic cholangiogram showing invasion of the intrahepatic bile ducts by carcinoma of the bile ducts after a choledochojejunostomy. **(B)** The liver of the same patient removed at postmortem shows infiltrating carcinoma. **(C)** Typical bile duct adenocarcinoma replacing the normal structure. H&E stain, x160. (From Misiewicz et al., 1987.)

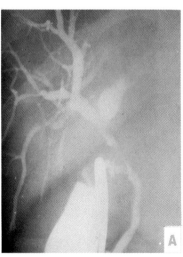
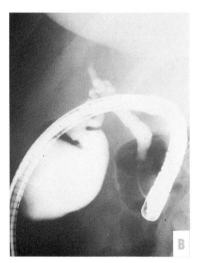

FIGURE 5.33 (A) Operative cholangiogram showing carcinoma of the common hepatic duct. **(B)** Endoscopic retrograde cholangiogram showing blockage of the common hepatic duct by a bile duct carcinoma. (From Misiewicz et al., 1987.)

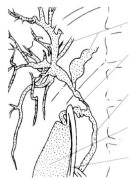
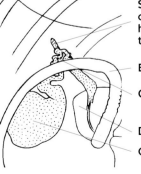

Dilated intrahepatic ducts

Carinoma

Normal common bile duct

Gallbladder

Clamp on cystic duct

Stricture of common hepatic duct due to carcinoma

Endoscope

Cystic duct

Duodenum

Gallbladder

Clinical Presentation

The major clinical presentation is painless obstructive jaundice (90 percent). Usually jaundice is severe as 50 percent of patients have a serum bilirubin level of greater than 13 mg/dl at the time of diagnosis (128). Weight loss and cholangitis are present in 50 percent and 30 percent of patients, respectively (129). Other possible symptoms are pruritus, diarrhea (steatorrhea), and anorexia. If only one hepatic duct is obstructed, jaundice may be absent and the presenting symptom may be only vague abdominal discomfort, associated with the finding of an elevated alkaline phosphatase and gamma glutamyl transferase.

The most common physical findings are jaundice and hepatomegaly. Courvoisier's sign (palpable gallbladder) is invariably present when the cancer is located in the lower duct, unless a cholecystectomy had been performed previously, or the gallbladder is thickened and contracted. Clinical deterioration proceeds rapidly after the onset of jaundice or biliary sepsis. Hepatocellar failure occurs within six months and is characterized by the appearance of ascites, spider nevi, palmar erythema, variceal and mucosal (vitamin K deficiency) bleeding, and malnutrition.

Diagnosis

Ultrasonography is the first and primary diagnostic test that should be used after obstructive jaundice is suspected on the basis of a history, physical examination, and laboratory tests (the serum alkaline phosphatase is increased in more than 95 percent of patients) (129). Ultrasonography is 90 percent sensitive for differentiating between malignant and benign obstruction and is accurate in detecting the level of obstruction and predicting resectability in 90 percent and 70 percent of patients, respectively (130). In these assessments, ultrasonography has a similar or greater accuracy than computed tomography.

The features of cholangiocarcinoma on ultrasonography are proximal duct dilatation, narrowing of the distal duct, and an intraluminal soft tissue mass characterized by intraluminal echos or echogenic transluminal bands. In addition, ultrasonography can often detect the size of the tumor, liver

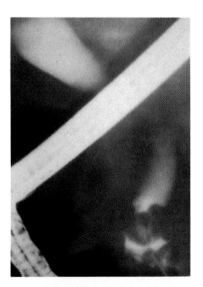

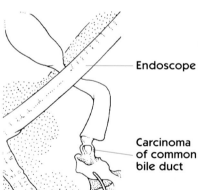

FIGURE 5.34 Endoscopic retrograde cholangiogram showing carcinoma of the common bile duct. (From Misiewicz et al., 1987.)

Endoscope

Carcinoma of common bile duct

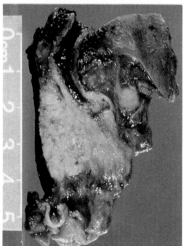

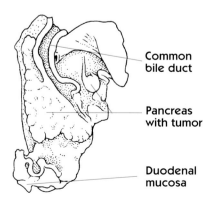

FIGURE 5.35 Most of this tumor was in the head of the pancreas extrinsic to the bowel wall. The secondary encroachment on the common bile duct resulted in its clinical presentation as an ampullary lesion. (From Mitros FA. *Atlas of gastrointestinal pathology.* New York: Gower Medical Publishing, 1988.)

Common bile duct

Pancreas with tumor

Duodenal mucosa

invasion, or metastases to the liver organ or lymph nodes. During localization of the tumor with an imaging technique, a fine-needle aspiration can be done which is 87 percent sensitive and 100 percent specific for the diagnosis of extrahepatic duct mass, more accurate than cytologic examination of the bile. The value of magnetic resonance imaging (MRI) in evaluating patients with suspected extrahepatic biliary tumors is evolving. MRI may prove to be extremely useful since it can demonstrate encasement, displacement, or involvement of vessels, soft tissue masses, and distant metastases to the liver and lymph nodes.

To determine resectability, percutaneous transhepatic cholangiography is better than endoscopic retrograde cholangiography because it provides information regarding intrahepatic ductal anatomy and extension of the tumor into the intrahepatic ducts. These data are critical to planning an operation, particularly a hepaticojejunostomy. Criteria of unresectability are: 1) extension of the tumor beyond the second order of intrahepatic ducts; 2) involvement of the portal vein, hepatic arteries, and portal veins in both lobes of the liver; or 3) involvement of the vessel(s) on one side of the liver with extensive involvement of the duct on the contralateral side (131). Resectability of tumors that do not involve secondary intrahepatic ducts should be determined by angiography (132).

Approach to the Patient

SURGICAL TREATMENT

At present, the only realistic chance for cure is resection of the tumor, as neither chemotherapy nor radiotherapy (nor both together) is associated with long-term survival. Several retrospective studies (133) have suggested that preoperative drainage decreases operative mortality and postoperative morbidity. Three prospective trials, however, have failed to show any decrease in operative mortality when preoperative percutaneous transhepatic drainage was used (134–136). Furthermore, preoperative drainage was associated with increased morbidity and increased hospitalization costs. Similarly, use of bile salts, lactulose, and hyperalimentation preoperatively have not been associated with more favorable postoperative outcomes (137).

The type and extent of curative resections depend on tumor location. Carcinomas of the distal bile duct are treated with a radical pancreaticoduodenectomy (Whipple procedure) or a pylorus-saving Whipple operation (74). Operative mortality of the Whipple procedure is less than 3 percent, and the average five-year survival rate has been reported as 42 percent but has ranged from 16 to 68 percent (138–142).

Carcinomas of the mid-duct (e.g., common hepatic and suprapancreatic common bile duct tumors) are resected by an en bloc cholecystectomy, with removal of the mid-duct and the cystic and choledochal lymph nodes. Biliary-enteric continuity is re-established by Roux-Y hepaticojejunostomy. Tumors in this location are usually unresectable as they spread into the portal vein and hepatic artery. In the few patients in whom resection has been performed, survival has not been reported beyond two years (138).

Sixty percent to 80 percent of patients with carcinoma of the proximal duct(s) have an unresectable tumor (138,143). The operation consists of an extension of the dissection described for mid-duct tumors to include the bifurcation of the common bile duct. Lobar resection of the liver and cholangiojejunostomy are performed if there is direct extension of the tumor into the liver. Operative mortality and mean survival time are 10 percent and 20 months, respectively (143). The results of the operation are superior to hepatic transplantation, followed by cyclosporine immunosuppression, which has been associated with a median survival of 9.7 months and a one-year survival of 32 percent (144).

Because of the high rate of unresectability and the poor survival rates of curative operations, palliative procedures are relied on to maintain quality of life. These procedures include incomplete removal of the carcinoma with a bypass operation, intraoperative decompression by transtumoral intubation, and either transcutaneous or endoscopic insertion of a transtumoral endoprosthesis. It is generally accepted that the quality of life after resection of the tumor and bilioenteric anastomosis is superior to biliary decompression alone, but mean survival after these procedures is likely similar and ranges from 12 to 16 months (145) for the former, and nine to 30 months (146) for the latter operation. Clearly, nonoperative decompression of the biliary tree by endoscopic means is superior to percutaneous methods because a variety of complications are associated with the former secondary to the liver puncture, including pain, bleeding, and intraperitoneal bile leakage (75). Although quality of life is better after surgical decompression, a recent randomized trial of surgical vs. endoscopic decompression showed that early mortality was significantly greater with surgical decompression (76).

RADIOTHERAPY

Palliation is the main goal of radiotherapy, but results have been disappointing as median survival has ranged between nine and 12 months. Several modalities have been investigated. External-beam orthovoltage radiation (average dose 4000 rads; range 3588 to 6000 rads) alone has been associated with median survival of 11 months (147,148). An occasional patient treated with nonoperative drainage of the biliary tract plus external beam radiation, however, may have long-term benefit; one of 25 patients so treated survived for more than five years (149).

In an attempt to increase the amount of radiation to the tumor and yet decrease radiation to surrounding healthy tissue, transcatheter administrations of iridium or intraoperative boost radiation have been used. These procedures have been associated with median survival of nine to 11.5 months and 10.9 to 12 months, respectively (145,147,150). It is important to recognize that complications may commonly follow radiation therapy; patients may have gastrointestinal bleeding (47 percent), sepsis (48 percent), cholangitis (38 percent), and recurrent obstruction (25 percent) (151).

CHEMOTHERAPY

No chemotherapeutic regimen has been shown to improve survival significantly. In trials with more than ten patients, 5-fluorouracil (5-FU) and mitomycin-C used as single agents have been associated with response rates of 23 percent and 42 percent, respectively (152). The combination of 5-FU and mitomycin-C administered intra-arterially (153), FAM (S-FU, doxorubicin, and mitomycin) (154), and M-AMSA (AmSacrine) (155) have been associated with response rates of 51 percent, 31 percent, and 9 percent, respectively.

Recently, other drugs such as interleukin-2, tumor necrosis factor, and interferon have become available and deserve evaluation. Recently, it has been reported that intra-arterial 5-FUDR (5-fluorodeoxyuridine) infusion, combined with radiation therapy, has been successful in locally controlling biliary obstruction in 40 percent of patients (156). Other treatments that may prove beneficial in the future are endoscopic laser therapy (157), and hematoporphyrin-derivation photodynamic therapy which has provided a 100 percent response rate in human cholangiocarcinoma transplanted into nude mice (158,159).

CANCER OF THE GALLBLADDER
Epidemiology

Although cancer of the gallbladder is rare, it is the most common malignant tumor of the biliary tract. The crude incidence of gallbladder cancer is 1.2 per 100,000 person years in Olmsted County, Minnesota (111). It causes 1 percent of cancer deaths and comprises 3 percent of gastrointestinal malignancies, but is two to three times more frequent in women than men. Seventy-five percent to 85 percent of gallbladder cancers occur in patients with gallstones. In American Indian women who have a 70 percent prevalence for gallstones, gallbladder cancer is five to ten times more frequent, and is the most common gastrointestinal malignancy.

In a case control study (160), gallstones were associated with an increased risk for gallbladder cancer in American Indian men and women, black American women, and Swedish men and women; black American men had no increased risk. Recently, we found in a prospective cohort study of 2583 Caucasian residents of Rochester, Minnesota, that the risk for gallbladder cancer was increased three-fold. This increase was significant only in men, however, and the absolute risk was low (161). Only two men and three women of the entire cohort developed gallbladder cancer. Thus, cholecystectomy or dissolution of gallstones is not indicated to prevent development of gallbladder cancer in patients with gallstones. In addition, the population of patients with gallstones in this study did not have an increased risk for colon cancer, or any other gastrointestinal malignancy, even after cholecystectomy.

Pathology

Most tumors arise in the fundus or neck of the gallbladder, but often the origin of the tumor is difficult to determine because at surgery or autopsy the fungating tumor usually fills the entire gallbladder. The tumors are usually adenocarcinomas. Squamous and anaplastic tumors, which are particularly malignant, only rarely occur. Some tumors are associated with mucoid change, grow rapidly, metastasize early, and cause gelatinous peritoneal dissemination.

In the majority of patients, the tumor is characterized by early metastasis to hilar lymph nodes and spread to the adjacent liver. Metastases to other hilar structures and more distant liver parenchyma occur later. More distant metastases and invasion into the duodenum, stomach, and colon occur very late; the late extensions to surrounding organs may be associated with external compression or fistulae. At the time of diagnosis 75 percent of patients have stage IV disease (serosal and regional lymph nodes) or stage V disease (extension into the liver or distant metastases) (162). Most long-term survivors have stage I disease (intramucosal) or stage II disease (submucosal and muscularis).

Clinical Presentation, Diagnosis, and Treatment

Gallbladder carcinoma has one of four clinical presentations: l) unremitting deep jaundice from involvement of the common bile duct and liver; 2) acute cholecystitis with a palpable mass; 3) chronic cholecystitis with intermittent right-upper-quadrant pain; and 4) advanced disseminated carcinomatosis. Two-thirds of patients have an abdominal mass, and one-third have localized right-upper-quadrant tenderness.

A gallbladder tumor can be seen as a polypoid intraluminal tumor with abdominal ultrasonography and is differentiated from gallstones because it does not move with changing body position. If an oral cholecystogram is performed, not currently a common procedure, the gallbladder fails to opacify more than 90 percent of the time, and if it does, the tumor will not be visualized. CT examination may show a gallbladder mass, a nonenhancing hilar mass, an intrahepatic mass of low attenuation, or an obstruction of the common intrahepatic duct near the bifurcation. Even with the development of these imaging techniques, the diagnosis is made preoperatively in only 10 percent of patients.

Resection is the only hope for cure since the tumor does not respond to chemotherapy or radiation therapy. Approximately 25 percent of tumors are resectable and should be treated with cholecystectomy and the removal of adjacent liver and common bile duct lymph chain. Even in this group, five-year survival is 5 percent (163). Mean survival of all patients is 4.5 months.

Benign Tumors of the Gallbladder

Benign tumors of the gallbladder are adenomyomatosis, cholesterol polyps, and adenomas. Rarely do these conditions cause symptoms or require treatment. Adenomyomatosis is hyperplasia of the mucosa with intraluminal diverticulae without neoplastic or inflammatory changes. Adenomyomatosis is usually diagnosed by oral cholecystography as a sessile filling defect and small peripheral opaque area representing diverticulae. They are asymptomatic, but it is possible that a few patients may have episodic pain that can be cured by cholecystectomy.

Cholesterol polyps are a focal form of cholesterolosis consisting of submucosal macrophages located at the villous tips and filled with cholesterol. Multiple polyps (5–19 mm in diameter) are present, and are attached to the mucosa by a fragile stalk. They are differentiated from gallstones during ultrasonography or oral cholecystography by their fixed positions. Possibly migration of polyps into the bile ducts causes biliary colic, which can be relieved by cholecystectomy.

Adenomas are papillary and nonpapillary. Most are pedunculated, and two-thirds are detected as multiple filling defects on oral cholecystography or as polyps during ultrasonography. It is doubtful that carcinoma of the gallbladder arises from adenomas, since the latter are much less common than the former.

REFERENCES

1. Silverberg E, Lubera JA. Cancer statistics 1988. *CA* 38: 5–22, 1988.
2. Gordis L, Gold EB. Epidemiology and etiology of pancreatic cancer. In: Go VLW, Gardner JD, Brooks FP, Lebenthal E, DiMagno EP, Scheele GA, eds. *The Exocrine Pancreas: Biology, Pathobiology and Diseases*. New York: Raven Press, 1986:621.
3. Edis AJ, Kiernan PD, Taylor WF. Attempted curative resection of ductal carcinoma of the pancreas. Review of Mayo Clinic experience 1951–1975. *Mayo Clin Proc* 55:531–536, 1980.
4. Kloppel G, Fitzgerald PJ. Pathology of nonendocrine pancreatic tumors. In: Go VLW, Gardner JD, Brooks FP, Lebenthal V, DiMagno EP, Scheele GA, eds. *The Exocrine Pancreas: Biology, Pathobiology and Diseases*. New York: Raven Press, 1986:649.
5. Castlemen B, Scully R, McNeely BU. Case records of the Massachusetts General Hospital, Case 25-1972. *N Engl J Med* 286:1353–1359, 1972.
6. Gross JB. Hereditary pancreatitis. In: Go VLW, Gardner JD, Brooks FP, Lebenthal E, DiMagno EP, Scheele GA, eds. *The Exocrine Pancreas: Biology, Pathobiology and Diseases*. New York: Raven Press, 1986:193.
7. Fitzgibbons RJ, Lynch HT, Stanslav GV, et al. Recognition and treatment of patients with hereditary nonpolyposis cancer (Lynch syndromes I and II). *Ann Surg* 206:289–295, 1987.
8. Turner HM, Grace HG. An investigation into cancer mortality among males in certain Sheffield trades. *J Hyg* 38:90–103, 1938.
9. Redmond CK, Strobino BR, Cypress RH. Cancer experience among coke by-product workers. *Ann NY Acad Sci* 271: 102–115, 1976.
10. Mancuso TF, El-Attar AA. A cohort study of workers exposed to betanaphthylamine and benzidine. *J Occup Med* 9:277–285, 1967.
11. Li FP, Fraumeni JF Jr., Mantel N, Miller RW. Cancer mortality among chemists. *J Natl Cancer Inst* 43:1159–1164, 1969.
12. Hoar KS, Pell SA. A retrospective cohort study of mortality and cancer incidence among chemists. *J Occup Med* 23:485–494, 1981.
13. Gold EB, Gordis L, Diener M, et al. Diet and other risk factors for cancer of the pancreas. *Cancer* 55:460–467, 1985.
14. Mack TM, Paganini-Hill A. Epidemiology of pancreas cancer in Los Angeles. *Cancer* 47:1474–1484 (6 Suppl), 1981.
15. Doll R, Peto R. Mortality in relation to smoking: 20 years' observations of male British doctors. *Br Med J* 245:147–152, 1981.
16. Hammond EC. Smoking in relation to the death rates of one million men and women. In: Haenszel W, ed. *Epidemiological Approaches to the Study of Cancer and Other Chronic Diseases*. U.S. Public Health Service, National Cancer Institute Monograph 19:126,1966.
17. Kahn HA. *The Dorn study of smoking and mortality among U.S. veterans: Report on eight and one-half years of observation*. [U.S. Public Health Service, National Cancer Institute Monograph 19:1–125, 1966.
18. Wynder EL, Mabuchi K, Maruchi N, Fortner JG. Epidemiology of cancer of the pancreas. *J Natl Cancer Inst* 50:645–667, 1973.
19. Wynder EL. An epidemiological evaluation of the causes of cancer of the pancreas. *Cancer Res* 35:2228–2233, 1975.

20. Segi M, Kurihara M, Matsuyama T. *Cancer mortality for selected sites in 24 countries*. No. 5, 1964–1965. Sendai, Japan: Department of Public Health, Tohoku University School of Medicine, 1960.

21. Cohen LA. Diet and cancer. *Sci Am* 257:42–48, 1987.

22. Schwartz SS, Zeidler A, Moossa AR, Kuku SF, Rubenstein AH. Prospective study of glucose tolerance, insulin, C-peptide and glucagon responses in patients with pancreatic carcinoma. *Am J Dig Dis* 23:1107–1114, 1978.

23. Kessler II. A genetic relationship between diabetes and cancer. *Lancet* 1:218–220, 1970.

24. Burch GE, Ansari A. Chronic alcoholism and carcinoma of the pancreas: a correlative hypothesis. *Arch Intern Med* 122:273–275, 1968.

25. DiMagno EP, Shorter RG, Taylor WF, Go VLW. Relationships between pancreaticobiliary ductal anatomy and pancreatic ductal and parenchymal histology. *Cancer* 49:361–368, 1982.

26. Hendricks JC, DiMagno EP, Dozois RR, Go VLW. Reflux of duodenal contents into the pancreatic duct of dogs. *J Lab Clin Med* 96:912–921, 1980.

27. Maringhini A, Moreau JA, Melton LJ, Hench VS, Zinsmeister AR, DiMagno EP. Gallstones, gallbladder cancer and other gastrointestinal malignancies. *Ann Intern Med* 107:30–35, 1987.

28. Maringhini A, Thiruvengadam R, Melton LJ, Hench VS, Zinsmeister AR, DiMagno EP. Pancreatic cancer risk following gastric surgery. *Cancer* 60:245–247, 1987.

29. Cubilla AL, Fitzgerald PJ. Tumors of the exocrine pancreas. In: *Atlas of Tumor Pathology*, Second series, fasc. 19. Washington, DC: Armed Forces Institute of Pathology, 1984.

30. Cubilla AL, Fitzgerald N. Pancreas cancer. 1. Duct adenocarcinoma. A clinical pathologic study of 380 patients. In: *Pathology Annual*, part 1. New York: Appleton-Century-Crofts, 1978:241.

31. Horie A, Yano Y, Kotoo Y, et al. Morphogenesis of pancreatoblastoma, infantile carcinoma of the pancreas: report of two cases. *Cancer* 39:247–254, 1977.

32. DiMagno EP, Malagelada J-R, Taylor WP, Go VLW. A prospective comparison of current diagnostic tests in pancreatic cancer. *N Engl J Med* 297:737–742, 1977.

33. Howard JM, Jordan CL Jr. Cancer of the pancreas. *Curr Probl Cancer* 2:1–52, 1977.

34. Gambill EE. Pancreatic and ampullar carcinoma: diagnosis and prognosis in relationship to symptoms, physical findings, and elapse of time as observed in 255 patients. *South Med J* 63:1119–1122, 1970.

35. Gullick HD. Carcinoma of the pancreas. A review of 100 cases. *Medicine* 38:47–84, 1959.

36. Perez MM, Newcomer AD, Moertel CG, Go VLW, DiMagno EP. Assessment of weight loss, food intake, fat metabolism, malabsorption, and treatment of pancreatic insufficiency in pancreatic cancer. *Cancer* 52:346–352, 1983.

37. Moosa AR, Levin B. Collaborative studies in the diagnosis of pancreatic cancer. *Semin Oncol* 6:298–308, 1978.

38. Regan PT, Malagelada J-R, DiMagno EP, Glanzman SL, Go VLW. Comparative effects of antacids, cimetidine, and enteric coating on the therapeutic response to oral enzymes in severe pancreatic insufficiency. *N Engl J Med* 297:854–858, 1977.

39. Fras I, Litin EM, Pearson JS. Comparison of psychiatric symptoms in carcinoma of the pancreas with those in some other intra-abdominal neoplasms. *Am J Psychiatry* 123:1553–1562, 1967.

40. Holland JC, Korzun AH, Tross S, et al. Comparative psychological disturbance in patients with pancreatic and gastric cancer. *Am J Psychiatry* 143:982–986, 1986.

41. Moertel CG. Exocrine pancreas. In: Holland JF, Frei E III, eds. *Cancer Medicine*. Philadelphia: Lea and Febiger, 1973:1559.

42. Go VLW, Taylor WF, DiMagno EP. Efforts at early diagnosis of pancreatic cancer: the Mayo Clinic experience. *Cancer* 3:1698–1703, 1981.

43. Piper CE, Remine WH, Priestly Jr. Pancreatic cystadenoma: report of 20 cases. *JAMA* 180:648–652, 1962.

44. Freeney PC, Weinstein CJ, Taft DA, Allen FH. Cystic neoplasms of the pancreas: new angiographic and ultrasonographic findings. *AJR* 131:795–802, 1978.

45. Dodds WJ, Margolin FR, Goldberg HI. Cavernous lymphangioma of the pancreas. *Radiol Clin Biol* 38:267–270, 1969.

46. Baltaxe HA, Leslie EV. Vanishing pancreatic calcifications. *AJR* 99:642–644, 1967.

47. Tucker DH, Moore IB. Vanishing pancreatic calcification in chronic pancreatitis. *N Engl J Med* 268:31–33, 1963.

48. Metzgar RS, Asch HL. Antigens of human pancreatic adenocarcinomas: their role in diagnosis and therapy. *Pancreas* 3:352–371, 1988.

49. Holyoke ED, Douglass HO, Goldrosen, et al. Tumor markers in pancreatic cancer. *Semin Oncol* 6:347–356, 1979.

50. Klavins JV. Tumor markers of pancreatic carcinoma. *Cancer* 47:1597–1601, 1981.

51. Moossa AR, Levin B. Collaborative studies in the diagnosis of pancreatic cancer. *Semin Oncol* 6:298–308, 1979.

52. Zamcheck N, Martin EW. Factors controlling the circulating CEA levels in pancreatic cancer. *Cancer* 47:1620–1627, 1981.

53. Podolsky DK, McPhee MS, Alpert E, et al. Galactosyltransferase isoenzyme II in the detection of pancreatic cancer: comparison with radiologic, endoscopic, and serologic tests. *N Engl J Med* 304:1313–1318, 1981.

54. Ritts R Jr, Jacobsen D, Ilstrup D, et al. A prospective evaluation of MoAb CA 19–9 to detect GI cancer in a high-risk clinic population. *Cancer Detect Prev* 7(5/6):525, 1984.

55. Ritts R Jr, Klug T, Jacobsen D, et al. Multiple tumor marker tests enhance sensitivity of pancreatic carcinoma detection. *Cancer Detect Prev* 7(5/6):459, 1984.

56. DiMagno EP, Regan PT, Clain JE, et al. Human endoscopic ultrasonography. *Gastroenterology* 83:824–829, 1982.

57. Fitzgerald PJ, Fortner JG, Watson, et al. The value of diagnostic aids in detecting pancreas cancer. *Cancer* 41:868–879, 1978.

58. Moossa AR, Levin B. The diagnosis of "early" pancreatic cancer: the University of Chicago experience. *Cancer* 47:1688–1697, 1981.

59. Gowland M, Kalantzis N, Warwick F, Braganza J. Relative efficiency and predictive value of ultrasonography and endoscopic retrograde pancreatography in diagnosis of pancreatic disease. *Lancet* 2:190–193,1981.

60. Faintuch J, Levin B. Clinical presentation and diagnosis of exocrine tumors of the pancreas. In: Go VLW, Gardner JD, Brooks FP, Lebenthal E, DiMagno EP, Scheele GA, eds. *The Exocrine Pancreas: Biology, Pathobiology and Diseases*. New York: Raven Press, 1986:193.

61. Ferrucci JF Jr, Wittenberg J. CT biopsy of abdominal tumors: aids for lesion localization. *Radiology* 129:739–744, 1978.

62. Yeh H. Percutaneous fine needle aspiration biopsy of intraabdominal lesions with ultrasound guidance. *Am J Gastroenterol* 75:148–152, 1981.

63. DiMagno EP, Malagelada J-R, Moertel CG, Go VLW. Prospective evaluation of the pancreatic secretion of immunoreactive carcinoembryonic antigen, enzyme, and bicarbonate in patients suspected of having pancreatic cancer. *Gastroenterology* 73:457–461, 1977.

64. DiMagno EP. Diagnosis of chronic pancreatitis: are noninvasive tests of exocrine pancreatic function sensitive and specific? *Gastroenterology* 83:143–146, 1982.

65. Shapiro TM. Adenocarcinoma of the pancreas: a statistical analysis of biliary bypass vs Whipple resection in good-risk patients. *Ann Surg* 182:715–721, 1975.

66. Trede M. The surgical treatment of pancreatic carcinoma. *Surgery* 97:28–35, 1985.

67. Grace PA, Pitt HA, Tomkins RK, et al. Decreased morbidity and mortality after pancreatoduodenectomy. *Am J Surg* 151:141–149, 1986.

68. Braasch JW, Deziel DJ, Rossi RL, et al. Pyloric and gastric-preserving pancreatic resection. Experience with 87 patients. *Surgery* 204:411–418, 1986.

69. Connolly MM, Dawson N, Michelassi F, Moossa AR, Lowenstein F. Survival in 1,001 patients with carcinoma of the pancreas. *Ann Surg* 206:366–373, 1987.

70. Crist DW, Sitzmann JW, Cameron JL. Improved hospital morbidity, mortality, and survival following the Whipple procedure. *Ann Surg* 206:358–365, 1987.

71. Brooks JR, Culebras JM. Cancer of the pancreas: palliative operation, Whipple procedure, or total pancreatectomy. *Am J Surg* 131:516–520, 1976.

72. Tsuchiaya R, Noda T, Harada N, et al. Collective review of small carcinomas of the pancreas. *Ann Surg* 203:77–81, 1986.

73. Fortner JG. Surgical principles for pancreatic cancer—regional, total and subtotal pancreatectomy. *Cancer* 47:1712–1718, 1981.

74. Traverso LW, Longmire WPJ. Preservation of the pylorus in pancreatoduodenectomy. *Surg Gynecol Obstet* 146:959–962, 1978.

75. Speer AG, Cotton PB, Russell RC, et al. Randomised trial of endoscopic versus percutaneous stent insertion in malignant obstructive jaundice. *Lancet* 2:57–62, 1987.

76. Dowsett JR, Williams SJ, Hatfield ARW, Houghton J, Lennon T, Russel RCG. Does stent diameter matter in the endoscopic palliation of malignant biliary obstruction? A randomized trial of 10 FG versus 12 FG endoprosthesis. *Gastroenterology* 96:A128, 1989.

77. Dowsett JF, Russell RCG, Hatfield ARW, et al. Malignant obstructive jaundice: a prospective randomized trial of bypass surgery versus endoscopic stenting. *Gastroenterology* 96:A128, 1989.

78. Huibregtse K, Katon RM, Coene PP, Tytgat GNJ. Endoscopic palliative treatment in pancreatic cancer. *Gastrointest Endosc* 32:334–338, 1986.

79. Barkin JS, Goldberg RI, Sfakianakis GN, Levi J. Pancreatic carcinoma is associated with delayed gastric emptying. *Dig Dis Sci* 31:265–267, 1986.

80. Schantz S, Schickler W, Evans TK, Coffey RS. Palliative gastroenterostomy for pancreatic cancer. *Am J Surg* 147:793–796, 1984.

81. Shivshanker K, Bennett RW, Haynie TP. Tumor-associated gastroparesis: correction with metoclopramide. *Am J Surg* 145:221–225, 1983.

82. Moertel CG, Engstrom P, Lavin PT, Gelber RD, Carbone PP. Chemotherapy of gastric and pancreatic carcinoma. *Surgery* 85:509–513, 1979.

83. Cullinan SA, Moertel CG, Fleming TR, et al. Comparison of three chemotherapeutic regimens in the treatment of advanced pancreatic and gastric carcinoma. *JAMA* 253:2061–2067, 1985.

84. Karlin DA, Stroehlein JR, Bennetts RW, Jones RD, Heifetz LJ, Mahal PS. Phase I–II study of the combination of 5-FU, doxorubicin, mitomycin, and semustine (FAMMe) in the treatment of adenocarcinoma of the stomach, gastroesophageal junction, and pancreas. *Cancer Treat Rep* 66:1613–1617, 1982.

85. Gastrointestinal Tumor Study Group. Treatment of locally unresectable carcinoma of the pancreas: comparison of combined-modality therapy (chemotherapy plus radiotherapy) to chemotherapy alone. *J Natl Cancer Inst* 80:751–755, 1988.

86. Roldan GE, Gunderson LL, Nagorney DM, et al. External beam versus intraoperative and external beam irradiation for locally advanced pancreatic cancer. *Cancer* 6:1110–1116, 1986.

87. Mohiuddin M, Cantor RJ, Biermann W, Weiss SM, Barbot D, Rosato FE. Combined modality treatment of localized unresectable adenocarcinoma of the pancreas. *Int J Radiat Oncol Biol Phys* 14:79–84, 1988.

88. Lanspa SJ, Chan ATH, Bell JS III, Go VLW, Dickson ER, DiMagno EP. Pathogenesis of steatorrhea in primary biliary cirrhosis. *Hepatology* 5:837–842, 1985.

89. Gray GM. Mechanisms of digestion and absorption of food. In: Sleisenger MH, Fordtran JS, eds. *Gastrointestinal Disease,* 2nd ed. Philadelphia: W.B. Saunders Co., 1978:241.

90. Regan PT, DiMagno EP. Exocrine pancreatic insufficiency in celiac sprue: a cause of treatment failure. *Gastroenterology* 78:484–487, 1980.

91. DiMagno EP, Malagelada J-R, Go VLW, Moertel CG. Fate of orally-ingested enzymes in pancreatic insufficiency: comparison of two dosage schedules. *N Engl J Med* 296:1318–1322, 1977.

92. Regan PT, Malagelada J-R, DiMagno EP, Glanzman SL, Go VLW. Comparative effects of antacids, cimetidine, and enteric coating on the therapeutic response to oral enzymes in severe pancreatic insufficiency. *N Engl J Med* 297:854–858, 1977.

93. DiMagno EP. Medical treatment of pancreatic insufficiency. *Mayo Clin Proc* 54:435–442, 1979.

94. DiMagno EP, Go VLW, Summerskill WHJ. Relations between pancreatic enzyme outputs and malabsorption in severe pancreatic insufficiency. *N Engl J Med* 288:813–815, 1973.

95. Foley KM. Pain syndromes and pharmacologic management of pancreatic cancer pain. *J Pain Sympt Manage* 3:176–187, 1988.

96. Foley KM, Inturrisi CE. Analgesic drug therapy in cancer pain: principles and practice. *Med Clin North Am* 71:207–232, 1987.

97. Maguire LG, Yon JL, Miller E. Prevention of narcotic induced constipation. *N Engl J Med* 305:1651, 1981.

98. Moore DC, Bush WH, Burnett LL. Coeliac plexus block. A roentgenographic, anatomic study of technique and spread of solution in patients and corpses. *Anesth Analg* 60(6):369–379, 1981.

99. Ischia S, Luzzani A, Ischia A, Faggion S. A new approach to the neurolytic block of the coeliac plexus: the transaortic technique. *Pain* 16(4):333–341, 1983.

100. Leung JWC, Bowen-Wright M, Aveling W, Shorvon PJ, Cotton PB. Coeliac plexus block for pain in pancreatic cancer and chronic pancreatitis. *Br J Surg* 70:730–732, 1983.

101. Thompson GE, Moore DC, Bridenbaugh LD, Artin RY. Abdominal pain and alcohol coeliac plexus block. *Anesth Analg* 56:1–5, 1977.

102. Galizea EJ, Lahiri SK. Paraplegia following coeliac plexus block with phenol. *Br J Anaesth* 46:539–540, 1974.

103. Compagno J, Oertel JE. Mucinous cystic neoplasms of the pancreas with overt and latent malignancy (cystadenocarcinoma and cystadenoma). A clinicopathologic study of 41 cases. *Am J Clin Pathol* 69:573–580, 1978.

104. Cullen PK, ReMine WH, Dahlin DC. A clinicopathological study of cystadenocarcinoma of the pancreas. *Surg Gynecol Obstet* 117:189–195, 1963.

105. Hodgkinson DJ, ReMine WH, Weiland LH. Pancreatic cystadenoma—a clinicopathologic study of 45 cases. *Arch Surg* 113:512–519, 1978.

106. Alguacil-Garcia A, Weiland LH. The histologic spectrum, prognosis, and histogenesis of the sarcomatoid carcinoma of the pancreas. *Cancer* 39:1181–1189, 1977.

107. Tschang TP, Garza-Garza R, Kissane JM. Pleomorphic carcinoma of the pancreas: an analysis of 15 cases. *Cancer* 39:2114–2126, 1977.

108. Burns WA, Matthews MJ, Hamosh M, VanderWeide G, Blum R, Johnson FB. Lipase-secreting acinar cell carcinoma of the pancreas with polyarthropathy—a light and electron microscopic, histochemical and biochemical study. *Cancer* 33:1002–1009, 1974.

109. Robertson JC, Ecles GM. Syndrome associated with pancreatic acinar cell carcinoma. *Br J Med* 2:708–709, 1970.

110. Osborne BM, Culbert SJ, Cangir A, Mackay B. Acinar cell carcinoma of the pancreas in a nine-year-old child: case report with electron microscopic observations. *South Med J*

70:370–372, 1977.

111. Riela A, Melton LJ, Zinsmeister AR, DiMagno EP. Carcinomas of gallbladder, bile ducts and ampulla, and ductal cancer of the exocrine pancreas in Olmsted County, MN, 1950-1988. Submitted to American Gastroenterological Association, May 13–16, 1990.

112. Lerut JP, Gianello PR, Otte JB. Pancreaticoduodenal resection: surgical experience and evaluation of risk factors in 103 patients. *Ann Surg* 199:432–437, 1984.

113. Maram ES, Ludwig J, Kurland LT, et al. Carcinoma of the gallbladder and extrahepatic biliary ducts in Rochester, Minnesota, 1935–1971. *Am J Epidemiol* 109:152–157, 1979.

114. Silverberg E, Lubera JA. Cancer statistics, 1989. *Cancer Journal for Clinicians* 39:3–20, 1989.

115. Sako K, Seitzinger GI, Gasside E. Carcinoma of the extrahepatic bile ducts. A review of the literature and report of six cases. *Surgery* 41:416–437, 1957.

116. Sons HU, Borchard F. Carcinoma of the extrahepatic bile ducts: a postmortem study of 65 cases and review of the literature. *J Surg Oncol* 34:6–12, 1987.

117. Nagorney DM, McPherson GAD. Carcinoma of the gallbladder and extrahepatic bile ducts. *Semin Oncol* 15:106–115, 1988.

118. Coffey RJ, Wiesner RH, Beaver SJ, et al. Bile duct carcinoma: a late complication of end-stage sclerosing cholangitis. *Hepatology* 14:1056 (abstract), 1984.

119. Flavell DJ. Liver fluke infection as an aetiologic factor in bile duct carcinoma of man. *Trans R Soc Trop Med Hyg* 75:-814–824, 1981.

120. Purtilo DT. Clonorchiasis and hepatic neoplasms. *Trop Geogr Med* 28:21–29, 1976.

121. Ritchie JK, Allan RN, Macartney J. Biliary tract carcinoma associated with ulcerative colitis. *Q J Med* 43:263–279, 1974.

122. Akwari OE, Van Heerden JA, Foulk WT, Baggenstoss AH. Cancer of the bile ducts associated with ulcerative colitis. *Ann Surg* 181:303–309, 1975.

123. Kagawa Y, Kashihara S, Kuramoto S, Maetani S. Carcinoma arising in a congenitally dilated biliary tract. Report of a case and review of the literature. *Gastroenterology* 74:1286-1294, 1978.

124. Dayton MT, Longmire WP Jr., Tompkins RK. Caroli's disease: a premalignant condition? *Am J Surg* 145:41–48, 1983.

125. Battifora HA. Thorotrast and tumours of the liver. In: Okuda K, Peters RL, cds. *Hepatocellular Carcinoma*. New York: John Wiley & Sons, 1976.

126. Neumann RD, Livolsi VA, Rosenthal NS, Burrell M, Ball TJ. Adenocarcinoma in biliary papillomatosis. *Gastroenterology* 70:779–782, 1976.

127. Frierson HG, Fechner RE. Pathology of malignant neoplasms of gallbladder and extrahepatic bile ducts. In: Wanebo HJ, ed. *Hepatic and Biliary Cancer*. New York: Marcel Dekker, 1987:281.

128. Tompkins RK, Thomas D, Wile A, et al. Prognostic factors in bile duct carcinoma. Analysis of 96 cases. *Ann Surg* 194:447–457, 1981.

129. Okuda K, Kubo Y, Okazaki N, et al. Clinical aspects of intrahepatic bile duct carcinoma including hilar carcinoma. *Cancer* 39:232–246, 1977.

130. Gibson RN, Yeung E, Thompson JN, et al. Bile duct obstruction: radiologic evaluation of level, cause, tumor resectability. *Radiology* 160:43–47, 1986.

131. Blumgart LH, Hadjis NS. Proximal bile duct cancer. Curative resection or palliative bypass. In: Wanebo HG, ed. *Hepatic Biliary Cancer*. New York: Marcel Dekker, 1987:375.

132. Voyles CR, Bowley NJ, Allison DJ, et al. Carcinoma of the proximal extrahepatic biliary tree. Radiologic assessment and therapeutic alternatives. *Ann Surg* 197:188–194, 1983.

133. Nakayama T, Ikeda A, Okuda K. Percutaneous transhepatic drainage of the biliary tract. *Gastroenterology* 74:554–559, 1978.

134. Hatfield ARW, Terblanche J, Fataar S, et al. Preoperative external biliary drainage in obstructive jaundice. *Lancet* 2:896–899, 1982.

135. McPherson GAD, Benjamin IS, Hodgson HJF, et al. Preoperative transhepatic biliary drainage: the results of a controlled trial. *Br J Surg* 71:371–375, 1984.

136. Pitt HA, Gomes MD, Lis JL, et al. Does preoperative percutaneous biliary drainage reduce operative risk or increase hospital cost? *Ann Surg* 201:545–553, 1985.

137. Foschi D, Cavagna G, Callioni F, et al. Hyperalimentation of jaundiced patients on percutaneous transhepatic biliary drainage. *Br J Surg* 73:716–719, 1986.

138. Warren KE, Choe DS, Plaza J, et al. Results of radical resection for periampullary cancer. *Ann Surg* 181:534–540, 1975.

139. Tarazi RY, Hermann RE, Vogt DP, et al. Results of surgical treatment of periampullary tumors: a thirty-five year experience. *Surgery* 100:716–723, 1986.

140. Grace PA, Pitt HA, Tompkins RK, et al. Decreased morbidity and mortality after pancreatoduodenectomy. *Am J Surg* 151:141–149, 1986.

141. Jones BA, Langer B, Taylor BR, et al. Periampullary tumors: which ones should be resected? *Am J Surg* 149:46–52, 1985.

142. Alexander F, Rossi RL, O'Bryan M, et al. Biliary carcinoma. A review of 109 cases. *Am J Surg* 147:503–509, 1984.

143. Blumgart LH, Benjamin IS. Liver resection for bile duct cancer. *Surg Clin North Am* 69(2):323–337, 1989.

144. Scharaschmidt BF. Human liver transplantation: analysis of data on 540 patients from four centers. *Hepatology* 4:95S-101S, 1984.

145. Broe PJ, Cameron, JL. The management of proximal biliary tract tumours. *Adv Surg* 15:47–91, 1981.

146. Ottow RT, August DA, Sugarbaker PH. Treatment of proximal biliary tract carcinoma: an overview of techniques and results. *Surgery* 97:251–262, 1985.

147. Johnson DW, Safai C, Goffinet DR. Malignant obstructive jaundice: treatment with external-beam and intracavitary radiotherapy. *Int J Rad Oncol Biol Physiol* 11:411–416, 1985.

148. Hanna SS, Rider WD. Carcinoma of the gallbladder or extrahepatic bile ducts: the role of radiotherapy. *Can Med Assoc J* 118:59–63, 1978.

149. Cady B, Macdonald JS, Gunderson LC. Cancer of the hepatobiliary system. In: DeVita VT Jr, Hellman S, Rosenberg SA, eds. *Cancer: Principles and Practice of Oncology*, 2nd ed. Philadelphia: J.B. Lippincott, 1985:741–770.

150. Fletcher MS, Dawson BJL, Nunnerley H, et al. Treatment of hiliar carcinoma by bile drainage combined with internal radiotherapy using ^{192}Ir wire. *Br J Surg* 70:733–735, 1983.

151. Hayes JJ, Sapozink M, Miller F. Definitive radiation therapy in bile duct carcinoma. *Int J Radiat Oncol Biol Phys* 15(3):735–744, 1988.

152. Gunderson LL, Martin JK, O'Connell MJ, et al. Local control and survival in locally advanced gastrointestinal cancer. *Int J Radiat Oncol Biol Phys* 12:661–665, 1986.

153. Bukowski RM, Leichman LP, Rivkin SE. Phase II trial of MAMSA in gallbladder and cholangiocarcinoma: a Southwest Oncology Group study. *Eur J Cancer Clin Oncol* 19:721–723, 1986.

154. Ravry MJR, Hester M. Combination chemotherapy of hepatocellular and biliary tract cancer with Adriamycin plus bleomycin (Abstr.). *Proc Am Soc Clin Oncol* 21:366, 1980.

155. Adolphson CC, Carpenter JP. Response to doxorubicin and mitomycin in cholangiocarcinoma: a case report. *Cancer Treat Rep* 66:209–210, 1982.

156. Wollner I, Prust R, Andrews J, Walker-Andrews S, et al. Combination chem-radiation therapy for jaundice due to focal malignant obstruction of the major bile ducts. *Sel Cancer Tel* 5(2):81–91, 1989.

157. Pietrafitta JJ. Laser therapy of cancer of the gastrointestinal and biliary tracts. *Semin Surg Oncol* 5(1):17–29, 1989.

158. Alexander G, Wang K, Ahlquist D, Pittelkow M. Development of an in-vivo model for photodynamic therapy of human cholangiocarcinoma. *Gastroenterology* 98:A269, 1990.

159. Alexander G, Wang K, Ahlquist D, Carpenter H, Pittelkow M, Wieand H. Hematoporphyrin derivative photodynamic therapy of human cholangiocarcinoma implanted into athymic mice. *Gastroenterology* 98:A268, 1990.

160. Lowenfels AB, Lindstrom CG, Conway MJ, Hastings PR. Gallstones and the risk of gallbladder cancer. *J Natl Cancer Inst* 75:77–80, 1985.

161. Maringhini A, Moreau JA, Melton LJ, Hench VS, Zinsmeister AR, DiMagno EP. Gallstones, gallbladder cancer and other gastrointestinal malignancies. *Ann Intern Med* 107:30–35, 1987.

162. Adson MA, Farnell MB. Hepatobiliary cancer—surgical considerations. *Mayo Clin Proc* 56:686, 1981.

163. Albores-Saavedra J, Manrique J, de J Angeles-Angeles A, Henson DE. Carcinoma in situ of the gallbladder. A clinicopathologic study of 18 cases. *Am J Surg Pathol* 8:323, 1984.

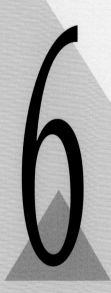

Endocrine Tumors of the Gastrointestinal Tract

Murray F. Brennan

In terms of functional endocrine mass, the gastrointestinal tract is the largest endocrine organ in the body. The endocrine tumors of the gastrointestinal tract include islet cell tumors of the pancreas and carcinoid tumors of the stomach and intestine. The distribution of gastrointestinal endocrine glands is ubiquitous; substance P and 5-hydroxytryptamine-producing cells can be found by immunohistochemistry throughout the gastrointestinal tract, while other polypeptide-producing cells are less widespread and may be found, as in the case of gastrin, in the more proximal gastrointestinal tract, particularly in the duodenum. Glucagon, depending on species, may be found with gut-like activity in the more distal intestine, whereas pancreatic glucagon is characteristically concentrated in the pancreas. Some of the gastrointestinal hormones and their localization are listed in Figure 6.1 (1).

The pancreas itself is the source of a large number of neuroendocrine cells of varying function. These can be divided into the endocrine cells (Fig. 6.2), the paracrine cells (Fig. 6.3), and the neurocrine cells (Fig. 6.4). In the endocrine cells, secretory granules are released systemically, as in the case of insulin. The paracrine cell has a direct effect on its surrounding and associated cells, as in the case of somatostatin. In the neurocrine cells the direct secretion of the endocrine cell is able to influence the neuron, as, for example, with vasoactive intestinal polypeptide (1). Pancreatic neuroendocrine tumors may be part of the multiple endocrine neoplasia syndrome (MEN-I).

This syndrome should be considered when evaluating patients for possible insulinoma or gastrinoma (Zollinger–Ellison syndrome, or ZES). Hypercalcemia due to hyperparathyroidism is seen in virtually all patients with MEN-I. Family members should also be evaluated, since the MEN syndromes are inherited in an autosomal dominant fashion.

THE PANCREATIC ENDOCRINE TUMORS: GENERAL FEATURES

Epidemiology

Neuroendocrine tumors of the pancreas are rare. Absolute prevalence rates are unknown, but it has been suggested from an analysis of the data collected by the National Institutes of Health that approximately 250 new islet cell carcinomas are

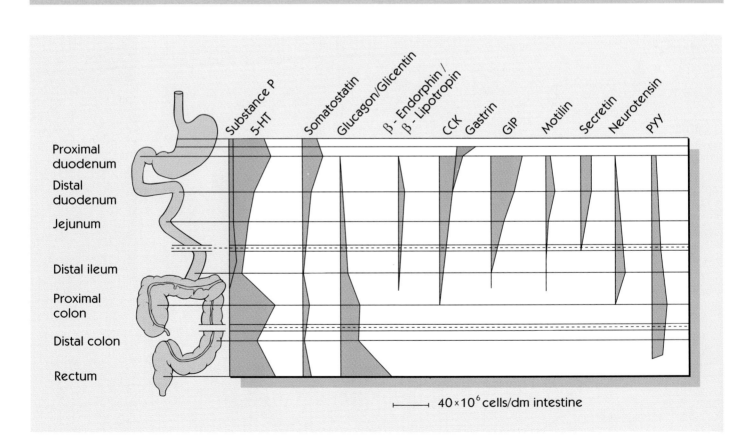

FIGURE 6.1 Distribution and frequency of distribution of human gastroenteropancreatic endocrine cells. (Adapted from reference 1.)

found in the United States each year. The true prevalence of benign tumors is even less well known; but, because islet cell adenomas may be found in as many as 1.5 percent of carefully performed autopsies, most of which are not diagnosed antemortem, one may conclude that islet cell adenomas are common and that most are nonfunctional. Overall, 200 to 1000 new endocrine pancreatic tumors will be diagnosed clinically each year in the United States, and many will be nonfunctional.

MEN-I can be found in approximately 25 percent of patients with ZES and about 10 percent of patients with insulinoma. The incidence of gastrinoma is not known, although it has been suggested that it occurs in one out of every 100,000 people in Denmark, and as many as one in 1000 patients with duodenal ulcer disease (2).

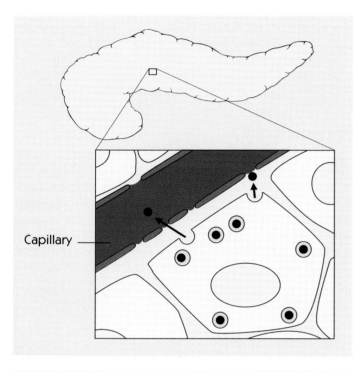

FIGURE 6.2 Neuroendocrine cells in the pancreas: the endocrine cells.

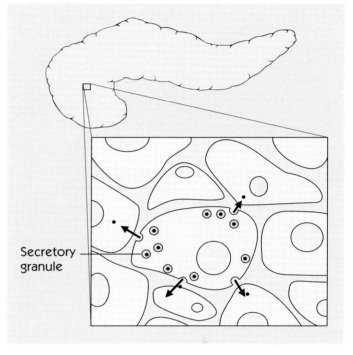

FIGURE 6.3 Neuroendocrine cells in the pancreas: the paracrine cells.

FIGURE 6.4 Neuroendocrine cells in the pancreas: the neurocrine cells.

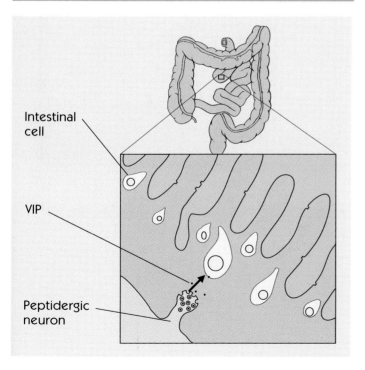

Histopathology

Neuroendocrine pancreatic tumors all look alike with the light microscope and in fact cannot be distinguished from carcinoid tumors. Unlike other solid neoplasms, pathologists cannot predict a benign from a malignant course solely on the appearance of the tumor (3). Immunohistochemistry has been able to utilize the unique production of polypeptides by these tumors to characterize possible function.

Immunohistochemistry has made major advances in the diagnosis of all neuroendocrine pancreatic tumors. Of great interest is the fact that even in tumors that are predominantly clinically functional with one hormone, multiple other hormones such as pancreatic peptide, gastrin, glucagon, and adrenocorticoptopic hormone (ACTH) are frequently identified by immunohistochemistry. Presumably the relative prevalence and quantitative secretion of such hormones are the factors that determine the symptom complex with which they present.

INSULIN-PRODUCING TUMORS
Pathophysiology

Insulin-secreting islet cell tumors are the most common of the functioning pancreatic neuroendocrine tumors, accounting for approximately 75 percent of these tumors. Insulinomas are usually benign, predominantly occur in the pancreas, and only rarely localize outside of the pancreas. Women are affected more than men, with a ratio of 3:2. The average age of presentation is in the mid-forties (4).

Clinical Presentation and Course

The classic presentation is that of symptoms of central nervous system hypoglycemia, with confusion, weakness, lethargy, and occasional loss of consciousness. These symptoms are responsive to the ingestion of carbohydrates. Often the patient is aware that the symptoms can be reversed by food ingestion and presents with associated obesity. The symptoms of insulinoma can continue for years before being correctly identified, and patients may carry inaccurate neuropsychiatric diagnoses.

Diagnosis

Diagnosis is suspected by a disproportionate elevation in insulin, inappropriate for the serum level of glucose (Fig. 6.5). The diagnosis is rapidly confirmed by the determination of fasting glucose and fasting insulin (Fig. 6.6) (5). True hypoglycemia is defined as a fasting blood sugar of less than 40 mg/dl. In patients for whom the diagnosis is not clear, a fast from 24 to 72 hours is almost always

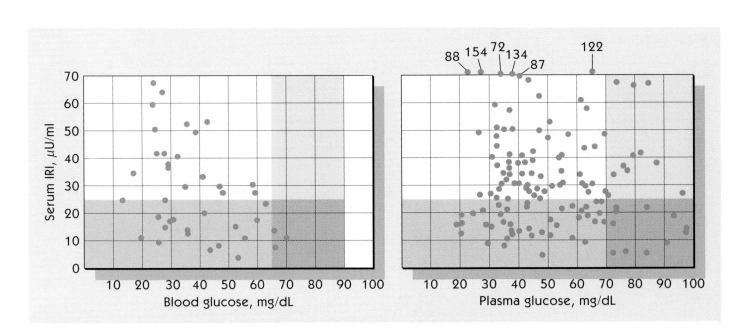

FIGURE 6.5 Blood plasma glucose and serum insulin levels for insulinoma patients. (Adapted from reference 4.)

diagnostic (Fig. 6.7) (6). A great majority of patients will become hypoglycemic within 24 hours, and over 95 percent of patients with insulinoma will become hypoglycemic within 72 hours (Fig. 6.8). Simplistic insulin-to-glucose ratios have been proposed, but, as a working rule, a ratio of insulin to glucose that is greater than 0:3 is highly suggestive of insulinoma.

Radioimmunoassay for insulin and its precursor proteins may also be helpful. Proinsulin, initially produced by the islet cell, consists of the A and B chains of insulin joined by a connecting peptide (C-peptide). Small amounts of proinsulin are secreted with insulin, whereas similar amounts of C-peptide and insulin are secreted. Therefore, patients with insulinoma, in addition to having increased serum

FIGURE 6.6: DIAGNOSTIC TESTS FOR INSULINOMA

TEST	% POSITIVE
Prolonged fast	95
Tolbutamide tolerance	80
Glucagon	72
Glucose tolerance	60
Leucine tolerance	50

From reference 5.

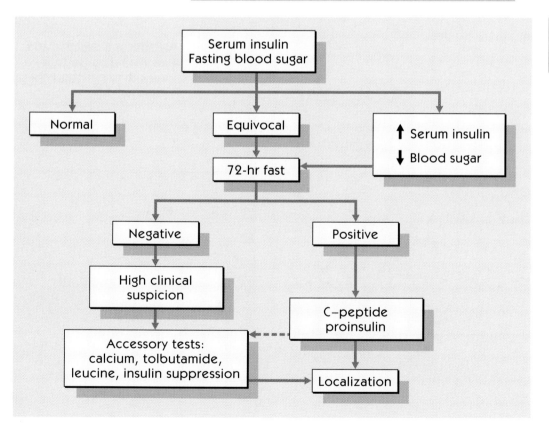

FIGURE 6.7 Flow chart for the diagnosis of suspected insulinoma.

insulin levels, usually also have elevated proinsulin and elevated C-peptide levels. These two determinations can help rule out factitious administration of insulin as the cause for the hypoglycemia and its associated symptoms. Although radioimmunoassay for C-peptide and proinsulin can aid in the diagnosis of insulinoma, the use of these measurements specifically to identify malignant insulinomas remains an issue of some debate. As with the other endocrine tumors, the ultimate diagnosis of whether an insulin-producing tumor is benign or malignant is quite difficult. The absolute indication, the presence of metastasis, cannot always be identified, and, as noted above, histologic evaluation of the lesion will not differentiate a benign from a malignant neuroendocrine tumor.

Because of the propensity for neuroendocrine tumors to secrete more than one polypeptide, malignant insulinomas may secrete the α subunit of human chorionic gonadotrophin. It has been suggested that this may be used as a marker for malignancy; however, the value of this determination is limited.

Once the diagnosis of insulinomas has been made, the next important issue is to determine whether the insulinoma is a component of the MEN-I syndrome. This association occurs in approximately 10 percent of patients. The presence of MEN-I syndrome can be ascertained by obtaining a serum calcium determination. No patient with an insulinoma should be considered for management without this determination. If the serum calcium is elevated, then one must suspect a multiple endocrine neoplasia syndrome, and the possibility of multiple pancreatic tumors must be considered.

TUMOR LOCALIZATION

Localization of the tumor can be most expeditiously performed by use of arteriography (Fig. 6.9). In selective arteriography, the frequently small (less than 1 cm) lesion can often be identified as a very vascular lesion within the pancreas (Fig. 6.10). In addition, it is important to determine, by careful arteriographic examination of the liver, whether metastatic disease is present. Neuroendocrine tumors are predominantly vascular and will show as multiple vascular defects within the liver (Fig. 6.11). In the patient in whom the insulinoma is not identified by selective arteriography or high-quality-contrast computed tomography (CT) (Fig. 6.12), further investigations are justified.

Selective venous sampling via the portal vein and its major tributaries is the next most appropriate study. In this test, a catheter is introduced trans-

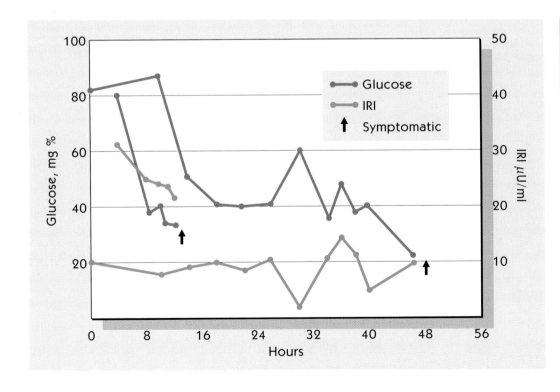

FIGURE 6.8 Glucose and insulin response to fasting in two patients with insulinoma.

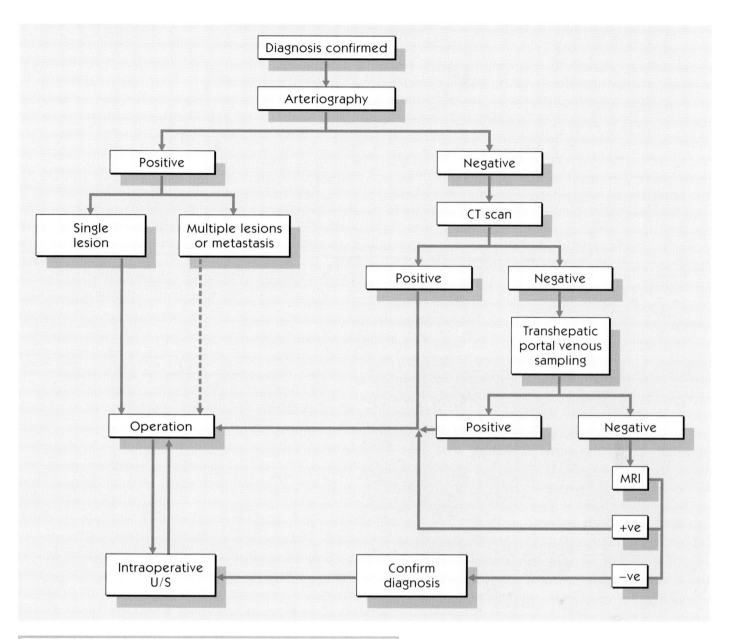

FIGURE 6.9 Management of insulinoma following diagnosis.

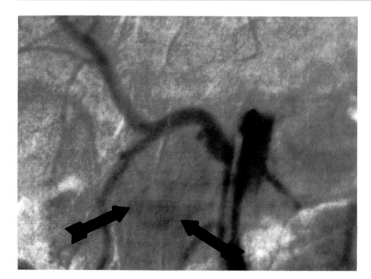

FIGURE 6.10 Identification of a small lesion by selective arteriography.

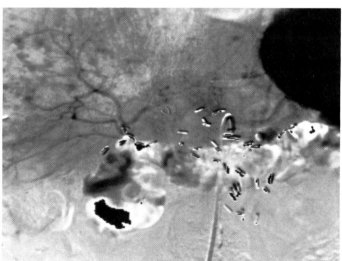

FIGURE 6.11 Neuroendocrine tumors are predominantly vascular which allows identification by arteriography of multiple small hepatic metastases.

hepatically to sample the portal venous tract (Fig. 6.13). It is most valuable in localizing an insulinoma as opposed to other functional neuroendocrine pancreatic tumors. A clear example is given in Figure 6.14 in a patient who has had a prior distal pancreatectomy, intraoperative ligation of the portal and splenic veins for the control of hemorrhage, and yet remains with symptoms of hypoglycemia. Here the pancreatic lesion can be identified by selective portal venous sampling for insulin.

Another clinical setting where selective portal venous sampling may be useful is in the patient with suspected MEN-I in whom arteriography has identified several different tumors. Portal venous sampling may localize the insulin-producing pancreatic lesion, enabling accurate surgical resection and correction of the hypoglycemic episodes (Fig. 6.15). It makes little sense in this situation to explore the patient and remove an obvious pancreatic tumor if it is not the one responsible for the clinical problem.

Another technique that has advanced the ability to localize these tumors is the use of intraoperative sonography which, in experienced hands, can further improve the results in patients not localized preoperatively. However, it is important to point out that even in the absence of preoperative localization, most tumors will be found by the experienced endocrine pancreatic surgeon.

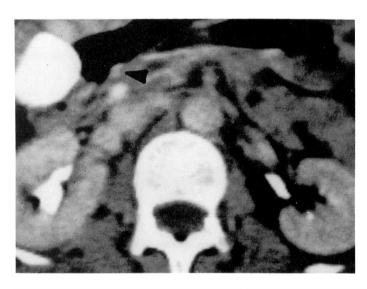

FIGURE 6.12 A patient in whom the insulinoma is identified by high-quality-contrast computed tomography. The proximity of the bile duct is also noted.

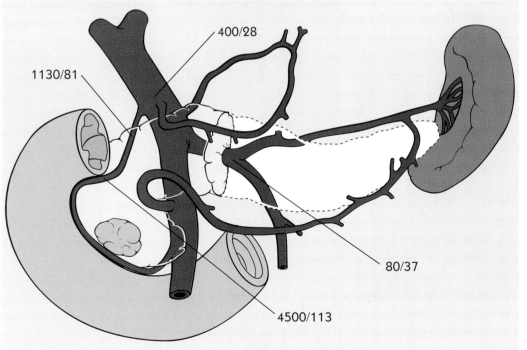

FIGURE 6.13 Selective venous sampling of the portal vein and its major tributaries can identify an insulinoma in a patient who has had a prior distal pancreatic resection without finding the lesion. The numbers refer to serum insulin in pg/ml contrasted with serum gastrin in pg/ml.

400/28

1130/81

80/37

4500/113

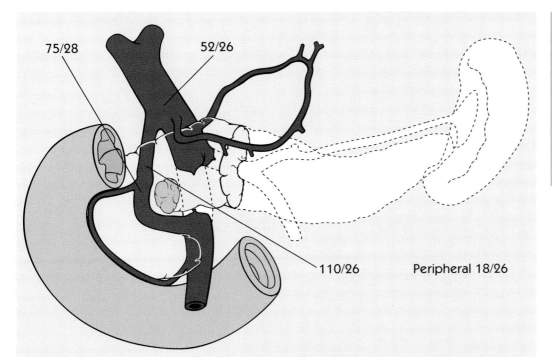

75/28   52/26

110/26   Peripheral 18/26

FIGURE 6.14 Selective transhepatic venous sampling in a patient who has had a prior distal pancreatectomy, intraoperative ligation of the portal and splenic veins, and yet remains with all the symptoms and signs of an insulinoma.

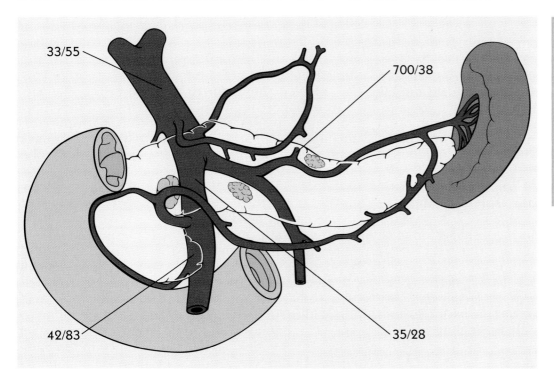

33/55   700/38

42/83   35/28

FIGURE 6.15 The offending insulin-producing tumor, identified by portal venous sampling in a patient with multiple endocrine neoplasia and more than one endocrine tumor. The numbers refer to serum insulin in pg/ml contrasted with serum gastrin in pg/ml.

Approach to the Patient

The primary management of all insulinomas that do not have evidence of metastatic disease on angiography and CT scan consists of the surgical resection of the tumor. Because the vast majority of insulinomas are benign, often small, isolated lesions, enucleation is usually possible (Fig 6.16). Even lesions in the pancreatic head, in intimate relationship to the common bile duct, if carefully localized, can often be removed without serious consequences to the patient (see Fig 6.12). The major potential morbidity of this approach is the development of a pancreatic fistula. This occurrence is usually recognizable intraoperatively and, if adequately drained, will almost always close, provided that there is no proximal pancreatic duct obstruction. Failure of a fistula to close over several weeks should raise the concern of an intraoperative technical error involving pancreatic duct ligation. Short-term fistula management with somatostatin analogues can often rapidly decrease drainage and allow nonoperative closure.

Intraoperative monitoring of blood glucose has not been valuable in practice. It is potentially risky to manage these patients intraoperatively without a glucose infusion; the immediate instantaneous glucose measurement, particularly if done "online," is cumbersome and difficult. Similarly, use of an efficient rapid radioimmunoassay capable of detecting levels of insulin within 20 or 30 minutes, while theoretically attractive, is not practical.

Metastatic disease from insulin-producing islet cell carcinoma is dominated by spread to the liver and local lymph nodes (Fig. 6.17) (7). In patients with metastatic disease, serious consideration must be given to surgical removal of the bulk of the tumor, followed by other methods for obliteration of functional endocrine mass. These methods can include embolization of the liver, since any decrease in the amount of functional tumor mass can markedly improve the symptomatic patient.

PHARMACOLOGIC MANAGEMENT

Pharmacologic management of excess insulin secretion is difficult. Primary drugs available are somatostatin and its current analogues, and diazoxide (Fig. 6.18). Somatostatin is a 14-amino-acid peptide, originally described as a hormone that inhibits growth-hormone release. However, it is widely distributed throughout the central nervous system, the exocrine pancreas, the endocrine pancreas, and the gastrointestinal tract, so it can no longer be solely associated with growth hormone release-inhibition. Natural occurring somatostatin has a very short half-life in the circulation (approximately three minutes) and early attempts using intravenous administration (8) made long-term clinical use impractical. An 8-amino-acid analogue, SMS-201-995 (Sandostatin), was synthesized by Bauer and associates (9). This analogue was originally shown to be 45 times more powerful than natural somatostatin in its effect on inhibiting growth hormone secretion in the monkey, 11 times more active in the inhibition of glucagon, and one to three times more active in the inhibition of some insulin secretion. In addition, it has a prolonged half-life in the circulation. Currently the agent is usually used as a subcutaneous injection of 50 µg and peak plasma levels will be found 15 to 30 minutes after injection, with a half-life of approximately two hours (10).

Use of the somatostatin analogue in treating the symptoms of functional endocrine pancreatic tumors and metastatic carcinoid tumors is now well established (11,12). Somatostatin analogue works in several ways. One effect is caused by a decrease in circulating tumor hormone. In addition, somatostatin analogue has a direct effect on extraintestinal motility and secretory disturbances.

The analogue can show this direct effect by slowing transit time, increasing electrolyte reabsorption, and reducing jejunal secretion while suppressing pancreatic exocrine secretion. This has allowed the agent to be used in the management of pancreatic fistula, independent of its function on suppression of pancreatic endocrine hormones. Reports that somatostatin decreases tumor size (13) have not been substantiated in the vast majority of patients. Some data do suggest that somatostatin can inhibit growth and cell proliferation of cultured cells in selected malignant human cancer cell lines (14).

Somatostatin itself can be secreted by certain neuroendocrine tumors of the pancreas, and also by medullary carcinoma of the thyroid and small cell carcinoma of the lung. The syndrome produced by a somatostatinoma includes weight loss, malabsorption, diabetes, gallstones, and hypochlorhydria (15). Somatostatin and its current analogues represent the most significant advance in the management of excess insulin secretion. Many patients can be effectively managed by outpatient subcutaneous injection of 50 µg of somatostatin analogue two or three times a day, increasing the dose as required.

Diazoxide is a nondiuretic benzothiadiazine, originally introduced for the treatment of hypertension. The side effect of hyperglycemia led to its use as an agent to control hypoglycemic symptoms (16). The mean dosage of diazoxide used in long-term maintenance of patients with insulinoma is approximately 400 mg/day (17). The main side effects observed in patients are hirsutism (56 percent), edema (50 percent), weight gain (40 percent), and nausea (11 percent). Hypersensitivity reactions have also been reported. Diazoxide inhibits insulin secretion by direct action on the β-

Single lesion

Preoperative

Localized → Not localized

Operation
Single palpable lesion
or
Positive intraoperative ultrasound

Head → Body–tail < 1.0 cm → Body–tail > 1.0 cm

Enucleation → Distal pancreatectomy

FIGURE 6.16 Intraoperative approach to a single, functional, pancreatic, islet-cell tumor.

FIGURE 6.17:
SITES OF METASTASES

SITE	NATIONAL INSTITUTES OF HEALTH CASES		LITERATURE CASES	
	n	%	n	%
Lymph nodes	5/29	17.2	7/16	43.8
Liver	8/47	17.0	30/67	44.8
Liver/lymph nodes	3/18	16.7	5/11	45.4
Liver/other distant sites	1/6	16.7	2/4	50.0
Distant sites alone	0/0	—	1/2	50.0

From reference 7.

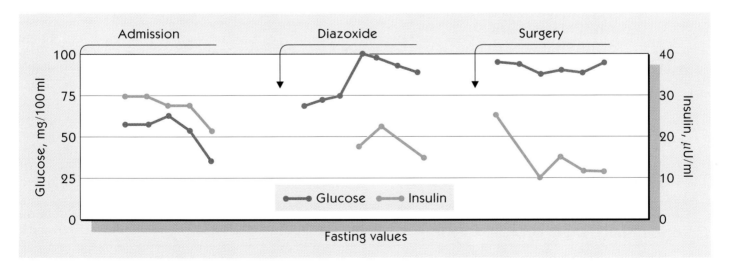

FIGURE 6.18 Pharmacologic management of excess insulin secretion, using diazoxide contrasted with the effect of operative removal of the lesion.

FIGURE 6.19:
PATHOLOGY, TUMOR LOCATION, AND TUMOR EXTENT IN PATIENTS WITH ZOLLINGER-ELLISON SYNDROME

TUMOR CHARACTERISTICS	% OF ALL PATIENTS	RANGE (%)
Pathology		
Gastrinoma	90	87–94
Malignant	—	61–90
Benign	—	10–39
Islet-cell hyperplasia	10	6–13
Tumor location		
Pancreas	42	21–65
Duodenum	15	6–31
Other	11	1–26
Metastases only	2	0–11
No tumor found	30	13–48
Extent of tumor		
Localized tumor	36	23–51
Metastatic tumor	34	13–52

From reference 26.

FIGURE 6.20:
CLINICAL FEATURES OF PATIENTS WITH ZOLLINGER-ELLISON SYNDROME

PATIENTS AND FEATURES	YEAR OF STUDY (REFERENCE)				
	1964 (21)	1978 (22)	1979 (23)	1986 (24)	1986 (20)
Total patients	260	40	34	144	80
Multiple endocrine neoplasia—type I (%)	21	23	24	24	21
Duration of symptoms before diagnosis (yr)	—	6.5	6.4	—	3.8
First symptoms (%)					
Abdominal pain	93	98	85	26	43
Pain and diarrhea	30	28	56	49	29
Diarrhea only	7	2	9	15	35
Dysphagia/pyrosis	0	0	6	0	13
Mean age at onset (yr)	—	50.5	50.4	47	45
Sex (% male)	60	60	62	68	64

From reference 26.

SUMMARY (BASED ON 400 PATIENTS)

- Approximately one out of four ZES patients has multiple endocrine neoplasia.
- Most patients have symptoms for years before diagnosis.
- The most common symptoms are abdominal pain and diarrhea accompanied by pain.
- ZES usually affects males between 40 and 50 years of age.

cell and probably by other mechanisms not clearly understood. Because of the prolonged half-life, significant accumulation of the drug can occur, with the primary side effect of fluid retention.

GASTRINOMA
Pathophysiology

Gastrinoma was first described by Zollinger and Ellison in 1955 (18). The syndrome is characterized by excessive secretion of gastric acid and a β-islet tumor of the pancreas. The cause of the excess acid was confirmed when a gastrin-like peptide was isolated from such tumors by Gregory in 1960 (19). Subsequently it was confirmed as being identical to human antral gastrin (20). The signs and symptoms of gastrinomas are all related to the excess gastric acid production and can be abolished by suppression of the excess acidity.

Clinical Presentation and Course (Figs. 6.19 and 6.20)

Epigastric pain is the classic symptom, but diarrhea is very common and may be the presenting symptom in the absence of pain (Fig. 6.21). The diarrhea is presumed to be due to the destructive nature of excess acid on small intestine mucosa, inactivation of pancreatic enzymes, and conceivably the precipitation of bile salts at very low intestinal pH levels. Certainly if the excess gastric acid secretion is controlled, then the diarrhea diminishes. Often the patient can titrate the dose of medication according to the presence or absence of liquid stool. This suggests that the role of gastrin by itself in the pathogenesis of the diarrhea is minimal.

Diagnosis

Gastric acid hypersecretion is one essential element in the diagnosis of Zollinger–Ellison syndrome (ZES). However, because the diagnosis is made earlier, gastric acid levels may be variable. The combination of an increased gastric acid output with an associated fasting hypergastrinoma strongly suggests the diagnosis.

Gastrin can be measured in plasma by radioimmunoassay. It is, however, important that the blood sample be collected properly. Gastrin is labile, and the sample should be mixed with a protease inhibitor immediately after venesection to avoid degradation.

When the diagnosis is suspected, it should be confirmed by a plasma gastrin level. In fact, plasma gastrin levels should be determined in any patient who is being considered for an operation for intractable peptic ulcer disease. In addition, patients with an unusual location of a peptic ulcer and those with associated diarrhea or an elevated serum calcium should be evaluated for ZES by plasma gastrin levels.

As with insulinoma and other pancreatic tumors, it is imperative that the patient with the familial variant be identified. About 21 percent to 37 percent of patients with MEN-I will have ZES (21–24). Determination of an elevated serum calcium must

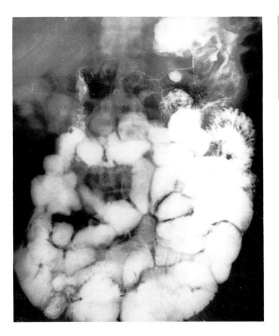

FIGURE 6.21 Diarrhea is very common in the Zollinger–Ellison syndrome and may be the presenting symptom in the absence of pain. Active fluid secretion and bowel changes are identified. (From Kassner EG. *Atlas of radiologic imaging.* New York: Gower Medical Publishing, 1989.)

raise again the concern that the tumors in the pancreas may well be multiple, and the important issue is to identify, as with insulinoma (see above), the functional tumor that is causing the patient's symptoms.

DIFFERENTIAL DIAGNOSIS

Elevated fasting plasma gastrin levels may be found in some patients in the absence of ZES. These patients may be divided into two groups: the first, with increased acid production, and the second, with hypochlorhydria or achlorhydria due to underlying causes such as gastritis, carcinoma, pernicious anemia, or after prior operations for peptic ulcer disease. In practical terms, if the patient has an elevated plasma gastrin level and the pH of a gastric aspirate is greater than 3, other causes of hypergastrinemia should be sought. Maximal stimulated gastric acid output can be obtained by such stimulants as intravenous calcium or pentagastrin. Ratios of maximal to basal gastric acid output have been used (Fig. 6.22), but they are rarely of more value in the diagnosis of the ZES than the measurement of the basal acid output alone (25). In the presence of marked elevations in basal acid output and hypergastrinemia, only two situations

may be present. One is ZES and the other is the so-called retained gastric antrum after a Billroth II gastroenterostomy. The gastric antrum, in this situation, remains in association with the duodenal stump and may be a source of high plasma gastrin levels. This situation has become rare and is now almost never seen.

In some patients with peptic ulcer disease and increased gastric acid output, lesser elevations of plasma gastrin concentrations (<1000 pg/ml) can be seen. In these patients provocative tests are necessary, and a number of these tests have been proposed. Calcium infusions (Fig. 6.23) and meal tests are relatively cumbersome to perform. The secretin infusion test is by far the one most favored (Fig. 6.24).

The most commonly used gastric acid secretory criteria for the diagnosis of ZES include a basal acid output (BAO) of >15 mEq/h. The mean BAO in five reported series varied from 34–53 mEq/h (26). If the patient has had a prior operation designed to decrease acid production, then a BAO >5 mEq/h is an indication of the presence of ZES. The mean BAO for patients in the five reported series, after an operation to decrease acid production, was 6–20 mEq/h (26). Requiring a BAO >15 mEq/h will

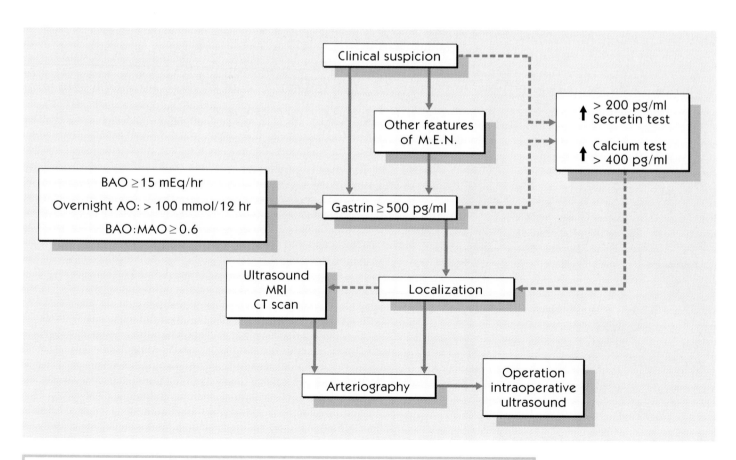

FIGURE 6.22 Diagnostic flow chart for suspected Zollinger–Ellison syndrome patients. (Modified from reference 6.)

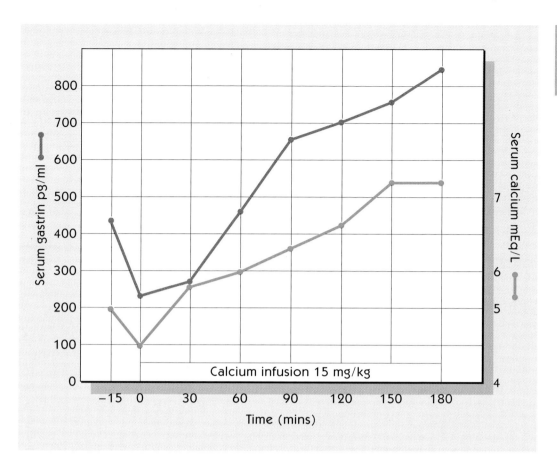

FIGURE 6.23 Gastrin response to calcium infusion in a patient with ZES.

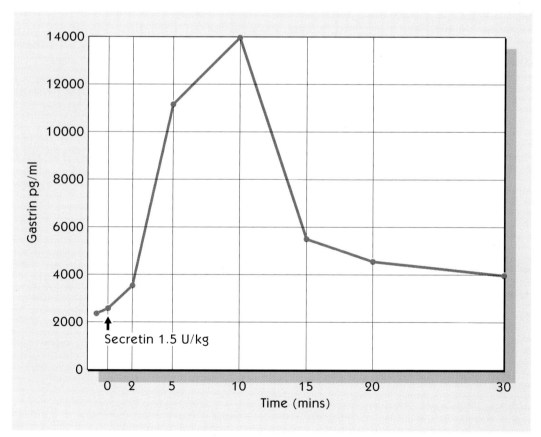

FIGURE 6.24 Gastrin response to secretin bolus in a patient with ZES.

include 66 percent to 99 percent of all patients with ZES. Approximately 40 percent of ZES patients will have gastrin >1000 pg/ml (27).

Once the diagnosis has been made, the site of the gastrin-producing tumor must be identified. The majority of gastrinomas occur in the pancreas, but they have been found in increasing numbers in the wall of the duodenum and in the peripancreatic and perigastric lymph nodes (28). Since the diagnosis is made earlier in the course of the disease, the prevalence of metastatic disease at the time of diagnosis appears to be falling. Debate continues about the source of the gastrinoma that arises in the true pancreas. Because classic gastrin cells predominate in the stomach and duodenum, reports suggest that the source within the pancreas involves the differentiation from some multipotent precursor cell.

TUMOR LOCALIZATION

Tumor localization in gastrinoma is much more difficult than in the patient with insulinoma. Arteriography is not as accurate. Arteriography, in the main, identifies metastatic disease, rather than finding the primary tumor (29). Portal venous sampling has been employed, and, although excellent results have been reported by some authors (30, 31), our experience and that of others is much less encouraging (32). Computed tomography is of little value except for very large lesions or in the presence of metastatic disease.

An important advance in tumor localization is use of endoscopic ultrasound, which can identify tumors close to the duodenum, either in the duodenal wall or in the nearby pancreas. This approach has been effective when all other localization tests, including intraoperative ultrasound, have failed

(Fig. 6.25) (33). Intraoperative ultrasound remains a powerful tool for all neuroendocrine tumors of the pancreas, but requires considerable experience and skill and is less effective in gastrinoma than in other tumors (32).

Approach to the Patient

Historically, management of gastrinoma revolved around end organ ablation, that is, using total gastrectomy as the treatment of choice. Little attempt was made to address the primary tumor. With the advent of medical control of the end organ, this approach can be modified.

CURRENT APPROACHES

With the availability of effective acid-reducing medications, operative end organ ablation is rarely required. Long-term management with cimetdine and ranitidine is very successful if adequate dosages are maintained, as determined by gastric acid output studies. Omeprazole, an H^+/K^+ ATPase inhibitor, may be used instead of cimetidine and ranitidine if the BAO can no longer be controlled or if side effects of the H_2-receptor antagonists, such as impotence and gynecomastia with cimetidine, are excessive. Only for those patients with established pyloric stenosis, or noncompliant patients, usually alcoholic, should gastrectomy be considered.

The long-term efficacy and safety of omeprazole in patients with Zollinger–Ellison syndrome has been recently documented (29). The mean daily dose required was 82 mg with 75 percent of the patients requiring only a single dose per day. Patients requiring higher doses, i.e., 120 mg once a day, could be controlled by giving 60 mg twice daily.

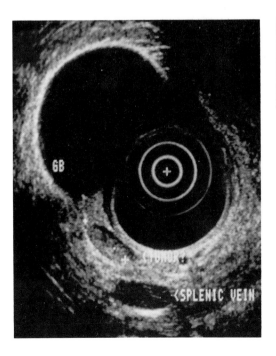

FIGURE 6.25 Endoscopic ultrasound image with the transducer in the duodenal bulb. The insulinoma is a relatively hypoechoic ovoid mass, 1.4 cm in size, seen anteriorly just above the splenic vein in the head of the pancreas near the gallbladder (GB). (Adapted from reference 33.)

No correlation of serum gastrin with omeprazole requirements was found, but the dosage was related to basal acid output, and prior use of H_2-receptor antagonists. More importantly, omeprazole appeared to be of value in patients with failed or incomplete acid secretory control on H_2-receptor antagonists. In the majority of patients, omeprazole was effective without requiring increasing doses, in contradistinction to cimetidine or ranitidine (34). Unfortunately, the current cost of omeprazole may preclude its use for many patients.

Once the consequences of the disease have been controlled, therapy can be directed to identification and removal of the tumor. Isolated reports have addressed the issue of gastrinoma resection with good long-term follow-up and no evidence of recurrence of disease (35). This requires identification of the small tumor, which is often not possible. An argument has been made that patients with ZES, in the presence of MEN-I, should not be operated on because of poor long-term results in respect to cure and decreased survival in the absence of operative resection (36). We have not taken this view and have on occasion resected patients with such tumors. An algorithm depicting perioperative management of a patient with ZES is illustrated in Figure 6.26.

The difficulty is that many of these patients will be expected to have multiple tumors of the pan-

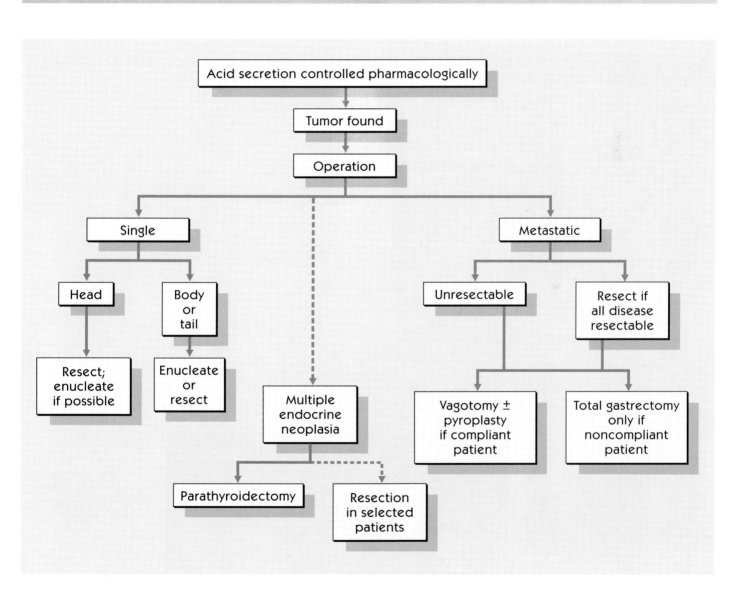

FIGURE 6.26 Perioperative management of patients with ZES.

creas, although on occasion these tumors do not appear to be dominant. Regardless, the only long-term cure for gastrinoma is identification and removal of the tumor. Tumor removal in patients with localized nonmetastatic ZES can be curative (6). Even in patients with isolated nodal metastases, long-term survival has been reported after resection. In patients with metastatic disease, an aggressive surgical approach to resection can be justified (Fig. 6.27) (37). In addition, resection of metastases from functional tumors can result in a marked decrease in the need for antisecretory medication. In some patients hepatic artery embolization can achieve a marked reduction in functional tumor mass (Fig. 6.28). Small lymph node

metastases should not be a barrier to this approach. The important issue at the time of operation is to expect that the tumor will not necessarily be confined or contained within the pancreas (28). Often the tumor is in the duodenal wall, either with or without metastases.

OTHER HORMONALLY ACTIVE TUMORS

With over 30 gastroenteropancreatic peptides reported in recent years, it is not surprising that numerous other pancreatic tumors have been described based on immunohistochemistry (38). The issue becomes even more difficult when it is realized that individual tumors may secrete a variety of

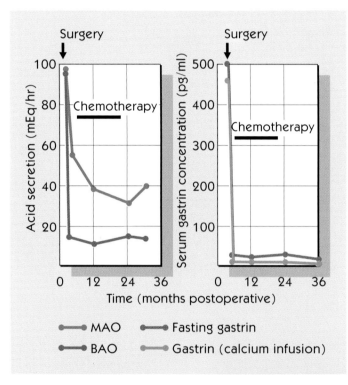

MAO   Fasting gastrin
BAO   Gastrin (calcium infusion)

FIGURE 6.27 "Cure" of metastatic Zollinger–Ellison syndrome. (Adapted from reference 37.)

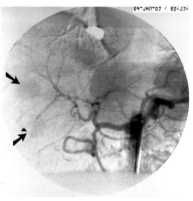

FIGURE 6.28 Hepatic artery peripheral embolization of vascular metastases in the Zollinger–Ellison syndrome.

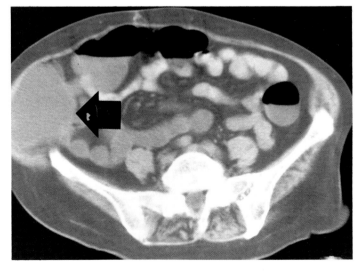

FIGURE 6.29 CT scan showing dilated fluid-filled colon (*arrow*) in a patient with VIP-producing tumor despite 1000 mg/day of somatostatin analogue.

end products, and that more than one peptide has been found not only in the same tumor but in the same cell, and even in the same secretory granule.

Vasoactive Intestinal Peptide (VIP)—VIPoma

PATHOPHYSIOLOGY

Verner and Morrison (39) described two patients with the syndrome of watery diarrhea, dehydration, and severe hypokalemia. They were subsequently shown to have a non-β-cell pancreatic islet-cell tumor. The syndrome was initially termed "pancreatic cholera" by Matsumoto (40), while Marks (41) suggested the acronym WDHA (watery diarrhea, hypokalemia, achlorhydria). The symptom complex includes fulminant secretory diarrhea and metabolic acidosis that can result in a life-threatening presentation. There is marked increase in pancreatic and biliary secretion and in jejunal fluid and electrolyte secretion. There is diminished fluid absorption in the ileum and colonic secretion, rather than active reabsorption (42,43). The patient can lose very large quantities (>300 mEq) of potassium in the stool within 24 hours.

Some patients will present with flushing caused by decreased peripheral resistance by vasodilating compounds and hypotension associated with fluid loss, as has been seen in infusions of VIP into normal subjects (44). Some degree of tachyphylaxis occurs when VIP is infused into normal man, and may well be the reason that the majority of patients with well-established VIP syndrome do not have persistent flushing.

Twenty to 50 percent of patients will have hyperglycemia, and a similar percentage will have hypercalcemia (43). The hypercalcemia is thought to be due to the effect of VIP on increasing osteolytic activity in the bone (45), although the multiple endocrine neoplasia syndrome with parathyroid hyperplasia must also be considered.

Peptides other than VIP may play a role in the watery diarrhea syndrome. A 27-amino-acid peptide (PHI: peptide-histidine-isoleucine) has been isolated from the submucosa of gut, brain, and other neural tissue (46), and elevated plasma levels have been seen in some VIP tumors (47). Of interest is that PHI is seen in tumor cells from VIP tumors and is produced by the same cells that contain the VIP. PHI in higher doses has also been shown to produce secretion of chloride and sodium in normal volunteers (48).

DIAGNOSIS

An important differentiation in the diagnosis is the persistence of diarrhea after fasting. For practical purposes, the patient secreting less than 700 ml of stool after fasting can have the diagnosis excluded; most patients with the disease will produce more than 3 l of stool (43). As mentioned previously, diarrhea can also be a manifestation of ZES, but ZES can easily be excluded from the differential by simple gastrin determination.

It is important that VIP levels be clearly demonstrated. The lowest initial VIP level reported in 29 cases of VIPoma was 225 pg/ml, while normal mean plasma VIP for 100 normal fasting samples in a selected reference laboratory was 62 ± 22 pg/ml (43). Elevated levels have been associated with other tumors, including pheochromocytoma, ganglioneuroma, and small-cell lung cancer. Of interest is that only four of the 29 reported patients did not have metastases at the time of operation.

TREATMENT

It is absolutely imperative that these patients be medically well prepared before any consideration of surgical operation. Since most patients will have metastases, the urgency for operation is minimal. The patient should be vigorously resuscitated with intravenous fluids, almost invariably begun on somatostatin (Fig. 6.29), and acidosis and hypokalemia corrected. After that, the extent of the tumor can be evaluated and a decision made as to resection. Most of the tumors occur in the tail of the pancreas, and a resection is often possible with minimal morbidity (Fig. 6.30), assuming that the bulk of the primary tumor is large and metastases can be removed.

Somatostatinoma

The diagnosis and management of somatostatinoma parallels that of other endocrine tumors of the pancreas. Diagnosis is usually suspected in the patient with mild to moderate diabetes, almost always with gallstones, who presents with a mass lesion of the pancreas. Because the effects of somatostatin are mild and clinically ubiquitous, patients tend to present late, often with metastases. Rarely have patients been cured of this disease. The patient's course can be measured in years, however, and therapy directed at palliation of the obstructive and diabetic symptoms is valuable (49). The number of cases reported is small and representative cases are illustrated in Figure 6.31 (49–55).

A recent report reviewed 31 cases from 1977–1984 (56). The predominant presenting symptoms were pain, weight loss, and diarrhea (Fig. 6.32). Nineteen (61 percent) of these patients were treated by pancreatic resection, and the majority had a tumor confined to the head of the pancreas. Of interest is that six patients (19 percent) were said to have a primary duodenal tumor. Metastases were present in 75 percent of the cases. In this total group there were four five-year survivors and 11 two-year survivors. Ten patients died within one year of diagnosis.

A recent review of 27 pancreatic and 21 intestinal somatostatinomas (38) confirmed many of these findings. The mean age was 53, and diabetes was common in the pancreatic group (95 percent) but less common in the intestinal group (21 percent). Similarly, gallbladder disease was more common in the pancreatic (94 percent) than in the intestinal (43 percent) tumors. Ninety percent of the pancreatic somatostatinomas presented with metastases. The patients with intestinal tumors had lower somatostatin levels in plasma than did the pancreatic group.

The frequent occurrence of gallbladder disease, not seen in other islet-cell tumors, suggests a cause-and-effect relation. Somatostatin infusion can cause delayed gallbladder emptying, consistent with the observation that some patients will have delayed emptying without stones. An underappreciated symptom has been diarrhea, often with steatorrhea, consistent with the action of somatostatin on pancreatic exocrine function.

An interesting association of duodenal carcinoids and more recently somatostatinoma with neurofibromatosis has been reported (57,58). In three patients duodenal carcinoid tumor was associated with neurofibromatosis and pheochromocytoma (58).

Glucagonoma

A glucagon-producing tumor results in the excess secretion of glucagon in association with an erythematous rash which can be necrolytic. There is mild diabetes, severe muscle wasting, and low levels of circulating amino acids on plasma determination. Once suspected, the diagnosis is established by determination of a markedly elevated plasma glucagon concentration. Again, localization of a glucagonoma is usually not difficult. Many patients present with large masses that are easily seen on CT scan or angiography and often have associated metastatic disease.

Pancreatic Polypeptide—PPoma

Within the islet cell, pancreatic polypeptide (PP) is located peripherally close to the site of neural innervation. PP cells are sensitive to autonomic stimulation. The actual biologic function of these cells and PP is unknown, although numerous stimuli such as prolonged fasting, meal ingestion, and exercise all increase circulating PP levels (36). PP-staining tumors are, therefore, thought to be clinically inactive. There are reports, however, of duodenal ulcer and diarrhea in association with increased PP levels. It may well be shown that PP is a valuable nonspecific marker for many other islet cell malignancies.

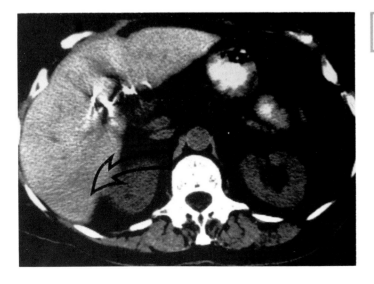

FIGURE 6.30 VIPoma treated palliatively in the presence of metastases with large doses of somatostatin.

Figure 6.31:
Somatostatinoma

REF.	AGE	SEX	GLU-COSE mg/dl	INSULIN µU/dl	GLUCAGON pg/ml	SRIF pg/ml	GTT	TREATMENT	OUTCOME
49	48	F	250	NR	NR	14,000	Diabetic	Pancreas resection	Alive after 2 yrs
50	70	F	NR	NR	NR	8,000	Diabetic	Pancreaticoduo-denectomy	Died post-operatively
51	46	F	169	5	0	NR	Diabetic	Pancreaticoduo-denectomy	Alive after 4 yrs
52	54	M	NR	NR	NR	NR	NR	Laparotomy	Died post-operatively
53	55	F	NR	3	10	107,000	Diabetic	Pancreaticoduo-denectomy	Died post-operatively
54	56	F	250	NR	110	30,800	Diabetic	Chemotherapy	Alive after 8 yrs with disease
55	52	M	163	224	70	20,000	Diabetic	Pancreaticoduo-denectomy	Alive after 1 yr with disease
[Normal range]			[60–90]	[4–24]	[70–200]	[80]			

GTT = glucose tolerance test; NR = not reported;
— = immunoreactivity present; SRIF = somatostatin.

Figure 6.32:
Symptoms and Presentation in Patients with Somatostatinoma

	SYMPTOMS	FREQUENCY SEEN CLINICALLY
A.	Abdominal pain Weight loss Diarrhea Polydipsia	22%–35%
B.	Jaundice Polyuria Steatorrhea	16%–19%
C.	Anorexia Abdominal distress/ distention Nausea Hypoglycemic symptoms	10%–13%

From reference 56.

Neurotensinomas

Neurotensin is another polypeptide with systemic effects that include hypotension, tachycardia, cyanosis, and increased secretion of small intestinal fluid (59,60). Seven cases have been reported (36) with predicted features based on known action of neurotensin. These include diarrhea, vasodilatation, edema, and diabetes.

Other Islet-Cell Tumors

Numerous other nonfunctional tumors can occur. They are usually large and present only because of the symptoms produced by their mass, obstruction, or metastases. Our recent experience with nonfunctional islet-cell carcinomas is shown in Figure 6.33. It should be emphasized that the term *nonfunctional* is arbitrary and usually refers to the absence of clinically identified function. By immunohistochemistry the majority of nonfunctional islet-cell carcinomas will show the presence of some peptides. Similarly, the ability to determine benignity vs. malignancy by histopathology of the primary lesion is difficult. In the absence of metastases this is usually done by histologic evidence of invasion of surrounding structures or intratumoral vascular invasion. Nevertheless, this may in part account for the apparent good results with islet-cell carcinoma in those patients able to be resected (see Fig. 6.33).

Carcinoid Tumors
EPIDEMIOLOGY

SEER data (from the National Cancer Institute's Surveillance, Epidemiology, and End Results program) report an annual incidence of 2.8 per million persons for small intestinal carcinoids, but an autopsy study at the Mayo Clinic found an incidence as high as 6.5 per 1000 (3,61). Most carcinoids will be asymptomatic, and the common presentation involves the bronchus, appendix, rectum, or small intestine (Fig. 6.34) (62–65). The isolated carcinoid tumor found in the resected appendix is often small (Figs. 6.35 and 6.36). If the tumor is less than 1 cm in diameter, without metastases and without mucosal invasion, no further treatment beyond appendectomy will be needed. When the appendiceal carcinoid is greater than 1 cm in diameter, the risk of invasion is real, and more aggressive surgical management may be warranted. Similarly, rectal carcinoids of 1 cm or less (80 percent) rarely metastasize and can be managed by local resection, while those greater than 2 cm require a true cancer operation. In the small intestine, spread to lymph nodes is common, and often a fibrous reaction leads to sclerosis, scarring, and symptomatic obstruction of the intestine (Fig. 6.37). Significant evidence suggests that gastrin is a trophic hormone for gastric carcinoids, such as those seen in patients with Zollinger–Ellison syndrome, in patients with pernicious anemia (Fig.

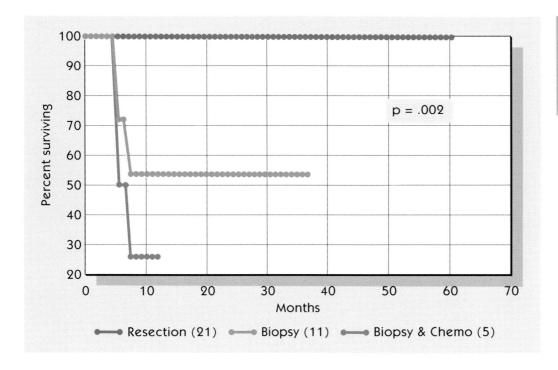

FIGURE 6.33 Recent experience with nonfunctional islet-cell carcinoma at the Memorial Sloan–Kettering Cancer Center.

p = .002

Percent surviving / Months

Resection (21) • Biopsy (11) • Biopsy & Chemo (5)

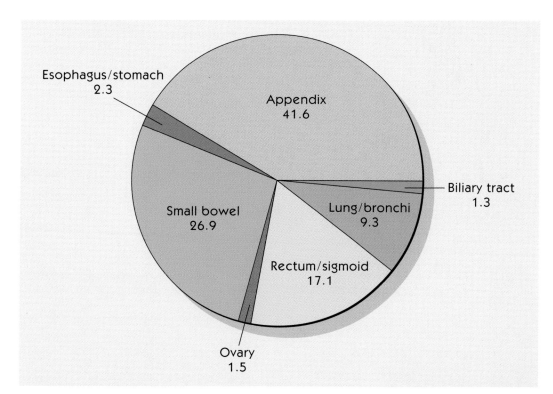

Esophagus/stomach
2.3

Appendix
41.6

Biliary tract
1.3

Small bowel
26.9

Lung/bronchi
9.3

Rectum/sigmoid
17.1

Ovary
1.5

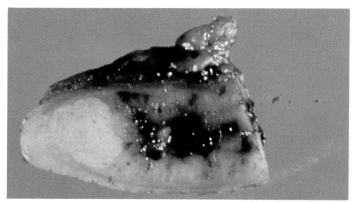

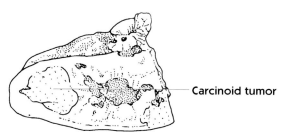

Carcinoid tumor

FIGURE 6.35 The isolated carcinoid tumor found in the resected appendix is often small. It is seen here as a yellow nodule at the appendiceal tip. (From Mitros FA. *Atlas of gastrointestinal pathology.* London: Gower Medical Publishing, 1988.)

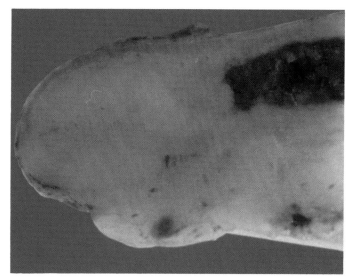

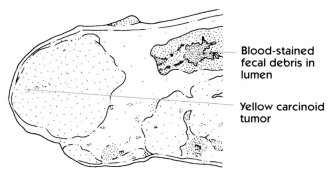

Blood-stained fecal debris in lumen

Yellow carcinoid tumor

FIGURE 6.36 Macroscopic appearance of a carcinoid tumor in the tip of the appendix. (From Misiewicz JJ, et al. *Atlas of clinical gastroenterology.* London: Gower Medical Publishing, 1987.)

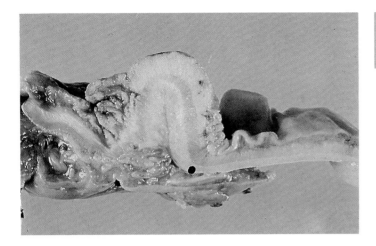

FIGURE 6.37 In the small intestine, a fibrous reaction leads to sclerosis, scarring, and symptomatic obstruction of the intestine. (From Mitros, 1988.)

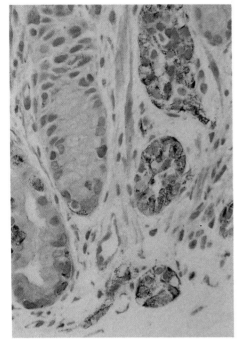

FIGURE 6.38 There is evidence that gastrin is a trophic hormone for gastric carcinoids, seen in patients with ZES, and pernicious anemia. (From Mitros, 1988.)

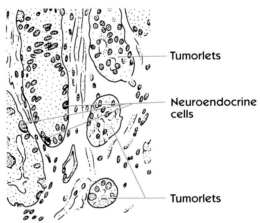

Tumorlets

Neuroendocrine cells

Tumorlets

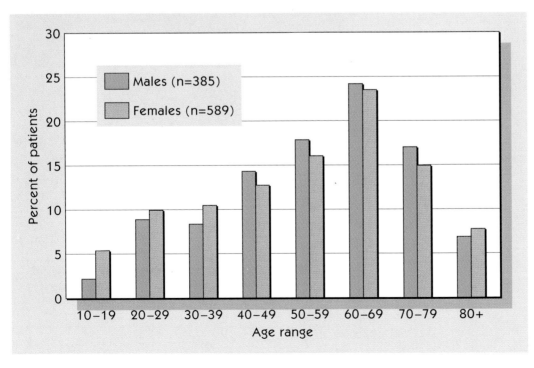

FIGURE 6.39 Age and sex distribution of malignant carcinoid tumors: data from 974 malignant carcinoids documented from 1973–1977 by the SEER program.

6.38), and in laboratory rats treated over long periods of time with omeprazole.

PATHOPHYSIOLOGY

The carcinoid tumor is another ubiquitous endocrine gastrointestinal tumor, which can occur at all sites in the gastrointestinal tract. Tumors have been found in adolescents and in patients in their eighties (Fig. 6.39). The tumors may be benign or malignant (Fig. 6.40), and in the absence of metastases, malignancy may be difficult to establish. Presentation is usually in response to intestinal obstruction or metastatic disease. Conventional classification of carcinoids into fore-, mid-, and hindgut was proposed by Williams and Sanders who found that foregut carcinoids had relatively low quantities of serotonin and the capacity to produce multiple hormones (Fig. 6.41). Clinical syndromes in foregut carcinoids were relatively uncommon, and many would be asymptomatic, particularly those arising in the stomach. The significance of these observations is debatable. Midgut carcinoids, including ileum and appendix, were more active in terms of serotonin production, but often produced less alternative peptide hormones (Figs.

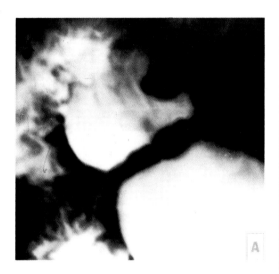

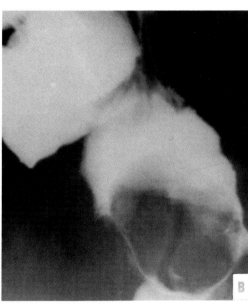

FIGURE 6.40 Carcinoid tumors may be (**A**) benign or (**B**) malignant.

FIGURE 6.41:
CHARACTERISTICS OF FORE-, MID-, AND HINDGUT CARCINOID TUMORS

LOCATION	STAINING	CHEMICAL TEST RESULTS	CARCINOID SYNDROME
Foregut	Argyrophil	5-HTP, 5-HT, histamine, gastrin, ACTH, PTH, urinary 5-HIAA	Frequent
Midgut	Argentaffin	5-HT and urinary 5-HIAA most common	Frequent
Hindgut	Nonreactive or argyrophil	Usually not detected	Rare

6.42 and 6.43). Hindgut tumors appeared in the rectum and the colon and had much less quantity of serotonin.

CLINICAL PRESENTATION AND CAUSE

The principal systemic features from the carcinoid syndrome are diarrhea, flushing, wheezing, and valvular heart disease.

Diarrhea and flushing are by far the most common symptoms, occurring in up to 80 percent of patients. Respiratory and cardiac disease usually occur in less than one-third of patients. The predominant primary lesion in patients with systemic symptoms occurs in the midgut. The severity of the carcinoid syndrome is related to tumor size and the resultant excess of tumor products entering into the systemic circulation. This occurs much more commonly in midgut carcinoids after development of distant metastases, usually to the liver.

DIAGNOSIS

Diagnosis of the carcinoid syndrome relies on the measurement of 5-hydroxytryptamine (5HTP) or 5-hydroxyindole acetic acid (5HIAA) in the urine. There are occasional false positive tests due to excessive ingestion of certain fruits and nuts, including walnuts, bananas, and pineapples. A number of reviews document medications that can interfere with the laboratory determination of 5HTP or 5HIAA (66). In cases where suspicion is high but 5HIAA is low, then other urine markers such as tryptophan can be measured.

APPROACH TO THE PATIENT

Operative resection remains the only curative possibility for carcinoid tumors at any site. Virtually no patient with appendiceal lesions less than 1 cm in size will go on to develop a recurrence or metastatic carcinoid (3,67,68). The extent of surgical resection can, therefore, be based on size and depth of penetration (Fig. 6.44.).

Resection of isolated hepatic metastases has been shown to be of some benefit (3). Palliation is obtained by resection of metastases when there is considerable evidence of the carcinoid syndrome. Resection is often also necessary to overcome the secondary effects of obstruction and bleeding.

Drug management is of limited value with the exception of the somatostatin analogues. These compounds can ameliorate flushing and diarrhea and, when used in the perioperative period, can prevent severe hypotension (Fig. 6.45). The 5HTP-

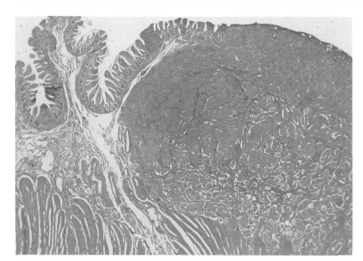

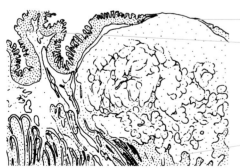

Involved mucosa
Intact mucosa
Tumor penetrating muscularis

FIGURE 6.42 Midgut carcinoids, including ileum and appendix, were more active in terms of serotonin production, but often produced less alternative peptide hormones. (From Mitros, 1988.)

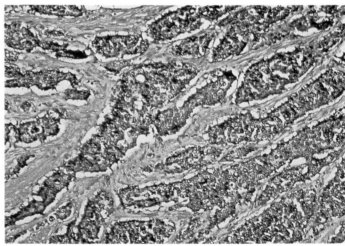

FIGURE 6.43 This higher power (x40) version of Figure 6.42 shows the prominent black granular staining of the tumor-cell cytoplasm, demonstrating striking argyrophilia in this terminal ileal carcinoid. (From Mitros, 1988.)

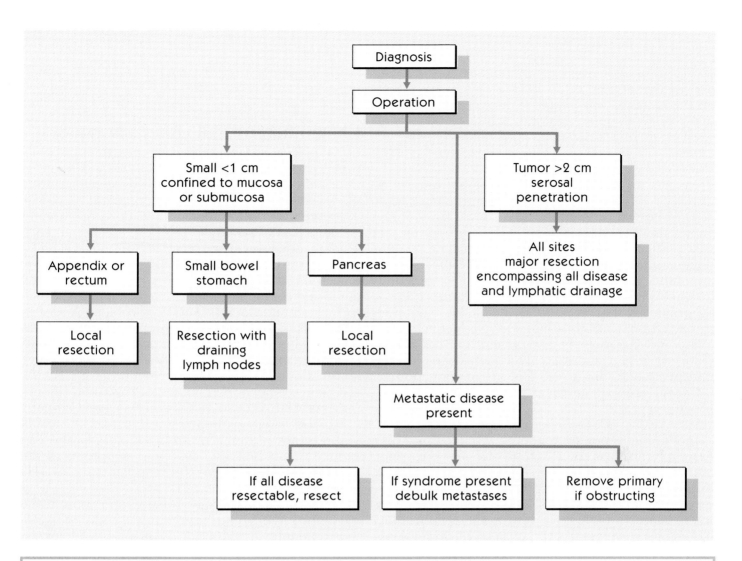

FIGURE 6.44 Algorithm for the perioperative management of carcinoid tumors.

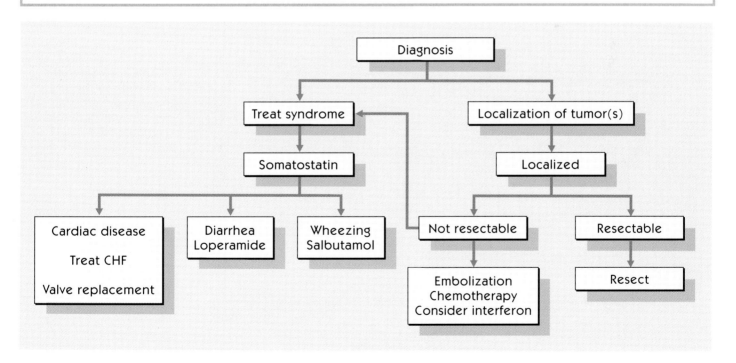

FIGURE 6.45 Management of patients with malignant carcinoid syndrome.

receptor antagonists, cyproheptadine, ketanserin, and methysergide, often have a significant effect on the diarrhea but limited, if any, effect on the 5-hydroxytryptamine excretion. Synthesis inhibitors such as α-methyldopa have only limited effects.

PROGNOSIS

Prognosis for the patient with carcinoid tumors is directly related to the extent of the primary tumor at the time of presentation. We have previously shown that the site of the primary tumor within the gastrointestinal tract has a major influence on outcome (67). Patients with incidentally discovered appendiceal carcinoids do best, while the worst prognosis is for those with pancreatic and colorectal primaries. The depth of invasion, i.e., confined to or through the intestinal wall, also affects outcome. Not surprisingly, the presence of nodal metastases, large tumors, or liver metastases are all bad prognostic features. The uncommon poorly differentiated or atypical tumors carry a poor prognosis.

Survival rates are dependent on both site and extent of the tumor. For patients with localized disease, a tumor less than 1 cm in size and not penetrating into the mucosa, long-term survival is excellent (Fig. 6.46) (67). Progressive increase in metastatic disease occurs as the tumor advances further into the intestinal lumen and lymph node metastasis develops. With subsequent disseminated disease, long-term survival diminishes, as might be expected. Survival is higher for tumors localized in the appendix; they are usually small with limited invasion.

Chemotherapy and Other Therapies

Chemotherapeutic antineoplastic treatment of functional islet-cell carcinoma and carcinoid tumors is poor although responses are clearly seen. In a study of 29 patients, 17 percent had complete response, 17 percent partial response (>50 percent), and 14 percent partial response (25 percent–50 percent). Median duration from start of treatment was 13 months (69). The most effective agent had in the past been streptozotocin (70), which has been used alone and in combination with cytotoxic drugs such as 5-FU (5 fluorouracil) and doxorubicin. A recently reported regimen of cisplatin and etoposide may be more effective for the poorly differentiated carcinoid tumors (71). A short trial of somatostatin should be used before chemotherapy is initiated since a small percentage of carcinoid tumors may stabilize or even regress on this agent alone.

Hepatic artery embolization deprives the metastatic tumor of much of its blood supply and can reduce tumor bulk and systemic symptoms of the syndromes. Here again, the response is relatively short lived (72).

Newer biologic therapies using interferon in the carcinoid syndrome have shown some symptomatic benefit, a reduction in urine 5HIAA levels, and stabilization of some carcinoid tumors, but they will require further serious evaluation (73).

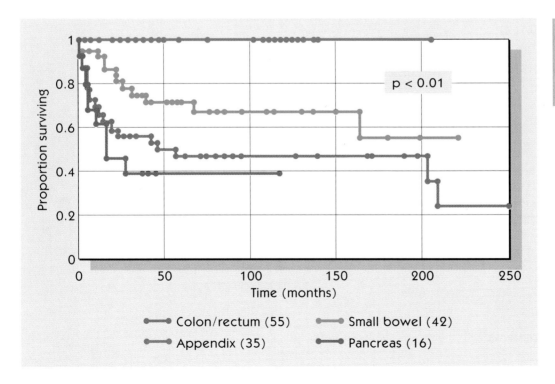

FIGURE 6.46 Survival according to the site of the primary carcinoid tumor. (Adapted from reference 67.)

REFERENCES

1. Sundler F. Bottcher G. Hakonson R, Schwartz TW. Immunocytochemical localization of the icosopeptide fragment of the PP precursor: a marker for 'true' PP cells? *Regul Pept* 8: 217–224, 1984.

2. Stadil F, Stage JG. The Zollinger–Ellison syndrome. *Clin Endocrinol Metab* 8:433–446, 1972.

3. Moertel CG. An odyssey in the land of small tumors. *J Clin Oncol* 5:1503–1522, 1987.

4. Service JF, Dale AD, Elveback IR, Jiang NS. Insulinoma: clinical and diagnostic features of 60 consecutive cases. *Mayo Clin Proc* 51:417–429, 1976.

5. Stefanini P, Carboni M, Petrasi N, et al. Beta islet cell tumors of the pancreas. Results of a study on 1,067 cases. *Surgery* 75:597–609, 1974.

6. Brennan MF, Macdonald JS. The endocrine pancreas. In: DeVita V, Hellman S, Rosenberg S, eds. *Principles and Practice of Oncology*. Philadelphia: J.B. Lippincott, 1982.

7. Danforth DN, Gorden P, Brennan MF. Metastatic insulin-secreting carcinoma of the pancreas: clinical course and the role of surgery. *Surgery* 96:1027–1036, 1984.

8. Mortimer CH, Carr D, Lind T, et al. Growth hormone release-inhibiting hormone: effects on circulating glucagon, insulin and growth hormone in normal, diabetic, acromegalic and hypopituitary patients. *Lancet* i:697–701, 1974.

9. Bauer W, Briner U, Doepfner W, et al. SMS 201–995: a very potent and selective octapeptide analogue of somatostatin with prolonged action. *Life Sci* 31:1133–1141, 1982.

10. delPozo E, Neufeld K. Schluter F, et al. Endocrine profile of a long-acting somatostatin derivative SMS 201–995. Study in normal volunteers following subcutaneous administration. *Acta Endocrinol* 111:433–439, 1986.

11. Wood SM, Kraenzlin ME, Adrian TE, Bloom SR. Treatment of patients with pancreatic endocrine tumors using a new long-acting somatostatin analogue symptomatic and peptide responses. *Gut* 26:438–444, 1985.

12. Maton PM, O'Dorisio TM, Howe BA, et al. Effect of a long-acting somatostatin analogue (SMS 201–995) in a patient with pancreatic cholera. *N Engl J Med* 312:17–21, 1985.

13. Kvols LK, Moertel OG, O'Connell MJ, et al. Treatment of the malignant carcinoid syndrome. Evaluation of a long-acting somatostatin analogue. *N Engl J Med* 315:663–666, 1986.

14. Lamberts SWJ, Koper JW, Reubi JC. Potential role of somatostatin analogues in the treatment of cancer. *Eur J Clin Invest* 17:281–287, 1987.

15. Bloom SR, Polak JM. Somatostatin. *Br Med J* 295:288–290, 1987.

16. Marks V, Samols E. Diazoxide therapy of intractable hypoglycemia. *Ann NY Acad Sci* 150:442–446, 1968.

17. Goode PN, Farndon JR, Anderson J, et al. Diazoxide in the management of patients with insulinoma. *World J Surg* 10: 586–592, 1986.

18. Zollinger RM, Ellison EH. Primary peptic ulcerations of the jejunum associated with islet cell tumors of the pancreas. *Ann Surg* 142:708–728, 1955.

19. Gregory RA, Tracy HJ, French JN. Extraction of a gastrin-like substance from a pancreatic tumor in a case of Zollinger–Ellison syndrome. *Lancet* 1: 1045–1048, 1960.

20. Gregory RA, Grossman MI, Tracy HJ, Bently PH. Nature of the gastric secretagogue in Zollinger–Ellison syndrome tumors. *Lancet* 2:543–544, 1967.

21. Bonfils S, Landor JH, Mignon M. Results of surgical management in 92 consecutive patients with ZES. *Ann Surg* 194: 692–697, 1981.

22. Townsend CM, Lewis BG, Gornley WK, Thompson JC. Gastrinoma. *Curr Probl Cancer* 7:1–33, 1982.

23. Friesen SR. Treatment of ZES: a 25-year assessment. *Am J Surg* 143:331–338, 1982.

24. Brennan MF, Jensen RT, Wesley RA, Doppman JL, McCarthy DM. Role of surgery in patients with ZES managed medically. *Ann Surg* 196:239–245, 1982.

25. Marshall WJ. The gastrointestinal tract. In: Marshall WJ, ed. *Textbook of Clinical Chemistry*. Philadelphia: J.B. Lippincott, 1988: 90–104.

26. Norton JA, Doppman JL, Jensen RT. Cancer of the endocrine system. In: DeVita V, Hellman S, Rosenberg SA, eds. *Cancer: Principles and Practice of Oncology*, 3rd ed. Philadelphia: J.B. Lippincott, 1989:1269–1344.

27. Jensen RT, Gardner JD, Raufman JP, et al. Zollinger–Ellison syndrome. NIH combined clinical staff conference. *Ann Intern Med* 98:59, 1983.

28. Fox PS, Hoffman JW, Wilson SD, et al. Surgical management of the Zollinger–Ellison syndrome. *Surg Clin North Am* 54:395–407, 1974.

29. Maton PN, Miller DL, Doppman JL, et al. Role of selective angiography in the management of patients with Zollinger–Ellison syndrome. *Gastroenterology* 92:913–918, 1987.

30. Roches A, Raisonnier A, Gillon-Savopure MC. Pancreatic venous sampling and arteriography in localizing insulinomas and gastrinomas: procedure and results in 55 cases. *Radiology* 145:621–627, 1982.

31. Burcharth F, Stage JG, Stadil F, Jensen LI, Fischermann K. Localization of gastrinomas by transhepatic portal catheterization and gastrin assay. *Gastroenterology* 77:444–450, 1979.

32. Cherner JA, Doppman JL, North JA, et al. Selective venous sampling for gastrin to localize gastrinomas. A prospective assessment. *Ann Int Med* 105:841–847, 1986.

33. Lightdale CJ, Botet JF, Woodruff JM, Brennan MF. Localization of endocrine tumors of the pancreas with endoscopic ultrasound. *Cancer* 68:1815-1820,1991.

34. Brennan MF, Jensen RT, Wesley R, Doppman JL, McCarthy DM. The role of surgery in patients with Zollinger–Ellison syndrome (ZES) managed medically. *Ann Surg* 196:239–245, 1982.

35. Horrman JW, Fox PS, Wilson SD. Duodenal wall tumors and ZES. *Arch Surg* 107:334–339, 1973.

36. Maton PN, Frucht H, Vinayek R, Wank SA, Gardner JD, Jensen RT. Medical management of patients with Zollinger–Ellison syndrome who have had previous gastric surgery: a prospective study. *Gastroenterology* 94:292–299, 1988.

37. Norton JA, Doppman JL, Gardner JD, et al. Aggressive resection of metastatic disease in selected patients with malignant gastrinoma. *Ann Surg* 203:352–359, 1986.

38. Vinik AI, Strodel WE, Eckhauser FE, Moattari AR, Lloyd R. Somatostatinomas, PPomas, neurotensinomas. *Sem Oncol* 14: 263–281, 1987.

39. Verner JV, Morrison AB. Islet cell tumor and a syndrome of refractory watery diarrhea and hypokalemia. *Am J Med* 25: 374–380, 1958.

40. Matsumoto KK, Peter JB, Schultze RG, Hakim AA, Franck PT. Watery diarrhea and hypokalemia associated with pancreatic islet cell adenoma. *Gastroenterology* 50:231–242, 1966.

41. Marks IN, Bank S, Louw JH. Islet cell tumor of the pancreas with reversible water diarrhea and achlorhydria. *Gastroenterology* 52:695–708, 1967.

42. Foster ES, Sandle GI, Hayslett JP, Binder HJ. Cyclic adenosine monophosphate stimulates active potassium secretion in the rat colon. *Gastroenterology* 84:324–330, 1983.

43. Mekhjian HS, O'Doriosio TM. VIPoma syndrome. *Sem Oncol* 14:282–291, 1987.

44. Modlin IM, Bloom SR, Mitchell SJ. Experimental evidence for vasoactive intestinal peptide as the cause of the watery diarrhea syndrome. *Gastroenterology* 75:1051–1054, 1978.

45. Bloom SR, Polak JM. VIP measurement in distinguishing Verner–Morrison syndrome. *Clin Endocrinol* 5 (suppl):223s–228s, 1976.

46. Tatemoto K, Mutt V. Isolation of two novel candidate hormones using a chemical method for finding naturally occurring polypeptide. *Nature* 285(1):417–418, 1980.

47. Bloom SR, Christofides ND, Yiangou Y, Blank MA, Tatemoto K, Polak JM. Peptide histidine isoleucine (PHI) and Verner–Morrison syndrome (abstr). *Gut* 24:A473, 1983.

48. Krejs GJ. Comparison of the effect of VIP and PHI on water and ion movement in the canine jejunum in vivo. *Gastroenterol Clin Biol* 8:868, 1984.

49. Kelly TR. Pancreatic somatostatinoma. *Am J Surg* 146:671–679, 1983.

50. Galmiche JP, Conlon JM, Srikant J, et al. Measurements of somatostatin like immunoreaction in plasma. *Clin Chiur Acta* 87:275–283, 1978.

51. Ganda OP, Weir GC, Soeldner JS, et al. Somatostatinoma. A somatostatin-containing tumor of the endocrine pancreas. *N Engl J Med* 296:963–967, 1977.

52. Kovacs K, Horvath E, Ezrin C, et al. Immunoreactive somatostatin in pancreatic islet-cell carcinoma accompanied by ectopic ACTH syndrome. *Lancet* i:1365–1366, 1977.

53. Larsson LI, Hirsch MA, Holst JJ, et al. Pancreatic somatostinoma: clinical features with pathological implications. *Lancet* i:666–668, 1977.

54. Pipcleers D, Somers G, Gepts W, et al. Plasma pancreatic hormone levels in a case of somatostatinoma. Diagnostic and therapeutic implications. *J Clin Endocrinol Metab* 49:572–579, 1979.

55. Krejs GG, Orci L, Conlon JM, et al. Somatostatinoma syndrome. Biochemical morphologic and clinical features. *N Engl J Med* 301:285–292, 1979.

56. Harris GJ, Tio F, Cruz AB Jr. Somatostatinoma: a case report and review of the literature. *J Surg Oncol* 36:8–16, 1987.

57. Swinburn BA, Yeong ML, Lane MR, Nicoholson GI, Holdaway IM. Neurofibromatosis associated with somatostatinoma: a report of two patients. *Clin Endocrinol* 28:353–359, 1988.

58. Griffiths DFR, Williams GT, Williams ED. Multiple endocrine neoplasia associated with von Recklinghausen's disease. *Br Med J* 287:1341–1343, 1983.

59. Hammer PA, Leeman SE. Neurotensin: properties and actions. In: Bloom SR, Polak JM, eds. *Gut Hormones*. Edinburgh: Churchill Livingstone, 1981:2:290–299.

60. Andersson S, Rosell S, Hjelmquist U, et al. Inhibition of gastric and intestinal motor activity in dogs by (Gln^4)-neurotensin. *Acta Physiol Scand* 100:231–235, 1977.

61. Black WC. Enterchromaffin cell types and corresponding carcinoid tumors. *Lab Invest* 19:473–486, 1968.

62. Wilson H, Cheek RC, Sherman RT, et al. Carcinoid tumors. *Curr Probl Surg* 11:1,1970.

63. Jager RM, Polk HG. Carcinoid apudomas. *Curr Probl Cancer* 1:11,1977.

64. Godwin JD. Carcinoid tumors. An analysis of 2837 cases. *Cancer* 36:560–569, 1975.

65. Marks C. *Carcinoid tumors. A clinicopathologic study*. Boston: G. Hall, 1979.

66. Young DS, Pesanter LC, Gibberman V. Effects of drugs on clinical laboratory tests. *Clin Chem* 21:1D–432D, 1975.

67. McDermott EWM, Gudrich B, Brennan MF. Prognostic variables in gastrointestinal carcinoid tumors. Submitted for publication.

68. Hajdu SI, Wanawer SJ, Myers WPL. Carcinoid tumors: a study of 204 cases. *Am J Clin Pathol* 6:521–528, 1974.

69. Schein PS. Chemotherapeutic management of hormone secreting endocrine malignancies. *Cancer* 30:1616–1626, 1972.

70. Obert K. Lundquist G, Bostrom H. The effects of streptozotocin in the treatment of endocrine pancreatic tumors and carcinoids. In: Grosbeck T, ed. *Streptozotocin*. New York: Elsevier Publishing Co., 1981.

71. Moertel CG, Kvols LK, O'Connell MJ, Rubin J. Treatment of neuroendocrine carcinomas with combined etoposide and cisplatin. *Cancer* 68:227-232, 1991.

72. Nobin A, Månson B, Lunderquist A. Evaluation of tempory liver dearterialization and embolization in patients with metastatic carcinoid tumor. *Acta Oncologica* 28:419-424, 1989.

73. Öberg K, Funa K, Alm G. Effects of leukocyte interferon on clinical symptoms and hormone levels in patients with mid-gut carcinoid tumors and carcinoid syndrome. *N Engl J Med* 309:129-133, 1983.

Index

Numbers in **bold** type indicate figures.